al Marketing
nd Public Health
Theory and practice

Social Marketing and Public Health

Theory and practice

Edited by

Jeff French with

Clive Blair-Stevens

Dominic McVey

Rowena Merritt

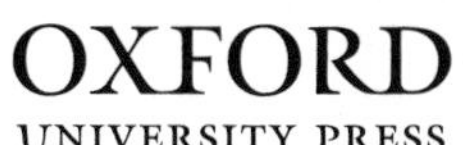

OXFORD
UNIVERSITY PRESS

Great Clarendon Street, Oxford OX2 6DP

Oxford University Press is a department of the University of Oxford.
It furthers the University's objective of excellence in research, scholarship,
and education by publishing worldwide in

Oxford New York

Auckland Cape Town Dar es Salaam Hong Kong Karachi
Kuala Lumpur Madrid Melbourne Mexico City Nairobi
New Delhi Shanghai Taipei Toronto

With offices in

Argentina Austria Brazil Chile Czech Republic France Greece
Guatemala Hungary Italy Japan Poland Portugal Singapore
South Korea Switzerland Thailand Turkey Ukraine Vietnam

Oxford is a registered trade mark of Oxford University Press
in the UK and in certain other countries

Published in the United States
by Oxford University Press Inc., New York

First published 2010

British Library Cataloguing in Publication Data
Data available

Library of Congress Cataloging in Publication Data
Data available

Typeset by Cepha Imaging Private Ltd., Bangalore, India
Printed in Great Britain
on acid-free paper by
The MPG Books Group, Bodmin and King's Lynn

ISBN 978–0–19–955069–2

10 9 8 7 6 5 4 3 2 1

Oxford University Press makes no representation, express or implied, that the drug dosages in this book are correct. Readers must therefore always check the product information and clinical procedures with the most up to date published product information and data sheets provided by the manufacturers and the most recent codes of conduct and safety regulations. The authors and publishers do not accept responsibility or legal liability for any errors in the text or for the misuse or misapplication of material in this work. Except where otherwise stated, drug dosages and recommendations are for the non-pregnant adult who is not breastfeeding.

Contents

Acknowledgements

I would very much like to thank Clive Blair-Stevens, Dominic McVey, and Rowena Merritt for their assistance in editing sections of this book, for their authorship of specific chapters. I would also like to thank all the other authors for their time and commitment to this project. A very big thanks must also go to Stephanie Allen for all her work in helping us polish and pull together the final manuscript of the book. I would also like to thank all the staff at the National Social Marketing Centre in England for their contributions and Oxford University Press for their support and encouragement.

Jeff French

Contributors List

Clive Blair-Stevens
Director of Strategy and Operations
National Social Marketing Centre
London, UK

Alex Christopoulos
Research Manager
National Social Marketing Centre
London, UK

Adam Crosier
Research and Insight
National Social Marketing Centre
London, UK

Jeff French
CEO Strategic Social
Marketing Ltd

Ross Gordon
Research Officer
Institute for Social Marketing
University of Stirling
Stirling, UK

Dean Hanley
Social Marketing Copywriter and
Editor
London, UK

Gerard Hastings
Director
Institute for Social Marketing and
Centre for Tobacco Control Research,
University of Stirling and
the Open University
Stirling, UK

Graham Lister
Fellow Judge Business School,
Cambridge
and Professor of Health and
Social Care
London South Bank University,
London, UK

Dominic McVey
Research Director
National Social Marketing Centre
London, UK

Rowena Merritt
National Programme Manager
National Social
Marketing Centre
London, UK

Robert Marshall
Assistant Director
Rhode Island Department of Health
and Clinical Associate Professor of
Community Health
Warren Alpert School of Medicine,
Brown University,
Rhode Island, USA

Denise Ong
Project Officer
National Social
Marketing Centre
London, UK

Lucy Reynolds
Project Manager
National Social Marketing Centre
London, UK

William A Smith
Innovations Management
Academy for Educational
Development
Washington DC, USA

Martine Stead
Deputy Director
Institute for Social Marketing
University of Stirling and the
Open University
Stirling, UK

Allison Thorpe
Senior Research Associate
Brunel University
Middlesex, UK

Aiden Truss
Marketing and New Media Manager
National Social Marketing Centre
London, UK

Lynne Walsh
Journalist and Campaigner
Walsh Media Ltd
UK

Paul White
Director
The Social Marketing Practice
Oxfordshire, UK

Introduction

Jeff French

For governments across the world, understanding human behaviour sits at the heart of developing interventions to tackle big social and health challenges across issues as diverse as HIV, obesity, smoking, and alcohol misuse through to climate change, crime, and active participation in the political process itself. Governments and civil society are constantly seeking to understand and influence how and why people behave as they do, to develop and implement social interventions that have the best possible chance of helping citizens have a positive life experience.

What we know is that our current approaches to tackling many of these huge challenges are not working, or at least are not at a rate to achieve the scale of improvement necessary to slow, and in some cases, ultimately reverse problems such as health inequalities or global warming. This book makes the case and explores much of what is known about what governments, public sector organizations, and others can do to work with people to tackle many of the big policy challenges we face more effectively. This book sets out to explore and define what social marketing is and how it can help with many of these challenges.

The term 'social marketing' was used for the first time in 1971 by Philip Kotler and Gerald Zaltman, who defined it as follows:

> Social marketing is the design, implementation, and control of programs calculated to influence the acceptability of social ideas and involving considerations of product planning, pricing, communication, distribution, and marketing research

Since the publication of this definition, a great deal of refinement of the concept of social marketing has occurred and much learning has been gained form field-level experience, which we explore in Chapters 6, 17, and 21. Social marketing has a number of defining principles (see Chapter 3) and concepts but is widely accepted to be a systematic planning and delivery methodology. Social marketing draws upon techniques developed in the commercial sector such as audience segmentation, but also draws on many-years experience of application in the public and not-for-profit sectors. The definition of social marketing used in this book is

> Social marketing is the systematic application of marketing alongside other concepts and techniques, to achieve specific behavioural goals, for a social good
>
> (French and Blair-Stevens, 2007)

Social marketing is focused on enabling, encouraging, and supporting behavioural change or maintenance among target audiences and the re-engineering of services and systems to support and facilitate change. Many of the central principles of social marketing and its techniques are applied in the mainstream public health and health promotion practice and in many other related fields without the label of social marketing being attached to them.

The aim of this book

The simple premise of this book is that we need to put a lot more effort into understanding why people act as they do and then ensure that this understanding is used in a systematic way to develop and deliver social improvement intervention programmes. We need to understand what people are prepared to buy into with their time, energy, beliefs, and values, and sometimes their money, if we are going to be able to make a significant impact. We also need to enable and empower people so that the energy, skills, and motivation that people already have to lead healthier, more productive, and satisfying lives is harnessed. At its core, the first theme of this book is that social marketing is an approach that recognizes that if we are to be successful, it is not about doing things to people but about working with and for them. This core idea, of starting from where people are and focusing on what support they say they need to make changes in behaviour, is the key shift towards a social marketing approach in the development and implementation of public service that we recommend in this book.

The second key theme of this book is the need for public sector programmes that are intended to help people live healthier and more fulfilled lives need to be more rigorously researched, designed, developed, implemented, and evaluated. Too many public policy interventions have unclear or unrealistic aims, poor pretesting and piloting, and often, weak evaluation. A key feature and strength of social marketing is its obsession with systematic programme development and implementation. Without clear measurable objectives and cogent development and implementation plans, it is clear that little will be achieved and little will be learnt about how to help people that can be used to further refine new interventions.

Why this book?

One of the key tasks in developing any social marketing programme is to understand the competition and also to identify and develop what is called in this book 'delivery coalitions'. There are a small but growing number of social marketing textbooks already in the market place; we consider these books to be our coalition partners in spreading understanding and helping people to apply social marketing rather than our competition. We urge the readers of this book to start to build their own library of key text by purchasing some of these other books. Our review of current textbooks, however, indicated that there was a need for a book that added to rather than just repeated what already existed and sought to clarify some of the questions and issues that are not fully worked through in some existing texts.

Social marketing, like every other multidisciplinary field of endeavour, is not static. It is a developing and dynamic concept; therefore, it was our intention in this book to add to the richness of social marketing's theory and practice. We have attempted in this book to take a globally relevant stance but inevitably, given the cultural and practical experience of the authors, do so from a largely UK perspective. We believe that a perspective from the United Kingdom is an important addition to the literature on social marketing, which up to this point has been with two exceptions, Hastings (2007) and Donovan and Henley (2003), dominated by a North American perspective.

In social marketing, another key task is to define clearly what you are trying to achieve, with whom, and what will count as success. In short, what we hope this book delivers is a compelling case about why social marketing should become an embedded approach to tackling many of the world's behavioural challenges—a rigorous examination of what social marketing is and is not, when to apply it, how to do it, and how to understand some of the ethical and practical tensions faced by those applying social marketing.

A single narrative but many voices

The chapters in this book have been authored by a range of people working in the field of social marketing. We deliberately wanted to assemble a collective work that draws on the many voices within the social marketing big tent. Our decision was based on a belief that social marketing is, like most other new transtheoretical multidisciplinary fields of endeavour, one that needs to embrace the tensions and disagreements that are markers of a vibrant field of study and application. This text is not then a single voice, as the vast majority of previous social marketing books have been, but a collection of views and analyses from a variety of perspectives. This collective work however does contain a single consistent narrative around the centrality of the importance of starting from a target audience perspective, and the need for systematic planning and reflective learning for the development and implementation of effective social marketing programmes.

Overview of the book

This book is intended to give the reader a structured learning experience that results in a good understanding of social marketing principles and techniques alongside examples of real interventions that have made a difference to people's lives. Each chapter starts with a brief overview and a set of learning objectives for the chapter. Some chapters also include brief case studies and review exercises to illustrate the concepts or techniques being described in the chapter.

The chapters in this book are set out in such a way as to lead the reader through a logical sequence of understanding and then applying social marketing.

The early chapters focus on making the case for social marketing as a key tool for most public sector policy. The nature of social marketing is explored in Chapters 2, 3, and 4, and a set of eight criteria for defining social marketing interventions and programmes is proposed. A theoretical framework for social marketing is described covering the contributions from a variety of theoretical traditions and fields of study together with what is termed an 'open theoretical framework'. The framework recognizes the need to draw on all relevant theoretical insights from a broad range of disciplines and the importance of setting social marketing in the context of a broad understanding of behavioural change theory and practice.

In Chapter 5, social marketing's actual and potential contribution to policy development is examined. This chapter explores how social marketing can assist with key political and policy challenges and examines why social marketing is increasingly being used by governments as part of their public health strategies and other forms of public sector interventions.

Chapter 6 sets out a review of the evidence base for social marketing, and a discussion of the nature of evidence and how we need to further build the evidence base for social marketing. Chapter 7 explores one of the most important theoretical principles of social marketing: the rationale and importance of segmenting target audiences and how this can be done.

Chapter 8 is aimed at managers and commissioners of social marketing interventions. The chapter covers issues such as effective commissioning and monitoring the progress of agencies who have been commissioned to deliver social marketing interventions or research. Chapter 9 explores some of the ethical issues in social marketing and the questions and considerations that should be addressed when developing social marketing interventions or programmes.

Chapters 10–15 set out a five-stage social marketing total process planning (TPP) framework that can be applied to most social marketing challenges. The TPP framework is a simple but powerful tool for ensuring that a systematic approach is taken to developing social marketing interventions.

The latter chapters of this book are intended to give the reader some additional practical and conceptual tools to aid in the development of social marketing programmes. Chapter 16 is called 'Social marketing on a shoestring', recognizing that many people who want to apply social marketing principles will not have a big budget to do so. The chapter provides some tips and suggestions about how in these situations it is the rigorous planning process that gives social marketing its power rather than just the amount of funding or other resources that can be deployed. Chapter 17 is called 'Critical social marketing', an aspect of social marketing that critically reviews commercial marketing, sales, and PR and advertising practices that can have a negative impact on people's health and well-being. In this sense, critical social marketing is a tool for understanding some of the competition that exists in most behavioural change arenas. Chapter 18 is focused on developing an understanding of the value of money and return on investment in social marketing. One of the strengths of social marketing is that it seeks to assess what investment delivers in a measurable and transparent way. This is clearly a key component of evaluation but also helps to build a case for investment and weed out inefficient practice. Chapter 19 reviews the skill base for individual and organizational competencies in social marketing. With the publication of the national occupational standards for social marketing, the United Kingdom has set out a clear benchmark for assessing competencies and building social marketing capacity. Chapter 20 explores the necessity and know-how about building coalitions across sectors to tackle difficult behavioural challenges that will be a feature of many social marketing programmes. Chapter 21 explores the lessons that can be learnt from a relatively long history of applying social marketing in developing countries. The final chapter is a summary of key learning and future challenges from many of the world's leading social marketing experts.

Conclusion

It is our intention in this book to capture in a single volume an up-to-date picture of the theoretical principles and concepts that underpin social marketing and to set them out in an open and accessible way. We have also sought to provide practical tools to assist the reader to scope, develop, deliver, and evaluate social marketing projects and programmes. We hope that you enjoy this book and that you will play an active part in further developing and refining our collective understanding of social marketing.

References

Donovan, R. and Henley, N. (2003). *Social Marketing: Principles and Practice.* East Hawthorn, Victoria: IP Communications.

French, J. and Blair-Stevens, C. (2007). *Big Pocket Book: Social Marketing.* London: National Social Marketing Centre.

Hastings, G. (2007). *Social Marketing: Why Should the Devil Have All the Best Tunes? Oxford:* Butterworth-Heinemann Ltd.

Kotler, P. and Zaltman, G. (1971). Social marketing: an approach to planned social change. *Journal of Marketing*, 35(3): 3–12.

Chapter 1

The case for social marketing

Jeff French

Social marketing is the systematic application of marketing, alongside other concepts and techniques, to achieve specific behavioural goals, for a social good.
French and Blair-Stevens

Learning points

In this chapter,

- The rationale and arguments for why social marketing will become a key tool for governments are reviewed;
- Key policy and other societal drivers for change in the way behavioural challenges are tackled are explored;
- The need for a new citizen-driven approach to addressing behavioural challenges is explored and the characteristics of effective practice reviewed.

Chapter overview

This chapter explores why social marketing is increasingly being applied by governments and public sector institutions when developing interventions to bring about social good. These themes are expanded in Chapter 5, which is a fuller exploration of the application of social marketing in policy development and strategy formulation. Nearly every big policy challenge facing governments around the world contains significant behavioural elements: for example, obesity, alcohol misuse, infection control, recycling, saving for retirement, and crime. At a population level limited progress is being made in many of these fields and the current approaches to tackling these challenges and others are being questioned. Conversely, questions relating to the legitimacy of state intervention in, what can be considered, private matters are often raised. A further challenge comes in the form of accusations that big state interventions breed dependence and sometimes even encourage people to behave in ways that are not good for them or society as a whole (Murray, 2006).

This chapter argues that citizens' views and wants will and should assume more prominence in planning and delivery of all social programmes. This transfer of power will lead to more effective interventions and increasingly empowered and demanding citizens. Such a change will mean that governments and their agencies will increasingly look to enhance legislation and education as well as other forms of state intervention with approaches that encourage, engage, and enable people to act to improve their own health and the well-being of others. Among such new forms of intervention, social marketing offers an approach that is citizen-centric and also focused on delivering measurable return on investment. It is probable, therefore, that social marketing will increasingly becoming an integral part of state-funded endeavours to promote health and social good.

Introduction

The world faces a number of key challenges as we move into the twenty-first century. We face a huge growth in chronic disease (WHO, 2008a), associated with both an aging population and behavioural choices such as overeating and smoking. We also face huge economic and social challenges associated with persistent and growing inequalities between regions, countries, and within countries (WHO, 2008b), in addition to the growing threats to the environment and sustainable development (Stern, 2007). At an individual level, a personal sense of self-worth and the search for meaning both act on the mental and physical health of millions of people, which are both contributory factors to and consequences of this complex web of challenges (Csikzentmihaly and Csikzentmihaly, 1992).

We also need to remember that the last hundred years of human development has seen remarkable progress in the well-being and material circumstances of much of the world's population. Governments, non-governmental organizations (NGOs), and the private sector in a growing number of countries are dealing with populations that are very different from those of even thirty years ago. Reduced absolute poverty, increased education, literacy, numeracy, mass access to information, and growing expectations are not universal, but they are becoming the expected and desired norm.

Until now, social marketing has been the province of a relatively few dedicated academics and practitioners around the globe. However, we are now witnessing the rapid adoption of social marketing by many public sector organizations, agencies, and governments. Why is this happening now? There are a number of drivers that have come together that are creating more interest in the application of social marketing to key policy and behavioural challenges. In a tautological and literal sense, human behaviour sits at the heart of all politics and subsequent policy formulation, strategy development, and operational delivery in the public sector. Due to the triumph of increasingly empowered populations, governments who want to stay in power, or parties seeking power, will in the future focus more on the development of policies and interventions that are not only supported by the electorate but also increasingly defined by, involve, and meet the needs of citizens. Social marketing, with its emphasis on understanding people as the starting point for developing interventions, is a powerful tool that needs to be more systematically applied. As a recent report by the King's Fund (Boyce et al., 2008) makes clear, much of what has been done to date to assist people to change behaviour has not been as effective as it could have been had a more systematic approach been taken to apply social marketing and the use of geodemographics. According to the King's Fund, these approaches can

> Give commissioners insights into the needs and behaviours of different kinds of people. Investment should be made in developing these skills among Primary Care Trust staff and in improving both the quality and the quantity of data on local public health needs that they use in their work. Understanding how to use social marketing tools and having reliable data on local needs are vital first steps to finding solutions.

People power: some key drivers

The new citizens

Since the Second World War, the populations of most countries in the developed world and an increasing number of developing countries have undergone dramatic transformations. Despite the continued existence of poverty and poor health, there have been great strides forward across countries. This is a remarkable transformation over two or three generations accompanied and sometimes driven by huge changes in global politics, trade, manufacturing, technology, human rights and a dramatically shifting demographic profile, increasing concerns about environmental and personal fulfilment, and growth in the policy impact of cultural and religious issues. However, the transient nature of the human condition also dictates that although many now lead better lives materially, suffering continues and will continue. As Illich (1977) argued, suffering and our experience of it is an essential element of what it is to be human and actually enriches our lives, and needs to be accepted as an essential part of what it is to be alive. Any policy goal that is dominated by impossibly high expectations of joyful living clearly has the potential to be pathogenic, as Philips (1999) states:

> Lives dominated by impossible ideals—complete honesty, absolute knowledge, perfect happiness, eternal love—are lives experienced as continuous failure.

There is always a tension when setting out the goals of social programmes between aiming high and being realistic and honest about what can be achieved. However, it is the case that we have succeeded in many parts of the world in generating a belief and reality that people can make their own history. As Anthony Giddens (1991) has pointed out, in the developed world, ours is the first mass generation to view life as other than just the playing out of fate; we have become the lead actor in the film of our own lives and are able to determine what happens to us to a larger extent than has ever been possible before.

This shift in emphasis for an increasing number of people away from just a daily grind to survive towards a situation where they are increasingly seeking higher levels of self-understanding, satisfaction, and happiness is a huge triumph. A consequence of this achievement is that the notion that your fate is determined by structural or mystic forces outside your control is being increasingly seen as untrue and even offensive to more and more people. This point is argued for by Paul Corrigan (2004) in the sphere of public health when it gets too focused on just the macrosocial and economic determinants of health to the exclusion of other explanations.

> Social determinants explains too much and leaves no dialectic for the importance of individual agency. The concept has to be reconsidered in the light of the fact that we now live in a world of consumption—a place where more people are able to have many more 'consumption experiences', or choices, than were available in previous eras. People enjoy consumption and the sense of being in control that it brings them. In these circumstances determining factors make a less powerful impact and the concept of external determining factors is itself less acceptable to people. Public Health cannot stand outside this world of consumption experience.

Julian Le Grand (2007) argues that there are four models for improving public services:

1. **Trust**—where professionals are trusted to deliver high-quality services
2. **Targets**, and performance management—where workers are directed to deliver by a higher authority who sets the targets and measures performance
3. **Voice**—where users are given a chance to say what they think about the service to the providers
4. The '**other invisible hand**' of choice and competition

Le Grand argues that although all of these models have their strengths and weaknesses, approaches to public service delivery that incorporate substantive elements of choice and competition have the best prospect of delivering services that make a positive contribution to people's lives. Le Grand also sets out extensive evidence that systems driven by choice and competition are not only more efficient and responsive but also better at providing people who have less voice and economic advantage with better services. It is also true that poor people want choice and competition just as much as the better off and stand to derive just as much if not more benefit from systems set up to emphasize these features. In short, there is a need for what Osborne and Gaebler (1992) argued for in their seminal work *Reinventing Government*—a customer-driven government. This means services and interventions being driven by a desire to meet customers' needs and not the needs of the bureaucracy.

People have in most areas of their lives increasing choice, and the private sector is very responsive to people's expressed wants and needs. Smart companies are increasingly focusing their business strategies around delighting their customers (NCC, 2007) and marinating long-term relationships with them. There is a need for public sector institutions to follow this lead, as Halpern et al. (2004) state:

> Ultimately, this is not just about the government and its agencies learning a few extra techniques to 'make people eat their greens'. Rather it is about helping individuals and communities to help themselves. A more sophisticated approach enables governments to do this in ways which command greater public engagement and therefore greater effectiveness.

In this situation, state approaches to behavioural change that emphasize telling people what to do, or restricting behaviour by the force of law, can be doomed to failure unless they have the popular support of the vast majority of citizens. People now need to be engaged, listen to, and helped to change, not hectored. It is also worth noting that as people are empowered they trust governments and state organizations less and become more resistant to what they perceive as interference by governments (OLR, 2002).

Halpern et al. (2004) have suggested that there is a case for moving towards what they call the 'full co-production' model, in which citizens are engaged in the design, implementation, and evaluation of policy and practice.

The fact of increasingly empowered citizens has huge implications for state-sponsored interventions intent on making the world a better place and improving health. It means that a focus on enabling and empowering people to do the right thing for themselves and others is increasingly a key part of the way forward. This means services and interventions being driven by a desire to meet citizens' needs and not needs defined solely by experts.

New paternalism and new individualism

During the twentieth century, the state's influence on the lives of populations grew in significance. The introduction of policies and legislation, universal education, universal suffrage, and the establishment of new health and social services and professional groups to provide them have had a large impact on the prevention of disease and promotion of well-being. It can be argued, however, that this 'big state' approach has now moved past its zenith. We may be at the beginning of a new phase in civic development, one that seeks to place the citizen as consumer at the centre of attempts to maintain and further improve health.

Governments are often rightly paternalistic: part of their function is to ensure that citizens are protected and live in environments in which they can flourish. However, paternalism can take many forms. The hallmark of new paternalism is a focus not only on tackling the determinants of ill health and punishing 'bad' behaviour but also on incentivizing positive choices and creating the conditions in which people feel able to and want to make healthy choices for their own and their families' and societies' benefit.

New paternalism locates responsibility with individuals, providers of public services, and private organizations to create the environments and social norms in which healthy choices can be made. Specifically, the responsibility of those delivering public services is to place the needs and wishes of individuals at the centre of their planning and provision. This rests on a new understanding of the individual and the role of the state. New individualism is about putting the responsibility on the shoulders of those who provide services or products to deliver what citizens require so that they can live healthy and self-actualizing lives. Individuals not only have the right to expect that services will be geared up to meet their needs but also have the responsibility within their sphere of influence to do all they can to protect their own health and to contribute to the development of wider social movement for health and well-being.

What we need is a concerted shift towards a more coordinated, sustained, evidence-, and intelligence-based[1] approach built on a deep understanding of the issues that impact on people's lives. This effort needs to be focused simultaneously upstream, in-stream, and downstream. Upstream policy that is designed to address the determinants of health, whereas in-stream actions and policy help people to cope with poor health and adverse conditions, and downstream efforts are those public health interventions designed to help people change behaviour to improve health.[2]

We do, of course, know that those with more power and resources can be more in charge of their experiences and also have more choices. These disparities in choice and control are some of the key reasons for health inequalities (Wilkinson and Marmot, 2003). However, less choice and less power are not the same as no choice and no power. It is well understood that choice systems are usually the most efficient way to distribute resources but that they can favour the better off and the more articulate (Giddens, 2003; Lent and Arend, 2004).

Creating an environment of maximum choice for the majority requires the coordinated application of all policy tools to influence the behaviour of individuals, organizations, and markets. In this way, we can shift to a more balanced view of the locus of power, to what Rothschild (2001) calls the 'apparent power' of government to the 'actual power' of individuals. We need to recognize the fact that both governments and individuals have power and responsibilities; public health strategy must explicitly acknowledge this.

Eighty-nine per cent of the people agree that individuals are responsible for their own health and 93% agree that parents are more responsible than anyone else for their children's health (King's Fund, 2004), whereas only 33% of the people think that the government has a key role to play in promoting health and less than 4% believe that it has the most important role (Ofcom, 2005). Eighty-four per cent of the parents feel that they have most responsibility for ensuring that their children eat a healthy diet, only 7% believe that the government has the most

---

1 Evidence alone is never the only stream of intelligence used to make policy, strategy, or operational decisions. Intelligence also includes information sources such as epidemiology, service uptake data, demographic data, competition analysis, horizon scanning, market research data, knowledge, attitude, and behavioural data. These data sources, along with evidence, are mediated by the need for policy coherence and understanding of political imperatives, and are ideally also informed by impact assessments and cost–benefit studies or modelling.

2 There is a need to focus upstream in policy terms on the determinants and risk conditions that impact people's health while focusing in-stream on how people can be helped to cope with the socio-economic circumstances that they find themselves in. It is also necessary to focus on what has often been termed as 'downstream health promotion', targeted at empowering and enabling people to protect their health.

responsibility, and less than 3% believe that food retailers have the most responsibility (Jebb et al., 2007). There is evidence of significant public demand for health information (Department of Health, 2004), but also strong support for state action to promote the health of the public (Lent and Arend, 2004). While people want public service professionals to make key judgements and give advice, they also want to be empowered to influence this process (Ipsos MORI, 2007; NSMC, 2008). This evidence suggests that public health interventions must in the future understand and engage people in delivering solutions. We need to recognize that policy that treats people as passive recipients of professionally determined solutions and simple exhortations to change behaviour will probably not bring about the large population-level change that is required to improve health.

User-defined value

The second driver for a more user-focused approach to tackling population behavioural challenges is essentially a public sector version of a switch from a product- or service-focused to a customer-focused strategy, which drives most successful for-profit organizations and many not-for-profit organizations who rely on user or donor support. The need for more responsive public services is illustrated by the results of research conducted by Ipsos MORI (2005), in which British people said the following words best described public service, with the highest-ranked words in descending order:

Bureaucratic

Infuriating

Faceless

Hardworking

Unresponsive

Unaccountable

The lowest-ranked words were as follows:

Friendly

Efficient

Honest

Open

An increasingly empowered and demanding citizenry represents a triumph rather than a problem for governments. This shift in power and expectation demands that governments and their institutions demonstrate that they are adding value to the lives of the people that they serve. Given this perception by the public, one of the challenges facing governments is to more clearly set out what value they are creating for the people they serve.

Moore (1995) and Kelly et al. (2002) have identified the concept of public value as having three dimensions: outcomes, the delivery of services, and trust. Kelly et al. (2002) also argue that public value only exists if people are willing to give something up in return for the service they get, such as granting coercive powers to the state in return for security and protection. This 'exchange' is a key feature of social marketing and requires reciprocal actions on the part of both the state and citizens, and is often called the 'social contract'. The state is required to understand the citizens' perspective about the nature and value of these trade-offs, and the citizen is required to accept limitations on behaviour for the collective good. In a world where public value will be measured and used by citizens to assess government and public sector performance, we require new approaches to both understand citizens and what they are prepared to exchange for different behaviour and change programmes that make changing behaviour easy and, where

Box 1.1 Shift in emphasis

To succeed we need to move from:

'Expert defined product' approach → 'Value to user' approach

possible, rewarding for people. This change in emphasis sits at the heart of this book and at the heart of social marketing (Box 1.1).

Case study: Don't just SAY they matter

An example of this shift in emphasis is the 'Don't just SAY they matter programme', run by Department of Health New Zealand 2008 which aimed to put Maori and Pacific women in New Zealand at the heart of a social marketing intervention that promotes the importance of cervical screening and facilitates its uptake (Fig. 1.1). The programme aimed to increase

- Awareness and understanding of cervical cancer and the benefits of cervical screening;
- Discussion about cervical screening, in order to get support from families, friends, and communities for women to have regular smears;

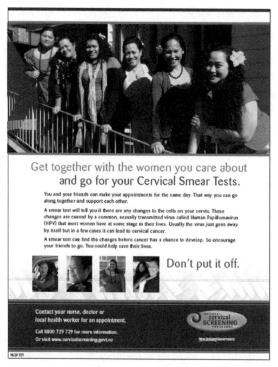

Fig 1.1 The 'Don't just SAY they matter programme', Department of Health New Zealand, 2008. *Source*: Reproduced with permission of the National Screening Unit, Ministry of Health (www.nsu.govt.nz)

- The number of women calling the programme 0800 number for more information;
- The number of Maori and Pacific women who make appointments and have smears.

The programme was built on deep user insights about how services needed to be changed. Women wanted the services to be offered in the community, from women's homes and involve peer recruitment. 'Don't just SAY they matter' was a $2 million per year, 3-year, ongoing programme of activity, evaluated through quantitative monitoring surveys at 12 monthly intervals, tracking call volumes to the 0800 number monthly, and conducting monthly reporting from the programme register to evaluating the impact on screening coverage. After 12-months participation in the programme, the increase in screening coverage was as follows: Maori, 6.8%; Pacific, 12.7%; Asian, 6.7%; others, 2.7%. Acknowledgments to Dr Hazal Lewis, Clinical Lead and Graham Bethune Ministry of Health New Zealand.

New technology and methodology

The technological revolution that the world has experienced over the last fifty years and is set to experience in the next fifty years is enormous. This revolution is generating a blurring of lines between producers and consumers, an explosion in access to information and opinions, and the development of new forms of communities. Our knowledge of how to develop policy, strategy, and intervention programmes is also being strengthened by new technology and new methodologies including interdisciplinary working. A host of academic disciplines are providing increasing understanding and evidence about what drives behaviour and how it can be influenced. The World Wide Web and electronic archiving and search technologies are also speeding up the collation, assessment, and synthesis of this knowledge at a speed that was simply not possible as little as ten years ago. We are also seeing more interdisciplinary synthesis of understanding. The growth in cross-disciplinary subjects such as behavioural economics, social psychology, and cultural and media studies indicates a new approach to understanding and addressing complex social issues. We know that there is rarely a single magic bullet that will create change in a complex environment. However, we do know a great deal about the kinds of characteristics that typify more successful programmes of action to bring about behavioural change. These are set out in summary form later in this chapter. The issue now is not what works but whether we are prepared to sustain investment in what we know works at a level that will have a demonstrable effect, and whether we can put in place the planning and systems to manage well-coordinated intervention strategies.

The acknowledgement that governments cannot do it alone

Kickbusch et al. (2005) have emphasized recognition of the need for co-production of solutions to complex social issues and challenges. Liberal democracy and regulated free market economies are generally recognized as forces for social good (Roberts, 1985; Fukuyama, 1992). These complex systems, with all their benefits, problems, and complexities, are the reality for many and an aspiration for more and more of the world's population. There is also increasing recognition that the power of civil society, the private sector, NGO sector, and the thousands of community groups and civil associations represents and has always represented the main bedrock of success in building better lives for people. Civil society provides more health and social care than the state, informs and educates more children and adults, creates more employment than the state, and provides the myriad of social networks that nurture and develop citizens. The well-being of society is intertwined with the well-being of individuals, their social networks, cultures, and the confidence and resources they have to choose and create the kinds of lives they want. It is also evident that the private sector and NGO sector have a vital part to play in tackling the big behavioural challenges that we face. The reach, expertise, and deep understanding of people that these sectors have needs to be harnessed in a far more coordinated way (Chapter 21 explores these issues).

State paternalism and the expert-defined product mentality

As argued so far in this chapter, most large behavioural issues faced by society stem from a combination of personal choice, environmental factors, cultural factors, and economic factors. Personal choices about issues such as healthy eating or reducing energy consumption are played out against a background of many powerful influences on individual behaviour. The issues of individual rights and responsibilities and those of free choice and compulsion are the everyday political and policy battlegrounds for those concerned with social issues. For social marketers, these are also key issues as policy derived through democratic means is the strongest starting point for the development of ethical social marketing practice.

There is evidence from many disciplines that people do not always act in an economically logical way, for example, by always acting in a way designed to maximize their own advantage. People often want to do the right thing and help others (NEF, 2005). People are concerned with fairness, equity, and generally do not wish to behave in ways that disadvantage or negatively affect others. The vast majority of the people also want to act in ways that result in a better collective experience for everyone (NSMC, 2008). The challenge is as much to encourage these deeply held beliefs in fairness and social justice as it is to drive out antisocial and entirely self-serving interest that negatively impacts on individuals and others.

The hallmark of this kind of paternalism is a focus not only on tackling the determinants of issues such as obesity, alcohol misuse, and lack of saving for retirement by punishing 'bad' behaviour but also on incentivizing positive choices and creating the conditions in which people feel able to and want to make constructive choices for their own and their families' benefit. This kind of paternalism locates responsibility with individuals, providers of public services, and private organizations to create the environments and social norms in which healthy choices can be made. Specifically, the responsibility of those delivering public services is to place the needs and wishes of individuals at the centre of their planning and provision.

Thaler and Sunstein's (2008) concept of 'nudging' people into different behaviours encompasses interventions that are

> Easy and cheap to avoid. Nudges are not mandates. Putting fruit at eye level counts as a nudge. Banning junk food does not.

Libertarian paternalism as advocated by Sunstein and Thaler (2003) seeks a middle ground between a state-dominated coercive paternalistic approach to creating social change and a more liberal approach that emphasizes free choice and the power of the market as the key driver. Although social marketing employs a lot of 'nudges' as defined by Thaler and Sunstein (2008), it goes beyond nudges to include more difficult interventions supported by both evidence that indicates it will help people change and research that shows people will value and be prepared to pay the price for the benefits they accrue with their time, money, attention, or by ceding some freedoms to governments. Social marketing can be considered a means through which libertarian paternalism can be delivered. Furthermore, social marketing is certainly rooted in the democratic tradition as it constantly seeks a mandate for action from the target groups it seeks to help in the form of insights gained from market research.

Social marketing often encompasses information giving, media advocacy, service change, legislation to incentivize or penalize behaviour, and measures designed to change the physical, economic, or social environments. The aim is to make the healthy and most socially positive choice of behaviour rewarding and if possible easy. Social marketing can inform and help develop a well-targeted policy intervention mix (see Chapter 5).

Change management in the public sector has been driven over many years by a focus on planning, service quality improvement, evidence-based practice, and systems and risk management. There has been a concerted effort to import such disciplines from the private sector as a way of increasing efficiency and effectiveness. The adoption of systematic business processes is however a second-order activity in most private sector organizations. The principle function of businesses is about winning customers, delighting them, and developing products and services that create an ongoing relationship with clients to realize what is often called the 'lifetime value' of the relationship.

The new citizen-driven business model

Many behavioural change interventions are based on evidence derived from published studies and analysis of demographic, service uptake, and epidemiological data. This information is vital but not sufficient to develop effective behavioural interventions. In contrast, the commercial sector invests heavily in market research to understand people's motivations, needs, wants, fears, aspirations about why they would purchase goods or services, or what goods and services they feel they need or would like. Public health and other forms of public sector interventions need to enhance their understanding of the target group's motivations if they are going to be able to develop more effective programmes.

> We must be relentlessly customer-focused. Many people want a single point of contact for a range of services. The public are not interested in whether their needs are met by Department X or Agency Y, they just want a good, joined up service where X and Y talk to each other and share the information the public have provided. We should strive to meet this demand.[3]
>
> If we don't understand what really matters to the people we are trying to reach, we will waste time and money and risk compromising our reputation by offering services which customers don't recognise as being for them and have difficulty accessing. We will base our management of those services on an illusion, recording as a triumph each duplicative and unnecessary phone call because it has been dealt with within the target time allowed. The complex social problems of exclusion, many of which can be alleviated by early intervention, will remain intractable.[4]

One of the main reasons people work in the public sector is because it provides them with a strong sense of satisfaction. In practice, however, they can sometimes find themselves dealing with the vagaries of working within a service verging on the edge of being, or at least perceived as being, institutionally dysfunctional and sometimes subject to public disquiet. Developing the means for sustained organizational change and service improvement through a process of satisfying customer needs is about building on the belief systems that already exist in public service. However, as argued earlier, this public sector ethos of service, care, collective responsibility, and social justice is often subjugated by a focus on meeting managerial or policy-defined targets pursued through what could be called mechanistic approaches to service improvement. The thinking is that if we can only get great planning, budgeting, HR, risk management, and quality assurance systems in place, everything will be just fine. The trouble is that this leaves the most important driver out of the solution—the user or client and what they think, feel, and do.

---

3 Sir Gus O'Donnell, Cabinet Secretary, quoted in the working paper on 'Customer insight in public services – "A Primer"' (Cabinet Office, October 2006).

4 Working paper on 'Customer insight in public services – "A Primer"' (Cabinet Office, October 2006, p. 2).

There is a case then for governments and those concerned with pursuing social good to move away from a purely 'expert-defined', systems-focused, mechanistic 'product' approach to change and service delivery towards a social marketing approach that places more emphasis on user or target audiences and needs. This simple but challenging switch in approach is illustrated in Fig. 1.2. In the citizen-driven model set out in the figure, views, beliefs, and suggestions from citizens are key streams of intelligence that are used to inform policy and strategy development.

The development of a citizen-driven model of service delivery and improvement in the public sector, through the rigorous application of social marketing, would result in public service organizations that are more motivated, progressive, ambitious, and constantly striving to improve services, not for the sake of managers or policymakers but for the benefit of the service users.

Such a 'user'-driven approach to service improvement would also gain new respect from the public for public services. If such an approach was universally applied, it would soon become clear to every user of public service that the service was geared up to providing them with the kinds of help they need and in a way that is most convenient for them. Health improvement interventions would be developed and delivered from a perspective of listening and understanding, and not telling and selling. Public service would be characterized by responsiveness and customer care, and would no longer be viewed simply as a once great but failing set of post-Second World War institutions whose staff has to put up with management chaos and chronic adversity. Rather, public services could be viewed as vibrant, responsive, and efficient, dedicated to satisfying people's needs.

Tackling the conspiracy of passive failure

Many traditional public health programmes that try to change behaviour are not effective or have such weak evaluation that it is difficult to tell if they are effective or not (Boyce et al., 2008). However, there has been significant growth in knowledge about what works and what does not in the field of behavioural change as well as how to plan and deliver such interventions over the recent years, but often this knowledge is not always used to shape national interventions or local community interventions.

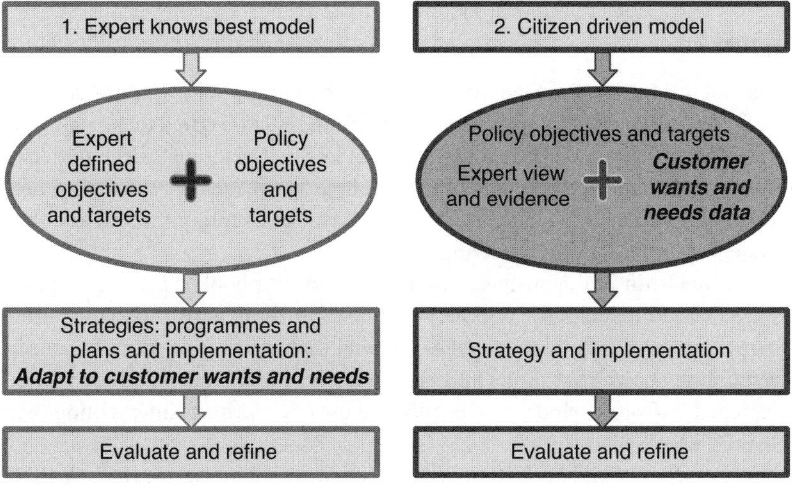

Fig 1.2 Expert-knows-best versus citizen-driven model.

There is also often political and policy pressure to 'be seen to be acting' on behavioural challenges and for action to happen rapidly. This means that advertising and other media promotions are often looked to as a quick way of demonstrating that action is being taken. This situation can be described as a conspiracy of passive failure. This conspiracy is not driven by a wish for programmes to fail but by more positive and understandable motivators such as a desire to do something and to do it quickly, or a belief that people need encouragement and information. There is also often a very real political need to be seen to be acting to give confidence to people that something can be done. It is a passive conspiracy because most politicians and senior officials that support these kinds of intervention know or have been advised that the predicted outcome will be minimal. Clearly, media promotions, advertising, and other forms of mass communication are extremely powerful tools that social marketers will want to deploy, and in the right circumstances, they have a major role to play (Hornick, 2002; Lannon, 2008). However, the point is that they should be used as part of planned and coordinated strategy, and not as the default solution. To end this passive conspiracy, a more transparent and systematic application of social marketing should be applied.

Does social marketing work?

Not withstanding the very real issues of proving cause and effect that are explored in Chapter 2, there has been developing over the last forty years a growing and compelling body of evidence about the effectiveness of interventions aimed at bringing about behavioural change, health improvement, and social change. There are now global networks of institutions that collaborate to review and collate evidence, and what is clear is that there are a number of common characteristics that are markers for the likely success of interventions in a variety of sectors across different issues and with different target groups. There is no formula that can be universally applied when developing and delivering social marketing programmes that will result in success every time in every situation, but there is a well-supported set of principles that can aid us in the development and application of interventions intended to develop health. There is also a well-proven set of planning steps and processes that have been developed. These principles are set out in Chapters 10–15. In addition to these key principles, social marketing is characterized by a systematic approach to planning. Box 1.2 sets out some of the characteristics that, if present in social marketing plans, have the potential to improve the impact.

Conclusion

This chapter and this book argue for a fundamental shift in how public sector organizations function. While we have developed impressive data-gathering systems related to mortality, morbidity, and health sector utilization, we have invested much less in developing a deep understanding of the wants, fears, needs, motivations, and barriers people face that either enhance or detract from their ability to live healthy lives. In short, we are fantastic at counting the sick and the dead but much less adept at understanding the living.

The fundamental shift in the business model set out in this book is from an approach where solutions are derived principally by policy annalists working with subject experts utilizing limited forms of evidence and data towards a model that is also influenced by a deep contextual understanding about what target audiences know, believe, value, and say will help them. This fundamental shift also includes the coordinated use of all forms of intervention that will help and enable people to change.

Social marketing is a highly systematic approach to social improvement that sets out unambiguous success criteria in terms of behavioural change alongside thorough and

Box 1.2 The 16 characteristics of social marketing plans

1. All plans are recorded in a published social marketing plan. This plan is based on a recognized planning template.
2. Clear aims and measurable behavioural objectives are set out and supported by policy-makers, programme commissioners, and managers—deliverers of the programme.
3. The target audience(s) and segments are explicit in the plan.
4. There is evidence that target group(s) are involved in needs assessment, target setting, delivery, and evaluation.
5. The plan sets out how prototype interventions or pilots will be tested and used to develop full-scale programmes.
6. The plan sets out a clear rationale for the programme and why the particular interventions have been selected.
7. The plan sets out how the programme will be funded to the level required to achieve impact and how it will be sustained over the recommended time scale for delivery.
8. The plan sets out how coalitions with other stakeholders, partners, and interest groups will be developed and coordinated.
9. The plan sets out the mechanism for coordinated action between international, national, regional, and local delivery, and how decision making, governance, and coordination of the programme will operate.
10. The plan sets out the political, policy, managerial, and institutional commitment to the programme.
11. Key barriers and enabling factors as well as other risks are identified in the plan together with what actions will be taken to address these factors.
12. The plan captures what evidence about effective practice from reviews and case studies, observational data, and target audience psychographic data is being used to formulate insight and interventions.
13. The plan indicates what theoretical perspectives have been used to inform planning that is congruent with the form, focus, and context of the intervention.
14. The plan sets out how funding and other resources will be applied and over what time period. A clear expected return-on-investment case is set out to justify the level of planned investment.
15. The plan sets out key milestones in developing and delivering the programme. These milestones should cover process, impact, and outcome elements.
16. Evaluation, performance management, learning, and feedback mechanisms are clear in the plan. Evaluation should encompass short-term impact measures for tracking purposes, process measures of efficiency, and outcome evaluation related to the specific objectives of the programme.

transparent planning about how to achieve it. This focus on measurable return on investment is a feature that many governments and other organizations trying to bring about change will value. Social marketing will also be attractive to governments because of its emphasis on developing deep customer insight and population segmentation enabling governments to develop interventions that can respond to a broad diversity of needs and target specific subgroups often with the most need (Prime Minister's Strategy Unit, 2006).

At a time of declining trust in civic institutions, fragmentation of society, and rising consumerism, social marketing offers a well-developed approach for tackling key behavioural challenges faced by society. Social marketing offers a methodology that embraces the reality of markets, choice, and mutual responsibility. Social marketing also offers a way to balance the rights and responsibilities of individuals and the rights and responsibilities of wider society through the exercise of choice and the provision of incentives and penalties to behave in a way that maximizes personal advantage and the well-being of others.

Authentic social marketing is not about telling people what to do or coercing them into doing it, but the art of understanding what will help people make choices and take action that will lead them to better lives. In short, those who seek to serve the public and make the world a better place have to learn how to make positive life choices the easy and natural choices for people.

In the coming years, it is highly probable that social marketing will become part of the standard operating systems for governments, public sector organizations, and not-for-profit organizations concerned with doing social good. This is because, it works, it can be shown to work, and it is a deeply democratic approach to social justice, well matched to the sophisticated cultural, social, and political environment of the twenty-first century. Public servants from politicians to practitioners will need to invest time and effort in developing their understanding of social marketing's principles so that they can become champions for the communities they serve.

References

Boyce, T., Robertson, R. and Dixon, A. (2008). *Commissioning and Behavioural Change: Kicking Bad Habits Final Report.* London: King's Fund.

Corrigan, P. (2004). *An Evening with Paul Corrigan, Government Advisor on Health.* Coventry: Warwick Institute of Governance and Public Management, Warwick University.

Csikzentmihaly, M. and Csikzentmihaly, I. (1992). *Optimal Experience. Psychological Studies of Flow in Consciousness.* Cambridge: Cambridge University Press.

DoH (2004). *Choosing Health: Making Healthy Choices Easier.* London: Department of Health.

Fukuyama, F. (1992). *The End of History and the Last Man.* London: Penguin.

Giddens, A. (1991). *Modernity and Self-Identity.* Cambridge: Polity Press.

Giddens, A. (2003). *Neoprogressivism: The Progressive Manifesto.* Cambridge: Polity Press.

Halpern, D., Bates, C., Mulgan, G., Aldridge, S., Beales, G. and Heathfield, A. (2004). *Personal Responsibility and Changing Behaviour: The State of Knowledge and Its Implications for Public Policy.* London: Cabinet Office.

Hornick, R.C. (ed.) (2002). *Public Health Communication: Evidence for Behavior Change.* New Jersey: LEA.

Illich, I. (1977). *Medical Nemesis.* London: Marion Boyars.

Ipsos MORI (2005). *Attitudes to health and health service improvement.* London: Ipsos MORI.

Ipsos MORI (2007). *Policy Review Citizens Forum: Emerging Conclusions.* London/Harrow: Ipsos MORI.

Jebb, S., Steer, T. and Holmes, C. (2007). *The Healthy Living Social Marketing Initiative: A Review of the Evidence.* MRC Human Nutrition Research, Department of Health. London.

Kelly, G., Mulgan, G. and Muers, S. (2002). *Creating Public Value: An Analytical Framework for Public Sector Reform.* London: Prime Minister's Strategy Unit, Cabinet Office.

Kickbusch, I., Maag, D. and Sann, H. (2005). Enabling healthy choices in modern health societies. Background paper for Parallel Forum F6 on 'Healthy Choices', presented at the *8th European Health Forum Gastein 2005 on Partnerships for Health*, Bad Gastein, Austria, October 6, 2005.

King's Fund (2004). *Public Attitudes to Public Health Policy*. London: King's Fund and Health Development Agency.

Lannon, J. (2008). *How Public Service Advertising Works*. London: World Advertising Research Centre.

Le Grand, J. (2007). *The Other Invisible Hand: Delivering Public Service through Choice and Competition*. Princeton and Oxford: Princeton University Press.

Lent, A. and Arend, N. (2004). *Making Choices: How Can Choice Improve Local Public Services?* London: New Local Government Network.

Moore, M.H. (1995). *Creating Public Value—Strategic Management in Government*. Cambridge, MA: Harvard University Press.

Murray, C. (2006). *In Our Hands*. Washington, DC: AEI Press.

NCC (2007). *The Stupid Company: How British Businesses Throw Money away by Alienating Customers*. London: National Consumer Council.

NEF (2005). *Behavioural Economics: Seven Principles for Policy Makers*. London: New Economics Foundation.

NSMC (2008). *Some Are More Equal Than Others: Public Attitudes to Health Inequalities and Social Determinants of Health*. London: National Social Marketing Centre.

Ofcom (2005). *Responsibility for promoting Health*, survey conducted by NOP. London: Office of Communications.

OLR (2002). *It's a Matter of Trust: What Society Thinks and Feels about Trust*. London: Opinion Leader Research.

Osborne, D. and Gaebler, T. (1992). *Reinventing Government: How the Entrepreneurial Spirit Is Transforming the Public Sector*. Reading, MA: Addison-Wesley.

Philips, A. (1999). *Darwin's Worms*. London: Faber and Faber.

Prime Minister's Strategy Unit (2006). *The UK Government's Approach to Public Service Reform*. London: Cabinet Office.

Roberts, J.M. (1985). *The Triumph of the West*. Boston, MA: Little, Brown.

Rothschild, M. (2001). Ethical considerations in the use of marketing for the management of public health and social issues. In A. Andersen (ed.), *Ethics in Social Marketing*. Washington, DC: Georgetown University Press.

Stern, N. (2007). *The Economics of Climate Change: The Stern Review*. Cambridge: Cambridge University Press.

Sunstein, C. and Thaler, T. (2003). Libertarian paternalism is not an oxymoron. *University of Chicago Law Review*, 70(4): 1159–1202.

Thaler, R. and Sunstein, C. (2008). *Nudge. Improving Decisions about Health, Wealth and Happiness*. New Haven and London: Yale University Press.

Wilkinson, R. and Marmot, M. (eds.) (2003). *Social Determinants of Health: The Solid Facts*, 2nd ed. London: World Health Organization.

WHO (2008a). *Now More Than Ever*. Geneva: World Health Organization.

WHO (2008b). *Closing the Gap in a Generation*. Geneva: World Health Organization.

Box 1.2 references

Andreasen, A. (1995). *Marketing Social Change: Changing Behaviour to Promote Health, Social Development, and the Environment*. San Francisco, CA: Jossey-Bass.

Australian Public Service Commission (2007a). *Changing Behaviour: A Public Policy Perspective*. Barton, ACT: Australian Government.

Australian Public Service Commission (2007b). *Tackling Wicked Problems: A Public Policy Perspective.* Barton, ACT: Australian Government.

Bate, P., Bevan, H. and Robert, G. (2004). *'Towards a Million Change Agents' A Review of the Social Movement's Literature.* London: NHS Modernisation Agency.

CDC (2005). Centres for disease control *CDCynegy, Social Marketing Edition.* CDROM. CDC Atlanta.

Darnton, A. (2008). *GSR Behaviour Change Knowledge Review.* London: Government Social Research Unit, Her Majesty's Treasury.

DoH (2003). *Tackling Health Inequalities: A Programme for Action.* London: Department of Health.

DoH (2007). *Health Challenge England.* London: Department of Health.

Donovan, R. and Henely, N. (2003). *Social Marketing: Principles and Practice.* East Hawthorn, Vic: IP Communications.

Elliot, B. (1988). The development and assessment of successful campaigns', Education co-ordinators' workshop on media skills, Brisbane. *Public Opinion Quarterly*, 37: 50–61.

French, J. (2004a). Nine steps for effective practice. *Community Practitioner*, February.

French, J. (2004b). *The Learning from Effective Practice Standard System (LEPSS) Outline Programme 2004–2007.* London: Health Development Agency.

French, J. and Mayo, E. (2006). *It's Our Health!* London: National Consumer Council.

Futerra (2005). The new rules new game. Communication tactics for climate change. The game is changing behaviours; the rules will help us win it. London: Futerra.

Goldberg, M., Fishbein, M. and Middlestat, S. (1997). *Social Marketing: Theoretical and Practical Perspectives.* Washington, DC: Academy for Educational Development.

Halpern, D., Bates, C., Mulgan, G., Aldridge, S., Beales, G. and Heathfield, A. (2004). *Personal Responsibility and Changing Behaviour: The State of Knowledge and Its Implications for Public Policy.* London: Cabinet Office.

Healthcare Commission and the Audit Commission (2008). *Are We Choosing Health? The Impact of Policy on the Delivery of Health Improvement Programmes and Services.* London: Health Care Commission.

Health Development Agency (2004). *The Effectiveness of Public Health Campaigns.* London: Health Development Agency.

Herron, D.B. (1997). *Marketing Nonprofits Programs and Services: Proven and Practical Strategies to Get More Customers, Members, and Donors.* San Francisco, CA: Jossey-Bass.

Hills, D. (2004). *Evaluation of Community-Level Interventions for Health Improvement: A Review of Experience in the UK.* London: Health Development Agency.

Iles, V. and Sutherland, K. (2001). *Managing change in the NHS: Organisational Change—A Review for Health Care Managers, Professionals and Researchers.* London: National Coordinating Centre for NHS Service Delivery and Organisation Research and Development.

International Union for Health Promotion and Education (2000). *The Evidence of Health Promotion Effectiveness*, 2nd ed. Brussels: European Commission.

Jackson, T. (2005). *Motivating Sustainable Consumption: A Review of Evidence on Consumer Behavior and Behavioral Change.* Surrey: Centre for Environmental Strategy, University of Surrey.

Kelly, G., Mulgan, G. and Muers, S. (2002). *Creating Public Value. An Analytical Framework for Public Sector Reform.* London: Prime Minister's Strategy Unit, Cabinet Office.

Kotler, P. and Roberto, W. (1989). *Social Marketing: Strategies for Changing Public Behaviour.* New York, NY: Free Press.

Kotler, P., Roberto, W. and Lee, N. (2002). *Social Marketing: Improving the Quality of Life*, 2nd ed. Thousand Oaks, CA: Sage Publications.

Manoff, R.K. (1985). Social *Marketing: New Imperative for Public Health.* New York: Praeger.

McGuire, W.J. (1986). The myth of massive media impact: savings and salvagings. *Public Communications and Behaviour*, 1: 173–220.

Michie, S., Jochelson, K., Markham, W. and Bridle, C. (2008). *Low Income Groups and Behaviour Change Interventions: A Review of Intervention Content and Effectiveness.* London: King's Fund.

Miller, M. and Ware, J. (1989). *Mass Media Alcohol and Drug Campaigns: Consideration of Relevant Issues*, monograph Series no. 9. Canberra: Australian Government Publishing Service.

Moodie, R. (2000). *Infrastructures to Promote Health: The Art of the Possible.* Victoria: Health Promotion Foundation.

Moor, M. (1995). *Creating Public Value: Strategic Management in Government.* Cambridge, MA: Harvard University Press.

National Social Marketing Excellence Collaborative (2004). *The Managers Guide to Social Marketing.* Seattle, CA: Turning Point.

NCCSDO (2001). *Managing Change in the NHS: Making Informed Decisions on Change.* London: NHS Service Delivery and Organisation Research and Development.

NEF (2005). *Behavioural Economics: Seven Principles for Policy Makers.* London: New Economics Foundation.

NESTA (2001). *Selling Sustainability: Seven Lessons from Advertising and Marketing to Sell Low-Carbon Living*, report suppl. 01. London: National Endowment for Science, Technology and the Arts.

NHS Centre for Reviews and Dissemination (1999). Getting evidence into practice. *Effective Health Care*, 5(1): 1–16.

NICE (2007). *Behaviour Change: Quick Reference Guide.* London: National Institute for Health and Clinical Excellence.

NSMC (2008). *The Total Process Planning Framework for Social Marketing.* London: National Social Marketing Centre.

Ogden, L., Shepherd, M. and Smith, W.A. (1996). *Applying Prevention Marketing. Atlanta, GA: Centers for Disease Control and Prevention, Public Health Service.*

OPM (2002). *The Effectiveness of Different Mechanisms for Spreading Good Practice.* London: Office for Public Management, Cabinet Office.

RCU (2003). *Review of Area Based Initiatives.* London: Regional Co-ordination Unit.

Roe, L., Hunt, P., Bradshaw, H. et al. (1997). *Health Promotion Effectiveness Reviews 6: Health Promotion Interventions to Promote Healthy Eating in the General Population: A Review.* London: Health Education Authority.

Rogers, E.M. and Storey, J.D. (1987). Communication campaigns. In C.R. Berget and S.H. Chattee (eds.) *Handbook of Communication Science.* San Francisco, CA: Sage Publications.

Rothschild, M. *(1999). Carrots, sticks and promises: a conceptual framework for the management of public health and social behaviours. Journal of Marketing*, 63(October): 24–37.

Ryan, M. (2001). *Overview of Practice Collections Relevant to Tackling Health Inequality.* London: Health Development Agency.

Schorr, L.B. (2003). *Determining 'What works' in Social Programs and Social Policies: Towards a More Inclusive Knowledge Base.* Washington, DC: Brookings Institution.

SMF (2008). *Creatures of Habit: The Art of Behaviour Change.* London: Social Market Foundation.

Solomon, D.S. (1982). Mass media campaigns in health promotion. *Prevention in Human Services*, 2(1/2): 115–123.

Solomon, D.S. (1984). Social marketing and community health promotion: the Stanford heart disease prevention program. In L.W. Frederiksen, L.J. Solomon, and K.A. Brehony (eds.) *Marketing Health Behaviour.* New York, NY: Plenum Press.

Strategy Unit (2008). *Cultural Change: A Policy Framework.* London: Cabinet Office.

Tones, K. and Whitehead, M. (1991). Avoiding the Pitfalls. London: Health Education Authority.

US DHHS (2003). *The Pink Book: Making Health Communication Programmes Work.* Washington, DC: National Institutes of Health National Cancer Institute.

WHO (1977). *Jakarta Declaration.* Geneva: World Health Organization.

WHO (2008). *Closing the Gap in a Generation.* Geneva: World Health Organization.

Chapter 2

A history of social marketing

Aiden Truss, Robert Marshall, and Clive Blair-Stevens

Do not believe in traditions because they have been handed down for many generations. But after observation and analysis, when you find that anything agrees with reason and is conducive to the good and benefit of one and all, then accept it and live up to it.
Buddha

Learning points

This chapter

- Encourages an appreciation of the historic development of social marketing;
- Introduces social marketing as a dynamic and integrative discipline;
- Explains the 'two parents' metaphor and the convergence of debates in marketing and social behavioural sciences;
- Provides an understanding of the ongoing dynamic nature of the social marketing debate; and
- Explains how social marketing fits alongside social advertising.

Chapter overview

To date, a great deal of writing on the evolution of social marketing has focused almost exclusively on describing its historical link to commercial marketing. In this chapter, we seek to challenge this narrow and only partial view by setting out the discipline's link to social and behavioural sciences. We will also look at the gradual establishment of social marketing in the UK government's health policy agenda.

Introduction

For many, social marketing is merely marketing used for health promotion or social good, and in general, this is a misunderstanding of the concept. It is also seen as something new and, perhaps most problematically, as something of a fad or buzzword in policy circles. In fact, social marketing has a pedigree stretching back at least forty years. Although government attempts at influencing public behaviour through interventions are dotted throughout history, it is only in the last decades of the twentieth century that there was any attempt to codify an effective means of achieving it.

The term 'social marketing' was first used in 1971 by Philip Kotler and Gerald Zaltman in an article that discussed the application of commercial marketing principles in health, social, and quality-of-life issues (Kotler and Zaltman, 1971). However it is increasingly being recognized that the discipline is better understood as derived from two 'parents': marketing and social sciences (as illustrated in Fig. 2.1). So, when we examine the evolution of social marketing, we really need to look at how these two distinct movements have converged to inform social marketing in the 21st century.

Although both parents come from different families, they do nevertheless start with the same primary concern: the challenge of how best to influence people's behaviour. The following text sketches out the family tree with the marketing story, the social sciences story, and even the anti-social marketing story.

The marketing story

Although we can trace the origins of consumerism as far back as the industrial revolution, it is only comparatively recently that consumer culture really took off. Henry Ford's pioneering production line for the Model T introduced in 1913 may have shown the way forward for mass production and mass marketing, but it took the industrial fallout from two world wars to really kick-start the movement.

By the 1950s, the West had a fully developed consumer culture, fuelled by social changes after the Second World War. The hope and optimism of an age where science offered new possibilities and promised much were seemingly being fulfilled. Fully mechanized economies that were used to churn out weapons and munitions on a huge scale were able to turn their energies from building tanks and bombs to building refrigerators and cars. Years of austerity were replaced by a new culture in which consumption took on almost ideological importance. Catalogues and stores were full of products, which were seen as iconic emblems of freedom and resistance to the conditions imposed by a new cold war enemy in the Soviet Union. In the United States, in particular, it was the citizen's patriotic duty to consume.

With a huge range of products available for every human need, marketing provided the mechanism through which to persuade consumers to buy a product. And if there was no real need for a specific product, marketing could stimulate one. A parallel growth in television sales provided a channel through which advertising could reach people, and the programme sponsorship that produced the 'soap opera' helped maintain a relentless stream of messages to encourage the public to spend.

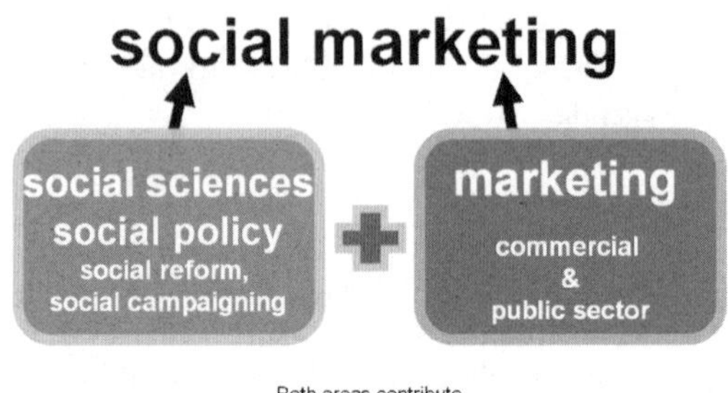

Fig. 2.1 The two parents of social marketing.
Source: French and Blair-Stevens (2007), with permission.

In 1960, the American Marketing Association (AMA) defined marketing rather conservatively as *the performance of business activities that direct the flow of goods and services from producer to consumer*, adding 20 years later *in order to best satisfy customers and accomplish the firm's objectives* (Manoff, 1985, p. 24). The British Institute of Marketing advanced the definition in 1966 by replacing the underlying notion of 'assessing consumer needs' with 'assessing and converting customer purchase power in effective demand for a specific product' (ibid.). By the 1980s, marketing on both sides of the Atlantic assumed the task of not only satisfying the demand but also *creating* the demand for goods and services.

From here, the concept of marketing grew or, as we shall see later, 'broadened' to include nearly the whole function of business (and other activities) as viewed from its results. One scholar went so far as to say it *integrated the use of all of a company's resources to aid and abet in supplying wanted goods and services at a profit to itself* (Adler, 1982, p. 653). In a final critical step, marketing redirected the task of the manufacturer from simply distributing its products to identifying and even creating customer wants and needs before inventing products and distributions systems to satisfy them.

Shaw and Jones (2005, p. 241) trace marketing thought as far back as ancient times, but they agree that it was only during the twentieth century that marketing ideas evolved into a systematic body of knowledge and an academic discipline. They define marketing thought as

- A substantial body of knowledge,
- Developed by a number of scholars,
- Which describes one aspect of performing marketing activities.

They divide the development of marketing thought into four periods:

- Pre-academic (prior to 1900)
- Traditional approaches (1900–1955)
- Paradigm shift (1955–1975)
- Following Kotler, paradigm broadening (1975–2000 and beyond)

During the paradigm shift period, researchers (e.g. psychologists) from fields beyond economy or business entered the discipline. Key scholars, such as Kotler, Levy, and Zaltman, split the field into three schools: marketing management, exchange, and consumer behaviour. This *expanded the boundaries of marketing thought from its conventional focus on business activities to a broader perspective embracing all forms of human activity related to any generic or social exchange* (ibid., p. 243).

Another development in marketing thought swept the field about the same time. This brought a focus on the role of 'marketing management and executive decision making'—as opposed to the previous focus on managing productions and sales. James Culliton (1948) was credited by some as describing the marketing executive as the *decider* or *mixer of ingredients*. Now, the marketer became instrumental in creating the 'marketing mix', later described as *decision area* by Howard (1957). In these decision areas, he included product, marketing channels, price, promotion (advertising), promotion (personal selling), and location decisions. Several similar works followed, but it was McCarthy's book (1960) that clearly established the four Ps of the marketing mix (see Chapter 12): product, price, place, and promotion.

According to Shaw and Jones, the decade following the 1960s witnessed a lively debate about whether marketing was *a set of management techniques applicable to all organizations and individuals or an economic institution designed to achieve social goals* (2005, p. 257). By the time Kotler's books emerged (1975, 1980), they (and by this point, the profession) were dominated by his advocacy of applying the marketing mix of techniques to any social or personal cause.

Two developments emerged from this 'broadening' of the field. First, the 'product' had been previously excluded from the marketing field as a production concept, similar to farming and manufacturing. The broadening brought the product back into the mainstream of marketing thought. Second, much marketing research today can focus on the product as a 'service' rather than a manufactured or agricultural item. Indeed, Vargo and Lusch (2004) argued that services are more fundamental because most consumers only want the service benefits that a product offers, or put another way, products only provide a delivery vehicle for service benefits.

Shaw and Jones go on to say that this broadening of marketing to generic exchange creates a dilemma for the field. Human behaviour is inherently social, and nearly all human social behaviour includes exchange relationships, even teenage kissing and mother–child affection. But to what end? If marketing applies to every instance of human behaviour, then its vagueness may obscure and obstruct its usefulness as a discipline. The sociologist George Homans (1958) inverted the dynamics and used the business analogy to explain interaction between individuals and groups. But although human interaction contains marketing behaviour, does the discipline of marketing (even under the guise of social marketing) contain all human behaviour? The answer to this question may be more conceptual than practical, but we have clearly reached the stage at which marketing ceased to be applied solely to business exchanges for profit and began to be applied to interactions resulting in 'social good'.

Marketing for social good

A small number of those instrumental for the fuelling and development of this consumer culture started to reflect and question the value of what they were doing. They knew they could sell cars, Coca-Cola, and baked beans for financial reward, but was there something more that could be achieved? Might marketing also be used to achieve social good?

In 1951, Weibe wrote what has become a seminal article for *The Public Opinion Quarterly*, in which he asked *Why can't you sell brotherhood and rational thinking like you sell soap?* (Weibe, 1951–52). He went on to articulate what he saw as the challenges presented by attempting to sell social good as if it were a commodity. Whereas commercial marketers aim to get as many people as possible to engage in the desired behaviour, this is rarely the aim of the social scientist: *cultural objectives cannot be purchased at your nearest drug or department store* (ibid., p. 680). He also recognized that advertising does not necessarily move people to act, but *moves them into interaction with social mechanisms* (ibid., p. 680). The article analysed several campaigns and attempted to test his hypothesis. He concluded by suggesting that in the right conditions and with suitable receptivity among the target audience there might be a measure of success.

The 1960s saw the introduction of pioneering social marketing-styled interventions, mainly in developing countries. International development initiatives sponsored by the World Health Organization (WHO) and the World Bank brought family-planning projects to Sri Lanka and oral rehydration initiatives to Africa. In developed countries, the first blood pressure and healthy-heart initiatives were established (Baker, 2002).

Introducing the term 'social marketing'

The next milestone in defining what we now know as social marketing came in 1971, with the publication of an article by Philip Kotler and Gerald Zaltman titled 'Social marketing: an approach to planned social change' (Kotler and Zaltman, 1971). This piece actually coined the term 'social marketing' and built upon Weibe's work. It suggested that social marketing was indeed a *promising framework for planning and implementing social change* and, further, that *the application of the logic of marketing to social goals is a natural development and on the whole a promising one* (ibid, p. 3). The article also included the first social marketing planning system, identified the conceptual distinctions between social and commercial marketing, and offered a definition:

> Social marketing is the design, implementation, and control of programs calculated to influence the acceptability of social ideas and involving considerations of product planning, pricing, communication, distribution, and marketing research.
>
> (ibid, p. 5)

The social sciences story

The view that social marketing is purely and simply the use of commercial-marketing skills for social good is countered by the integration of social and behavioural theory into its framework. It is, therefore, important that we examine the other parent of social marketing and look at the parallel and much older social (including behavioural) sciences story. After all, long before commercial marketers were beginning to question the application of their skills, people in the social sciences (and the connected disciplines of sociology, psychology, anthropology, and the political sciences) were asking questions about how best to understand people. The social sciences allied scientific methodologies with qualitative and quantitative analyses to gain insight into motivational and cultural currents, which are in turn informed by a growing body of behavioural theory.

The social sciences ask human questions such as

- What are people's behaviours and what are the key influences upon them?
- What is the relationship between individuals within communities and within the networks of which they are part?
- What is the fundamental relationship between the individual and the state?

Weibe's emphasis on the value of insight into the interaction of people with social mechanisms is where social science and marketing coalesce into something really valuable. It helps effect change with many contemporary issues that have behavioural causes: *the spread of AIDS, traffic accidents, and unwanted pregnancies are all the result of everyday, voluntary human activity* (MacFadyen et al., 1999, p. 1).

Because many health issues are influenced by social as well as individual behaviours, social marketing recognizes that policymakers and organizations need to be targeted in order to successfully effect change. MacFadyen et al. (1999) illustrate this point with their examination of the epidemiological data that shows the clear correlation between poverty and ill health.

The marriage between the 'social' and 'marketing' parents has for many been a problematic one, and this is as true today as it has always been, as the comments of our interviewees in Chapter 22 demonstrate. Writing on the ethical dimensions of social marketing, Laczniack worried that this convergence would be used for manipulation and social control rather than social good (Laczniack et al., 1979). In the United Kingdom, some expressed a resistance to the inclusion of 'marketing' in the terminology, due to its resonances with commercial practices and exploitation. Ironically enough, in the United States, it is the word 'social' that can raise hackles for some, due to its misplaced cultural associations with socialism. To a degree, the nomenclature is an irrelevance and a distraction from the real value of what can be achieved. Social marketing has never claimed to be a theoretically distinct discipline. In many ways it is better to approach it as a conceptual framework and a confluence of disciplines, skills, and approaches.

There is also the perception of the social sciences by some as 'soft science' to consider. This is really the fallout of having to deal with the constantly changing and unpredictable set of variables within which people frame their lives. But this accusation is being made less and less as the social sciences become increasingly quantitative in nature and the so-called hard sciences pay more attention to human behaviour, particularly with a view to environmental issues.

Marketing and social sciences should not, however, be thrown together without an awareness of the consequences. Lazer and Kelly (1973, p. 26) call for caution:

> Marketing has a key role to play in the drive for increased efficiency within our economy. It also has an opportunity to play a significant role in the drive for social justice[,] which is replacing the drive for security or affluence among many members of our society. There is a need for more vigorous action in both of these areas, efficiency and social justice. There also is a need [...] for truly responsible marketing practitioners and educators to vigorously resist action proposed in the cause of either efficiency or social justice[,] which is likely to damage the economy and to do more harm than good in the long run.

Like ripples in a pond, any changes to social structures and behaviours can have an unintended detrimental effect, although the continuing evolution of planning and ethical frameworks for social marketing seek to avoid such undesired outcomes.

So, when we come to considering the social sciences, and particularly the behavioural sciences, it is important to have a wider appreciation and perspective. Science, whether physical or social, is not something rigid or fixed that contains immutable truths. It is a dynamic and evolving framework with orthodoxies established and subjected to observation and empiricism. But, although the scientific process of systematic examination and testing is a fundamentally important process, it is not something that avoids the impact of human failings and flaws. Indeed, the very way 'evidence' is conceived and understood is a symptom of the way the physical and social sciences are understood and perceived.

The convergence of marketing techniques with social theory and social science really highlights the fact that social marketing is not merely marketing with a degree of altruism or social responsibility tacked on to it. Many of the tools of commercial marketers, particularly in the area of segmentation, are a part of the skill set, but their effectiveness is bolstered by research and theoretical methodologies that commercial marketers would never normally turn to. This does mean, however, that the outcomes of most social marketing interventions are much less predictable and more challenging to quantify.

Social advertising versus social marketing

There is a further distinction to be made between social marketing and social advertising. Social advertising is simply the use of advertising to inform the public about a social issue or to influence their behaviour. It generally lacks the stronger focus on consumer insight (see Chapter 7) that is vital to social marketing. Although many social advertising campaigns are successful in raising awareness, they are often used in far too indiscriminate a fashion to truly offer any sustained benefit.

Kotler and Zaltman offer a good explanation of the difference between sales and marketing: sales is simply *finding customers for existing products and convincing them to buy these products*; marketing is *discovering the wants of a target audience and then creating the goods and services to satisfy them* (Kotler and Zaltman, 1971, p. 5). This difference reflects the difference between social advertising and social marketing: in social marketing, the consumer's needs are the starting point for any intervention.

Education and communication have their place in health-promotion and social campaigns, and obviously, not every behavioural challenge needs a social marketing intervention. It is, however, important to make a clear distinction between social advertising and marketing, as mistaking one for the other often leads to criticism about social marketing's effectiveness and ethics.

Box 2.1 Example: The difference between social advertising and social marketing

After decades of campaigning and bans on advertising, there can be very few, if any, who do not know that smoking is an unhealthy activity. Habitual smokers know that they are actively harming themselves and first-time smokers know that they run the risk of addiction and health problems later in life. In these circumstances, campaigns to raise awareness of the damaging effects of smoking are of limited value. They may indeed reach a number of people and change opinions, but on the whole, they take a scattergun approach to the issue. Quite simply, even with the best of intentions, these campaigns make a whole raft of assumptions about their audience that is not informed by insight and research.

Social advertising may form a part of a social marketing intervention. Stead and Hastings argue that this is often more down to expediency than intention where, *in the absence of a tangible product and of an actual trade between marketer and market, mass media is perceived to be the only channel where social marketers can exert influence* (Stead and Hastings, 1997, p. 36).

Antisocial marketing

Case study: the tobacco industry and 'antisocial' marketing

Interestingly (perhaps even perversely) enough, the American tobacco industry was among the first to make the leap between production and sales to designing a product to fit the 'hopes and dreams' of a target population—although one could hardly call its motivation 'social good'. In fact, as a result of this transformation, the consumption of cigarettes as a proportion of all tobacco consumed in the United States rose from only 27% in 1900 to 81% in 1952. And it accounted for 1.4% of the gross national product and 3.5% of all consumer spending in the United States (Brandt, 2007). So pervasive and horrendous has been the impact of the cigarette on the health of Western populations (and now the populations of developing countries) that one might, at least from a public health perspective, refer to this as the era of 'antisocial marketing'.

As consumer culture grew during the 1920s, some questioned whether marketing had developed a sinister side. The overwhelming success of the 'Reach for a Lucky [cigarette] instead of a sweet' campaign grew out of its new approach designed to

- Target women
- Associate the product with beauty, fashion, women's rights, and above all, slimness
- Tap into the cult of personality, especially the growing celebrity of movie stars, socialites, and other famous people

According to Brandt (2007, p. 97), *psychologists catalogued a wide range of drives and desires, ranging from hunger and thirst to sexuality and beauty that individuals could 'satisfy' in the market-place of consumer goods.* One cigarette advertiser put it this way:

> You know a large part of the public really doesn't know what it wants. Our big task in recent years has been to dig up new likes or dislikes which we think might strike the public's fancy and sell them to the public ... The public must be given ideas as to what it should like ... The old sales bywords 'know your customer's needs' have been remolded to 'know what your customer should need and then educate him on those needs'.
>
> (Andrews, 1936, p. 27)

For women, this meant that the cigarette became the symbol of both a product and a behaviour that offered social attractiveness, physical beauty, and equality.

The cigarette, perhaps more than any other product of its day, suggested that demand could be generated and shaped by marketing and advertising—even for a product that not only had no 'practical' use but also actually exposed the consumer to disease and death. It embodied a crucial aspect of consumer culture, in which promoters manipulated meaning and experience, creating needs and consumer loyalties. Some, such as Brandt, viewed this phenomenon as a new and dangerous element of marketing: *the artificial creation of desire for purposes of profit* (2007, p. 79). Brandt goes on to say:

> The process by which the cigarette came to 'fit' within the parameters of American culture was anything but 'natural' or serendipitous. Produce and culture were brought into conformity by specific and often purposeful economic and social forces, a process that required 'adjustment' of traditional boundaries and social expectations as well as the deployment of new techniques that structured both produce and market. It is perhaps its remarkable range of meanings—and their successful definition and construction through advertising and promotion—that makes the cigarette such a powerful symbol of the consumer culture.
>
> (ibid., p. 98)

Brand loyalty represented a second perversity of cigarette marketing. Although most brands of cigarettes were undistinguishable by contents or taste, overwhelming advertising and promotion created what Brandt calls the *invention of choice* (ibid., p. 80). In fact, a standardized product was used to promote 'individualism'. Consider how consumers were convinced to express individual choice by selecting a standardized product, materially undifferentiated from all other tobacco products except for the notion that the individual consumer, along with millions of others, chose it. This paradox of asserting individuality through 'market choice' was not lost on the tobacco industry or other marketers during that era or since (ibid.)

This concept came to be known as the 'engineering of consent'. It was coined by Edward Bernays, a Viennese nephew of Sigmund Freud, brought in by the American Tobacco Company to alter the 'fit' between a product and cultural values by changing and exploiting those values. Through Bernays' efforts, starting in the early 1920's, the tobacco industry learned how to shift mass behaviour by shaping the news, using pseudo-educational information to overcome criticism and cast doubt on health fears related to tobacco use, linking tobacco use in public with feminist freedom, and placing cigarettes in film as a way of 'conveying dramatic meaning'. By engineering of consent, he meant the precise manipulation of individual autonomy: in other words, the *illusion* of free choice in the face of massive, corporate contrivance (Brandt, 2007, p. 88). So, through these techniques and others, the cigarette rose to prominence in America's emerging mass consumption culture. A relatively undifferentiated product, *it traded on identities fashioned not through any intrinsic qualities, but through advertising, public relations, [manipulation of public wants and needs] and design* (ibid., p. 89).

Social marketing and policy

Social marketing-based interventions are being adopted all over the world to tackle a growing range of behavioural issues. In particular, in the United States, Canada, Australia, and New Zealand, there are a growing number of programmes in place that are demonstrating its effectiveness. In Europe, the WHO is now employing social marketing to its tobacco-control work and 'Healthy Cities' programme, which is running in 1200 cities and towns in over 30 countries. To date, however, it is only in the United Kingdom that social marketing has been firmly embedded as a part of the government policy agenda.

In 2006, the National Consumer Council (NCC) launched an independent report entitled *It's Our Health!* This was the first ever national review of health-related campaigns and social marketing in England. Commissioned by the Department of Health (DH) as part of its *Choosing Health* white paper, the report set out strategic and operational recommendations on how social marketing could be applied to improve the effectiveness of health promotion at both national and local levels. These recommendations provided a framework for the first National Social Marketing Strategy for Health in England, a key part of which was the creation of the National Social Marketing Centre (NSMC).

The NSMC was launched with a remit to build skills and capacity in social marketing at both strategic and operational levels. In 2008, the DH launched its 'Ambitions for Health' framework with the aim of embedding social marketing principles into *all* health-improvement programmes. This commitment was underlined in the same year with the 'Change4Life' (http://www.nhs.uk/Change4Life/Pages/default.aspx) initiative, which uses social marketing techniques with the aim of catalyzing a 'society-wide movement' to reduce obesity levels by promoting better diet and more healthy activities.

Although its strategic partnership with the DH meant that the focus of most its work was in the public health arena, it was also mandated to work across government and sectors. This has meant that a growing number of governmental departments and organizations are now adopting social marketing approaches. A raft of policy documents and reports now reference and recommend social marketing in order to effect positive behaviour change in targeted population groups.

Conclusion

We have looked at the development of social marketing from the seemingly disparate disciplines of commercial marketing and the social sciences, and briefly explored its inverse opposite in what has been termed 'antisocial marketing'. And, although there are still debates around what actually constitutes social marketing as a concept, and even what it should be called, the growing evidence base for its effectiveness has gradually seen its framework adopted in behavioural interventions all over the world. Building on the set of tools that the commercial sector has used to sell its products, it has now been used effectively to tackle such wide-ranging issues as smoking cessation, obesity, and the screening of sexually transmitted infections to addressing urban transport problems, environmental issues, and the reduction of prison numbers.

Although there is a growing community of social marketing experts and institutions around the world, the UK government has been the first to employ social marketing within public health policy. The UK Marketing and Sales Standards Setting Body (MSSSB) has also codified its first ever set of occupational standards to ensure a consistent approach to its employment. There have also been significant efforts to get social marketing onto academic courses, with a growing number of universities now offering courses and modules in the subject (see Chapter 20).

There are still those who need persuading that the 'marketing' part of the name does not necessarily mean turning to the 'dark side' in order to achieve results, but as a concept, social marketing is increasingly gaining recognition as a legitimate toolset for tackling a huge range of societal problems.

Review exercise

What important tools do social sciences bring to the field of social marketing that commercial marketing would not typically include?

References

Adler, L. (1982). *Marketing: The Encyclopedia of Management*. New York, NY: VanNostrand Reinhold.

Andrews, P.B.B. (1936). The cigarette market, past and future. *Advertising and Selling*, Jan 16, p. 37.

Baker, M.J. (2002). *The Marketing Book*. Oxford: Butterworth-Heinemann.

Brandt, A. (2007). *The Cigarette Century*. New York, NY: Basic Books.

Culliton, J.W. (1948). *The Management of Marketing Costs*. Cambridge, MA: Harvard University Press.

French, J. and Blair-Stevens, C. (2007). *Big Pocket Guide: Social Marketing*. London: National Social Marketing Centre.

Homans, G. (1958). Social behavior as exchange. *American Journal of Sociology*, 63: 597–606.

Howard, J. (1957). *Marketing Management: Analysis and Decision*. Homewood, IL: Richard D. Irwin.

Kotler, P. (1975). *Marketing for Non-profit Organizations*. Upper Saddle River, NJ: Prentice-Hall.

Kotler, P. (1980). *Marketing Management: Analysis, Planning, and Control*. New Jersey: Prentice-Hall.

Kotler, P. and Zaltman, G. (1971). Social marketing: an approach to planned social change. *Journal of Marketing*, 35(3): 3–12

Laczniack, G., Lusch, R. and Murphy, P. (1979). Social marketing and its ethical dimensions. *Journal of Marketing*, 43: 29–36.

Lazer, W. and Kelley, E.J. (1973). *Social Marketing: Perspectives and Viewpoints*. Homewood, IL: Richard D. Irwin.

MacFadyen, L., Stead, M. and Hastings, G. (1999). *A Synopsis of Social Marketing*. Available at: www.ism.stir.ac.uk/pdf_docs/social_marketing.pdf (Accessed 30 January 2009).

Manoff, R. (1985). *Social Marketing*. Chicago, IL: American Marketing Association.

McCarthy, E.J. (1960). *Basic Marketing: A Managerial Approach*. Homewood, IL: Richard D. Irwin.

Shaw, E. and Jones, B. (2005). A history of schools of marketing thought. *Marketing Theory*, 5(3): 239–281.

Stead, M. and Hastings, G. (1997). Advertising in the social marketing mix. In *Social Marketing: Theoretical and Practical Perspectives*. Mahwah, NJ: Lawrence Erlbaum Associates.

Vargo, S. and Lusch, R. (2004). Evolving to a new dominant logic for marketing. *Journal of Marketing*, 68(1): 1–17.

Wiebe, G.D. (1951–52). Merchandising commodities and citizenship on television. *Public Opinion Quarterly*, 15(4): 679–691.

Chapter 3

Key concepts and principles of social marketing

Jeff French and Clive Blair-Stevens

The customer is never wrong.
Cesar Ritz

Learning points

This chapter

- Explains social marketing and its key features and concepts;
- Sets out the differences in people's understanding of social marketing;
- Introduces the 'customer triangle' as a device for remembering its key features;
- Introduces the national 'benchmark criteria' as robust set of core features that cut through different views of social marketing; and
- Explains the link between social marketing and the diverse ways of seeking to influence human behaviour.

Chapter overview

With the growth in political and practitioner interest in social marketing, this chapter seeks to provide a balanced view and understanding of the discipline. It starts from a premise that, as with all methods and approaches, it can be understood in a range of different ways. For those new to the discipline, this can sometimes make it difficult to understand what social marketing is.

However, it is in fact a positive thing that there is a dynamic debate about what social marketing actually is. It helps ensure that there is reflection and discussion rather than rigid and fixed considerations. This is the best position from which to consider and examine the potential benefit of any discipline.

The chapter also introduces key tools that have been introduced by the UK's National Social Marketing Centre (NSMC) to help people remember social marketing's most important concepts and to provide some consistency of approach among the various approaches to the discipline.

Introduction

Social marketing is viewed differently by different people. To some, it is a mindset that informs every aspect of their work, and to others, it is a practical tool they apply as and when needed.

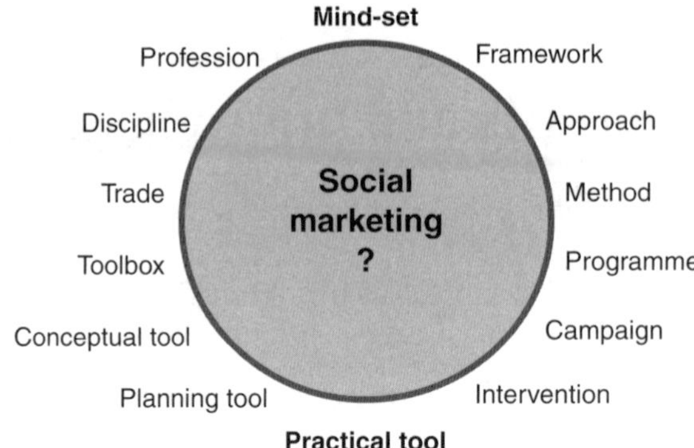

Fig. 3.1 The continuum of ways in which people approach social marketing.

Fig. 3.1 illustrates the continuum of ways in which people approach the discipline. It is not intended to be exhaustive, and in reality, social marketing can be any or all of the featured approaches. But it is important to be able to recognize the different ways that someone may approach, conceptualize, or present social marketing. How you view the discipline really depends on where you start from in examining and considering it. For some, it is the overarching framework or paradigm through which behavioural challenges can be viewed and addressed. For others, it is simply a tool that can be used (or not used) in a given situation, potentially integrated with other approaches or paradigms.

Seeking a definitive approach to social marketing is one of the 'bear traps' that some writers or commentators have fallen into. In our view, the most important thing is that those considering its potential are clear about how they are approaching it, are aware that it can be approached in different ways, and are as clear as possible about this in their discussions with others. Having a discussion about the strategic use of social marketing to inform policy formulation and strategy development (see Chapter 5) will be difficult if the person you are discussing it with sees social marketing simply as a 'campaign development tool'.

A parallel can be drawn here with the historic development of health education, which can be, and has been, approached in a range of quite different ways. Indeed, as Box 3.1 illustrates, the very development of health education 'language' illustrates the dynamic and changing way in which the discipline has been approached over time.

While undertaking a two-year independent review to examine current social marketing and other behavioural interventions (French, Blair-Stevens, 2006), it was found that people

Box 3.1 The different ways of framing health education

Health education → Health communications → Health promotion → Health development → Health improvement → ...

In setting this process out in a linear fashion, we seek to illustrate that the understanding and language of health education has developed over time, reflecting dynamic debate and discussion. In reality, the process is not as simplistic or linear.

tended to assess social marketing's potential in relation to their own academic and professional background and experience—something that is not unreasonable. However, some people were getting caught up in circular arguments and discussions for which there was no single or simple answer. Some of the different ways we found people approaching social marketing are set out in Box 3.2.

Again, in practice, any or all of these can be true. Interestingly, many people coming from marketing into social marketing often did the reverse and simply saw social marketing as including health promotion, sustainable development, and a whole range of other methods. This reveals that the debate about whether social marketing is unique or forms part of another discipline can be futile and counterproductive. You will see throughout this book that we take the view that social marketing is essentially a dynamic and integrative discipline. It is not rigid and fixed and, like other disciplines, it houses a range of active voices and debates. This is a positive thing, and our central concern in writing this book is to help people gain a robust and broad understanding of the discipline's potential, so that people can then ask what it can do for them, irrespective of their academic or professional background.

Box 3.2 Views of social marketing revealed by the independent review

Social marketing is *different to* 'health promotion' or 'sustainable development' or ...

For those who saw social marketing as different to their existing academic or professional background, two different approaches tended to occur. With the first, people saw that there might be something that they could learn from social marketing to help strengthen and enrich what they were doing. However, the second approach led to respondents rejecting it, because they viewed it not only as 'different' but in some ways 'counter to it', or 'in competition with it'. This understanding was often based on a misreading of social marketing's underpinning values and evidence base.

Social marketing is *the same as* 'health promotion' or 'sustainable development' or ...

The implication for some here was that we do not really need another term for the discipline they believed social marketing was replicating. During the independent review (NSMC, 2006), some of these people were described as the 'underwhelms': those who felt that what was being described in social marketing was the same as their own academic or professional training and therefore could not really see any difference or 'added value' in something called 'social marketing'.

Social marketing is *part of* 'health promotion' or 'sustainable development' or ...

Those who approached social marketing in this way tended to see it as a discrete, often 'specialist' activity that might or might not be used in a given situation or as a component of their existing methods or paradigm. Consequently, for some, social marketing is not seen as offering anything new to their discipline.

Defining social marketing

At its core, social marketing is a behavioural approach that is increasingly being used to achieve positive impacts on the lives of individuals and groups, and to help sustain these over time. This section seeks to explore some of the definitions of social marketing. Clearly, there is a need to recognize that all descriptions and definitions are subject to the time and context in which they are developed and the values, experience, and professional training of the writer. Three questions can help analyse the nature of social marketing:

- What is social marketing's primary purpose?
- How should we formally define it?
- What are the concepts and principles at its core?

What is social marketing's primary purpose?

In the simplest of terms, social marketing's primary purpose is to achieve a particular 'social or public good'[1] (i.e. there is some benefit to individual, groups, communities, and society). This social good could relate to health and well-being, environmental sustainability, reduction in crime and fear of crime, or any one of a range of social policy objectives. Social marketing, therefore, is not simply confined to health: it can be used to achieve and sustain a diverse range of social benefits.

This primary focus on 'social good' helps us to distinguish between social marketing and commercial marketing. However, the key word here is 'primary'. Simply seeing commercial marketing as concerned with financial and shareholder value is to fail to acknowledge the growing links between commercial value and social good. Indeed, even a cursory glance at the literature on marketing will reveal a range of different types of marketing in which there can be a social good component. However, in social marketing, 'social good' is the primary purpose rather than a secondary or complementary one.

Fig. 3.2 further illustrates these connections and differences between various forms of marketing. The three main forms of marketing for social good in the for-profit sector are as follows:

Cause-related marketing —where the marketing approach includes a per cent of profits going to a good cause

Prosocial marketing—where the marketing approach includes providing a profile for a social issue

Societal marketing—where the marketing approach promotes the companies commitment to positive and responsible business practices and policies (e.g. recycling)

The main types of marketing in the public or non-governmental groups (NGOs/third sector/charity/not-for-profit sector) are as follows:

Social marketing—where marketing is used to help achieve and sustain positive behaviours for social good

Service or organizational marketing—where marketing is used to promote a public or third sector service or organization, and can include generating an income, but where monies raised go directly back into the organization's 'social' aims

[1] 'Good' is defined both in an economic sense as anything that produces a benefit, be it a service or a physical commodity, and in the moral sense as something that is collectively supported by citizens as the 'right' thing to do.

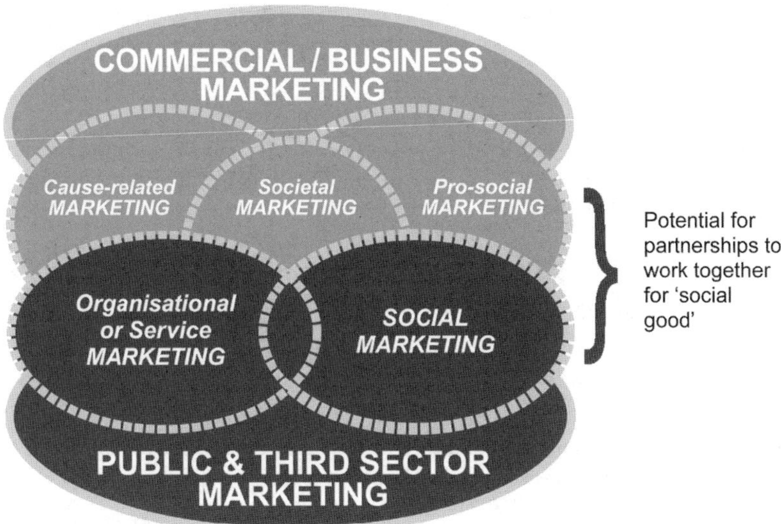

Fig. 3.2 Linking marketing strategies and developing partnerships to contribute to a social good.

It is clear that commercial and private sector development can be a critical component of many important social interventions such as health programmes, environmental programmes, and regeneration programmes. Therefore, simply seeing the public sector as 'good' and the private sector as 'bad' detracts from the fact that business can and does contribute crucial social benefits for individuals and communities. The potential for successful partnerships is explored in Chapter 21.

How should we formally define social marketing?

Like all developing concepts, it is artificial to articulate a simple linear development of social marketing as a concept. Concepts and the language used to articulate them form and develop in different ways with different influences and factors affecting them over time.

There are many definitions of social marketing, for example:

> ... the design, implementation and control of programs calculated to influence the acceptability of social ideas and involving considerations of product planning, pricing, communication, distribution and marketing research.
>
> (Kotler and Zaltman, 1971)

> ... concerned with the application of marketing knowledge, concepts, and techniques to enhance social as well as economic ends. It is also concerned with analysis of the social consequences of marketing policies, decisions and activities.
>
> (Lazer and Kelly, 1973)

> ... a programme planning process that promotes the voluntary behaviour of target audiences by offering benefits they want, reducing barriers they are concerned about, and using persuasion to motivate their participation in program activity.
>
> (Kotler and Roberto, 1989)

> … the use of marketing principles and techniques to influence a target audience to voluntarily accept, reject, modify or abandon behaviour for the benefit of individuals, groups or society as a whole.
>
> (Kotler et al., 2002)

> … the application of commercial marketing technologies to the analysis, planning, execution and evaluation of programmes designed to influence the voluntary behaviour of target audiences in order to improve their personal welfare and that of their society.
>
> (Andreasen, 1995)

> … the adaptation of commercial marketing theory and practice for social change programmes, campaigns and causes.
>
> (Dann, 2006)

> … a means for creating voluntary exchange between a marketing organisation and members of a target market based on the mutual fulfilment of self-interest.
>
> (Maibach et al., 2002)

> … a process that applies marketing principles and techniques to create, communicate and deliver value in order to influence target audience behaviours that benefit society as well as the target audience.
>
> (Kotler and Lee, 2007)

> … about making what we offer people fun, easy and popular.
>
> (Smith, 2006)

It is clear from the definitions that different writers place emphasis on different aspects of social marketing; however, it is possible to recognize core common ground, that is, a focus on

- Social good
- Behaviour
- Harnessing power of marketing (in all its forms)
- The importance of target audience- or customer-defined value

It is also useful to consider that some definitions try to focus on the overall purpose and aim of social marketing, whereas others move into the territory of trying to describe its key elements or components.

A review of the different methods and approaches being used by social marketers in different countries and organizations appears in the NSMC's report *It's Our Health!* (2006). The review suggests that social marketing has moved on from early definitions that imply that social marketing is simply the application of commercial marketing know-how to social issues. Social marketing is now a much more mature and integrative discipline, as explored by Andreasen (2006). Therefore, to see social marketing simply as 'commercial marketing in the public sector' is to fail to recognize the way it has grown and integrated social, political, and behavioural sciences into its development. It needs to be recognized that in parallel with the development of thinking about the nature of social marketing, there has been a growing debate across the social sciences focused on wider social policy, social reform, and social justice issues, and in particular, on the role citizens should have in informing policy and the most effective and ethical ways to influence individual and social

Social marketing is:

the systematic application of marketing, alongside other concepts and techniques, to achieve specific behavioural goals, for a social good.

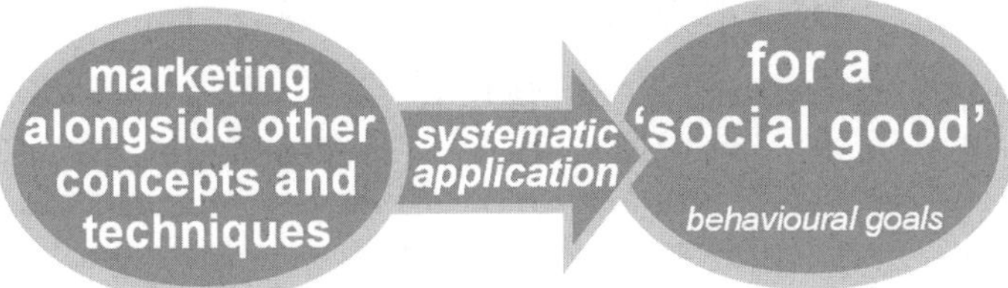

Fig. 3.3 The definition of social marketing.
Source: French and Blair-Stevens (2007), with permission.

behaviour for social good. Some of this debate is reviewed in Chapter 1. In 2007, French and Blair-Stevens finalized a descriptive definition of social marketing, shown in Fig. 3.3.

As with all formal definitions, this one incorporates a range of issues and debates. It is perhaps useful to explain and expand on the language used in the definition.

Social good: As discussed in the preceding, this is included to represent the primary purpose of social marketing. But inevitably, as with any behavioural intervention approach, seeking to positively influence people's lives presents a range of ethical issues and challenges (see Chapter 9). Good social marketing practice proactively helps to examine and understand 'how' social good is being defined and 'who' is actively involved in the defining what social good is. It also recognizes that although public sector interventions might have the intention of 'doing good', there is always the possibility that they will inadvertently cause harm. Effective social marketing, therefore, seeks to examine and consider this possibility before an intervention is implemented, so that it can eliminate or reduce the potential for harm and maximize the potential for good.

Marketing alongside: Marketing offers a great deal to enrich and strengthen public sector activity. However, the term 'alongside' has been included to clearly indicate that social marketing is not marketing in isolation. Instead, to achieve its aims, effective social marketing works to connect marketing with other behavioural interventions, theories, methods, and approaches. In this sense social marketing is an integrative discipline.

Systematic: This highlights that effective social marketing, as with any effective approach, involves being systematic and rigorous in its analysis, development, and application.

Behavioural goals: This is included to indicate clearly that social marketing is essentially a behavioural intervention approach and not solely a communications one. Social marketing is focused specifically on achieving and sustaining behaviour over time. In this way, it is much more than a communications or social advertising approach, which (although necessary in some contexts) tend to place greater emphasis on communicating and transmitting 'messages' rather than on achieving and sustaining specific behaviours. Effective social marketing begins with the identification of specific behavioural goals at the start of an initiative and then assesses and measures the extent to which these are achieved through the intervention mix and marketing mix used.

What are the concepts and principles at the core of social marketing ?

Social marketing concepts and principles can support policymakers and practitioners at all levels. At its very core, there are two key factors we consider when assessing if an initiative is consistent with social marketing. These are

- A driving concern with developing robust understanding and insight into the customer; and
- A clear focus on achieving and sustaining specific behaviours.

Strategic and operational social marketing

To date, the most common way social marketing has been used and applied is operationally, as a specific process to achieve something with a particular audience in relation to a specific topic. However, it is increasingly recognized that the customer understanding and insight focus of social marketing, and its clear behavioural focus, can be applied just as beneficially at the policy and/or strategy level.

Rather than assuming a campaign is required, it is helpful to use a social marketing mindset to inform policy formulation and strategy development. This is particularly important in that it helps question a default position where social advertising or communications becomes associated as the primary product. Instead, strategic social marketing seeks to examine all of the potential interventional options and assess them based on what the customer insight indicates would be most beneficial and effective.

Social marketing's 'customer triangle'

Social marketing's 'customer triangle' was developed at the NSMC (French and Blair-Stevens) as a simple way to highlight and promote key features of social marketing. In many respects, it has increasingly been used to 'market' social marketing features. Rather than simply listing the features, the triangle device provides a memory aid (Fig. 3.4).

There are a number of key features to social marketing. It is fair to say that writers on social marketing have perhaps inevitably tended to comment on and highlight different aspects and issues. However, a review of the development of social marketing discourse does reveal a fairly robust set of core features, about which there is consensus that they are key to understanding and using social marketing. It is these that the customer triangle helps to highlight.

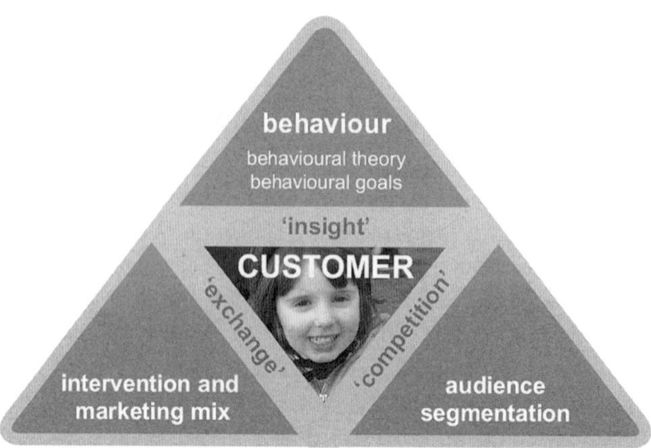

Fig. 3.4 Social marketing's customer triangle.
Source: French and Blair-Stevens (2007), with permission.

Social marketing's eight-point benchmark criteria

Social marketing's benchmark criteria are essentially those elements you should look for to determine whether your initiative is consistent with effective social marketing. They were developed by French and Blair-Stevens during the NSMC's two-year independent review, which examined social marketing methods and approaches and built on the previous work by Andreasen, who set out an initial six-point set of criteria in 2001. The benchmarks provide a way to help readily communicate key elements of social marketing while encouraging and supporting greater consistency of approach.

During the independent review, French and Blair-Stevens (2006) identified two different issues. The first was a great variability in initiatives that were being labelled 'social marketing', some of which did not appear to be consistent with basic social marketing principles. A simple example of this would be interventions that had no specific behavioural goal or focus but were focused just on communicating information. Having the eight-point benchmarks, therefore, provides a simple and straightforward way to focus on the substance of social marketing and help to bring greater consistency to the approach (Box 3.3). This also helps in reviewing and capturing learning and evidence from interventions. The second issue was effectively the opposite: French and Blair-Stevens found some excellent interventions that were consistent with effective social marketing principles (e.g. they had clear customer understanding and insight, strong behavioural focus, and a well-constructed exchange principle) but which did not necessarily describe themselves as social marketing. This meant that good work was often being overlooked. The eight-point benchmark criteria, therefore, helps bring greater consistency to the field and also helps identify and validate good practice wherever it exists.

Box 3.3 Purposes of the benchmark criteria

The eight-point benchmark criteria were developed to

- Increase understanding of core social marketing concepts and principles;
- Help focus attention on the substance of social marketing and go beyond the term;
- Increase consistency of approach and thereby potential impact and effectiveness;
- Maintain maximum flexibility and creativity to craft and develop interventions to address different needs;
- Assist more systematic capture and sharing of transferable learning between interventions; and
- Assist effective review and evaluation of different types of intervention.

The eight-point benchmark criteria

1 Customer orientation—'seeing the customer in the round'

Develops a robust understanding of the audience, based on good market and consumer research, combining data from different sources.

- A broad and robust understanding of the audience or customer is developed, which focuses on understanding their lives in the round, avoiding the potential to only focus on a single aspect or feature.

- Formative consumer or marketing research is used to identify audience characteristics and needs, incorporating key stakeholder intelligence and understanding.
- A range of different research analyses, combining data (using synthesis and fusion approaches wherever possible) and, if available, drawing from public and commercial sector sources, is used to develop a robust and rounded understanding of people's everyday lives.

2 Behaviour and behavioural goals

Has a clear and unequivocal focus for achieving impact on people's behaviour, and is based on a strong rounded behavioural analysis and development of specific behavioural goals.

- A broad and robust behavioural analysis undertaken to gather a rounded picture of the current behavioural patterns and trends, making sure to examine both
  - The 'problem behaviour'; and
  - The 'desired behaviour'.
- Intervention developed to clearly focus on specific behaviours (going beyond just focusing on addressing information, knowledge, attitudes, and beliefs).
- Specific actionable and measurable behavioural goals and key indicators have been established in relation to the specific issue or 'social good' being addressed.
- The intervention considers and addresses following four key behavioural issues:
  - *Formulation and establishment of the behaviour*—understanding what helps trigger and establish the behaviour in the first place (making sure to look at both the problem and the desired behaviour)
  - *Maintenance and reinforcement of the behaviour*—understanding what helps to maintain and sustain the behaviour over time (again making sure to look at both the problem and the desired behaviour)
  - *Behavioural change*—understanding what will move and motivate people to make changes and what barriers need to be addressed
  - *Behavioural controls*—understanding where voluntary approaches may not work and where ethical criteria can justify the use of requirements or controls to influence the behaviour in the given context

3 Theory based

Draws on and incorporates the use of behavioural theory to inform and steer development, drawn from an integrated theory framework (see chapter 4).

- Theory is used transparently to inform and guide development, with theoretical assumptions being tested as part of the developmental process.
- An open integrated theory framework is utilized to systematically examine which theory base offers the greatest utility in a given context, while avoiding the tendency to simply apply the same 'preferred' theory to every situation and context.

- Takes into account behavioural theory across four key domains:
  - Biological and physical factors — the biophysical
  - Psychological factors — the psychodynamic
  - Social factors — the social
  - Environmental/ecological factors — the wider environment

4 Insight

Based on work to develop a deeper 'insight' into peoples lives, with strong focus on what will move and motivate people.

- Focus is clearly on developing a deeper understanding and insight into what is likely to move and motivate the audience or customer in a given context.
- Drills down from a wide understanding of the customer (customer orientation) to focus on identifying key factors and issues relevant to positively influencing particular behaviour.
- The approach is based on identifying and developing 'actionable insights' using considered judgement, going beyond collation of data and intelligence.

5 Exchange

Incorporates a compelling 'exchange' proposition and analysis, while really understanding what the person has to give in order to get the benefits proposed.

- Clearly analyses the full cost to the customer in achieving the proposed benefit (e.g. financial, physical, social, and time spent).
- Analyses the perceived and actual costs versus perceived and actual benefits.
- Incentives, recognition, reward, and disincentives are considered and tailored according to specific audiences, based on what they directly value.

6 Competition

Incorporates a robust competition analysis to ensure that all those things competing for the time, attention, and behaviour of the audience are addressed.

- Examines both internal and external competition and seeks to address these.
  - Internal (e.g. psychological factors, pleasure, desire, risk taking, and addition)
  - External (e.g. wider influences and influencers competing for the audience's attention, time, and behaviour, promoting and reinforcing alternative or counter behaviours)
- Strategies aim to minimize the potential impact of competition by considering positive and problematic external influences and influencers.
- Factors competing for the time and attention of a given audience are considered.

7 Segmentation

Uses a developed segmentation approach, going beyond more simple targeting approaches, and avoids the use of generalized 'blanket' communications.

- Traditional demographic and (where relevant) epidemiological data are used for targeting but not relied on exclusively.
- Deeper segmented approaches that focus on what 'moves and motivates' the relevant audience are applied, while drawing on the greater use of psychographic data and insights.
- Interventions are directly tailored to specific audience segments rather than relying on 'blanket' approaches.
- Future lifestyle trends are considered and addressed.

8 Methods mix—intervention or marketing mix

Examines and uses an appropriate mix of methods to achieve the goals: at the strategic social marketing level, the 'intervention mix'; at the operational social marketing level, the 'marketing mix'.

- A range of different approaches are examined and used to establish an appropriate mix of methods.
- Avoids reliance on single methods or approaches used in isolation.
- Methods and approaches are developed, while taking full account of any other interventions in order to achieve synergy and enhance overall impact.
- Five primary interventional domains are systematically examined and an appropriate balance is reached; the DICES intervention domains:
  - Design—to alter the environment
  - Inform—to communicate facts and attitudes
  - Control—to regulate and enforce
  - Educate—to enable and empower
  - Service—to provide support services

The benchmark criteria are not a process. It is important that these criteria are not confused with a process of how to do social marketing. There are specific process models for this (see the Total Process Planning framework in Chapter 10). Instead, the benchmarks are essentially the key elements that indicate if something is consistent with effective social marketing.

The benchmarks have been framed in such a way as to ensure that they do not restrict the ability of planners and practitioners to develop flexible, creative, and imaginative solutions to the different types of behavioural challenges they face. However, these criteria provide a robust framework to assist those planning and developing interventions to ensure that they are consistent with the best evidence-based principle and practice in the social marketing field.

Recognizing there are other separate success criteria

The eight-point benchmark criteria should not be confused with other essential criteria for success. It is, therefore, important to note that there are a range of other important factors that are critical to the success of any intervention—whether social marketing or not. Obvious examples would include strategic planning, partnership and stakeholder engagement, review, and evaluation (to name just a few). These are all clearly important in their own right, and key to developing and delivering successful interventions. The reason that they are not part of the benchmarks is that they do not help people in identifying and distinguishing something as social marketing. Their presence (or absence) does not indicate if something is social marketing or not. The eight-point criteria, however, are the things that we would look for to indicate if something is consistent with effective social marketing.

The benefit and use of the benchmark criteria

The benchmark criteria can be used in a variety of ways to support effective practice, some examples of which are listed in the following.

Those contracting or commissioning interventions

Those commissioning work can use the eight-point benchmarks as a practical support in the tendering process.

Inclusion within the tender brief: The criteria can be included in the tender brief, along with a request that all those submitting tenders should indicate in their bid how they will ensure that their work is consistent with the eight-point criteria.

Used during short-listing and tender panel interviews: They can be used to guide questioning during the interviews, to see if those bidding have genuinely understood and incorporated the criteria into their proposals.

Those tendering or bidding for work—agencies, consultants, and other contractors

Those tendering can use the benchmarks in the preparation of their tender proposals to indicate to commissioners that they will be consistent with effective social marketing principles and practice. They can then also be highlighted during any interview panel process to indicate to the commissioners that what they propose is consistent with the best available principles and evidence.

Intervention planners and developers—projects or programmes

The criteria can be used as a robust guide throughout the development process to ensure that as work develops it is consistent with the core criteria. They are designed to allow greatest flexibility and creativity in being able to develop interventions. They cannot be used as a 'how to' list but rather as a steer to ensure the principles are reflected in the developing work and approach being adopted.

Evaluators and researchers

Those reviewing and evaluating the impact of interventions can use the benchmarks to reinforce the focus on determining the extent to which specific behavioural impacts have been achieved. They can also be used by those seeking to compare and contrast learning from different interventions and programmes and, therefore, to help in identifying relevant transferable learning and sharing this more widely.

Educators, trainers, and developers

Those educating or training others can use the benchmarks as a simple and systematic guide to highlight the key principles and concepts involved when trying to explain or debate how social marketing can be used and applied.

'The customer'—the public, professionals, or politicians

It is also important to make clear why a generic term such as 'the customer' is being used here. In practice, 'the customer' can be any person/people who is/are the target audience for the intervention. This means that social marketing is not just concerned or focused on the public (or specific groups within the public). Instead, social marketing can be used to engage and influence any group of people, including the public, key professionals or decision makers, and politicians.

The most important point is to focus on those whose behaviour it is important to influence for the given intervention to have a positive social benefit. This immediately challenges one of the common misunderstandings about social marketing—that it only focuses on the individual. Instead, effective social marketing, while considering the individual (public, professional, or politician), also considers their wider social context and is often focused on changing the way policy and strategic decisions are made, how budgets are allocated, and how services are delivered. In this sense, the customer or target audience for social marketing can be the public, professionals, or politicians.

Conclusions

As Stead et al. (2007) argue, social marketing is not a theory in itself; rather, it is a *framework or structure that draws from many other bodies of knowledge such as psychology, sociology, anthropology, and communication theory*. Social marketing is a dynamic interdisciplinary cross-sector approach to creating social good. Like marketing and many other public sector endeavours such as education, public health, and environmental development, social marketing needs to draw on a very broad range of disciplines, theories, and methodologies. In this sense, social marketing is an example of a new multidisciplinary whole systems approach to solving social issues.

The brief exploration of definitions in this chapter has demonstrated that social marketing is not simply the application of commercial marketing know-how to social problems; it is not simply like selling soap. Social marketing is fundamentally a user- or citizen-focused activity that seeks to develop deep contextual understanding about what will help people to choose to behave in ways that will benefit them and wider society. However, social marketing is also a process that can be applied at the most strategic level to refocus the delivery of public service from an overdominance of expert opinion to one that is also informed and shaped by the public's view and what users of public services and interventions say will help them. In this sense, strategic social marketing is just like great commercial sector marketing: it is not what the marketing department does but what the whole organization does.

References

Andreasen, A. (1995). *Marketing and Social Change: Changing Behaviours to Promote Health, Social Development and the Environment.* San Francisco, CA: Jossey-Bass.

Andreasen, A. (2006). *Social Marketing in the 21st Century.* Thousand Oaks, CA: Sage Publications.

Dann, S. (2006). Social marketing in the age of direct benefit and upstream marketing. *Third Australasian Non-profit and Social Marketing Conference,* August 10–11, 2006.

French, J. and Blair-Stevens, C. (2006). *Social Marketing: National Benchmark Criteria.* London: National Social Marketing Centre. Available at: http://www.nsmcentre.org.uk/images/CoreFiles/NSMC_Social_Marketing_BENCHMARK_CRITERIA_Sept2007.pdf [Accessed March 2009].

French, J. and Blair-Stevens, C. (2007). *Big Pocket Guide: Social Marketing.* London: National Social Marketing Centre.

Kotler, P. and Lee, N. (2007). *Social Marketing: Influencing Behaviours for Good.* New York, NY: Sage Publications.

Kotler, P. and Roberto, E. (1989). *Social Marketing: Strategies for Changing Public Behaviour.* New York, NY: Free Press.

Kotler, P., Roberto, E. and Lee, N. (2002). *Social Marketing: Improving the Quality of Life.* Thousand Oaks, CA: Sage Publications.

Kotler, P. and Zaltman, G. (1971). Social marketing: an approach to planned social change. *Journal of Marketing,* 35(3): 3–12.

Lazer, W. and Kelly, E.J. (1973). *Social Marketing: Perspectives and Viewpoints.* Homewood, IL: Richard D. Irwin.

Maibach, E., Rothchild, M. and Lee, N. (2002). Social marketing. In K. Glanz, B. Rimer, and F. Lewis (eds.) *Health Behaviour and Health Education,* 3rd ed. San Francisco, CA: Jossey Bass, pp. 431–461.

NSMC (2006). *It's Our Health!* London: National Social Marketing Centre.

Smith, W.A. (2007). Social marketing—making it fun, easy, and popular. Paper presentated at the *2nd National Social Marketing Conference on From Rhetoric to Reality,* Oxford, September 24–25, 2007.

Chapter 4

Behavioural theory: understanding the key influences on human behaviour

Clive Blair-Stevens, Lucy Reynolds, and Alex Christopoulos

Learning points

This chapter

- Provides an understanding of how behavioural theory can practically support effective intervention development and delivery;
- Discusses the different types of influence on human behaviour;
- Sets out the strengths and limitations of different disciplinary contributions to understanding what influences behaviour; and
- Stresses the value of bringing people from different disciplines together to help examine and consider key behavioural challenges.

Chapter overview

Having an understanding of the use of theory (particularly behavioural theory) is important, as it can strengthen and enhance the development and delivery of social marketing interventions and, therefore, ultimately improve and strengthen their potential impact and effectiveness. However, all too often people say that they find literature explaining different theoretical perspectives dense and hard to read and understand. As a result, many feel alienated from discussions about theory and do not always appreciate its practical value.

A key word in considering theory, as elsewhere with social marketing, is 'utility'. Here, therefore, we seek to help people appreciate how theory can be a practical aid in their work. In discussing it, we do not want to leave the impression that people necessarily need to become expert behavioural theorists—unless, of course, that is their interest. Rather, we aim to set out some broad frameworks and ideas that can help to support and assist people, and to help encourage people to develop a broad overview of theory and how different theoretical ideas can be integrated into intervention design and development.

It is also important to recognize that although people may not be able to officially name the particular theories that they use or drawn from in everyday practice, we all do have underpinning ideas, beliefs, or theories about what influences and impacts on people's behaviour.

Effective social marketing, therefore, is concerned with helping people recognize the ideas or theories that may underpin any assumptions they hold about what influences individuals or communities. This helps to ensure that such assumptions or ideas are more transparently acknowledged, allowing people to reflect on them and consider if they are indeed helpful or not.

Problems can sometimes occur when stakeholders or partners hold very different underpinning ideas to us about what will influence people, and if these ideas are not brought into the open and reflected on, they can undermine the potential of the relationship in question.

Finally, the other value of a more open understanding of theory in our work is that it can directly enhance the review and evaluation process. Setting out the theoretical assumptions that have informed the development of an evaluation helps to ensure that the right review and evaluation questions can be framed. All too often, in intervention design, researchers and evaluators have to 'retrofit' theory to their evaluations because they have not considered and addressed theory early in the process.

Introduction

What is meant by theory?

In answering this question, there is a risk of getting very technical and caught up in semantics. However, 'theory', in its simplest sense, is the underpinning ideas about why something is the way it is and the key factors influencing this. In everyday life, we are all theorists, in the sense that we have ideas about why things are the way they are, why people do what they do, why children do what they do, why a government does what it does, and so on.

Theory is about finding ways to look at complex issues and weave these together in a way that can bring deeper understanding and insights. Theory is best viewed as 'a means' rather than 'an end' in itself (unless you are a professional or academic theorist). Theory is useful if it helps people to understand and manage complex issues and act in a more systematic way on that understanding. It thus provides a potential 'frame of reference', helping people to think through how best to approach different issues.

Which theory should you use?

Every discipline generates ideas and theories (some at an alarming rate!). So even a basic reading in any particular area will reveal that some theories challenge or contradict others. Even within one specific discipline, there may be a wide range of theories that compete with each other for currency at any given time. There can be fads and fashions in theory. This all acts to further distance and alienate people, so that they do not recognize theory's potential value. Each individual theory can potentially offer something to help explain a given situation or context. However, few, if any, really help to explain 'the whole' of the complex and dynamic social and societal systems and contexts of which we are all a part.

A 'theoretical framework' has therefore been developed to help people more systematically consider and reflect on theory across a range of areas. This is sometimes referred to as an ecological or environmental approach to theory, although we refer to this as an 'integrated theory framework' (ITF), the purpose of which is to help people recognize that theoretical ideas from every discipline can potentially assist in developing a wider appreciation and understanding of people and their communities, and what influences them.

The integrated theory framework (ITF)

At the heart of the framework, and at the centre of the diagram, are four key 'domains', each of which can be approached in isolation:

- The biological (or biophysical)
- The psychological (or psychodynamic)

- The social
- The environmental context

However, in practice, domains interlink, overlap, and influence each other, as shown in Fig. 4.1, where the relationship between the three initial domains is shown in the centre of the diagram:

For example, a physical factor such as hormonal changes in adolescence can clearly influence young people's moods and their general psychological functioning, and ultimately influence their behaviour. Similarly, a psychological factor such as feelings of self-worth and esteem will be directly affected by the social context and reactions of those around the person, again having a combined influence on their behaviour.

However, in the wider environmental or ecological context in which we all live, there are many factors that will lie outside an individual's control and which are critical to the options and choices people have and the decisions they make. As Fig. 4.1 shows, we can add 'environmental' as the fourth domain around the three initial domains in our diagram to reflect this. As with the other domains, environmental factors can have a direct impact while influencing the other domains. For example, the combination of poor educational opportunities and lack of employment prospects can obviously have a significant effect on both psychological and social functioning.

Taking this basic integrated theory model, we can widen it out past environmental factors to look at the wide range of 'disciplines' that can potentially contribute and help to inform any particular domain. Clearly, there are a huge number of disciplines or professions such as psychology, genetics, or marketing that can potentially contribute. The diagram indicates the breadth and diversity of such disciplines. Apologies to any disciplines that we have not shown—the examples shown are illustrative and so the list is not exhaustive.

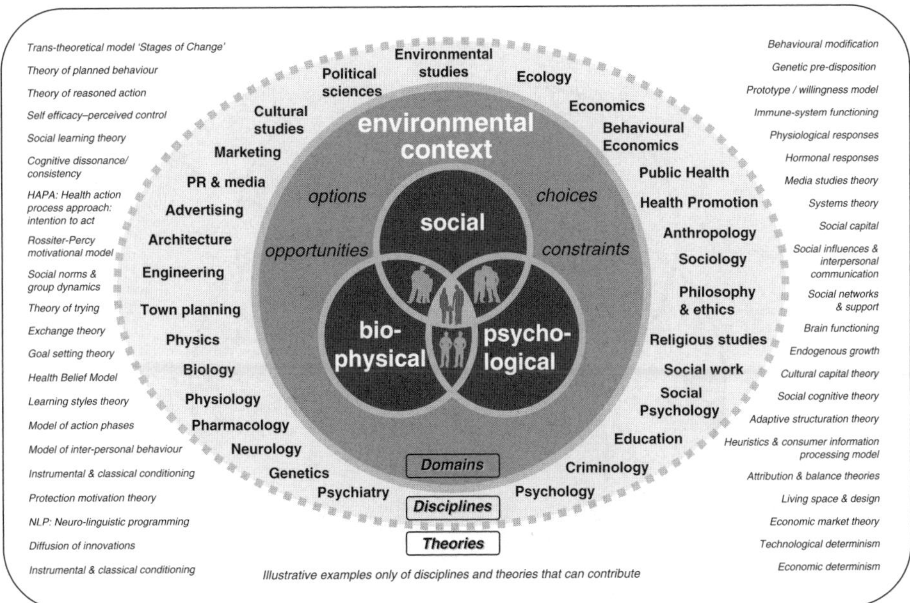

Fig. 4.1 The integrated theory framework (ITF).
Source: French and Blair-Stevens (2007), with permission.

In turn, each individual discipline has generated, and continues to generate, ideas and theories. There are, therefore, many hundreds of 'theories' that can potentially be drawn from. The outer circle of the diagram seeks to illustrate this by highlighting a selection of them. Again, this diagram cannot be comprehensive, but we have included many of those theories that people discussed with us when we undertook our two-year independent review. A brief overview of several key theories is provided at the end of this chapter.

Looking at the range of theories shown can be quite daunting. Our intention is not to suggest that you necessarily need to have a detailed understanding of each theory. However, appreciating the range of different theories involved is important.

The interventions framework

While considering the 'integrated theory framework', it is also useful to be aware of a related DICES 'interventions framework'. This helps provide an overall framework for considering the diverse and sometimes diametrically opposed ways of intervening to influence behaviour. This framework therefore moves beyond the issue of trying to assess what theory can help to explain the factors influencing behaviour in any given context to looking at what 'package' or 'mix' of interventions might achieve a positive impact.

As illustrated in Fig. 4.2, it is possible to identify five primary domains for influencing the DICES behaviour of others. The **DICES** intervention mix model;

1. **Design:** Creates the environment and procedures that support self and community development, and safety.
2. **Inform:** Informs and communicates facts and attitudes, and may seek to persuade and suggested behaviours.
3. **Control:** Using the power of the law and regulation as a body of rules and having binding force to incentivize and penalize the behaviour of individuals, organizations and markets for social good.

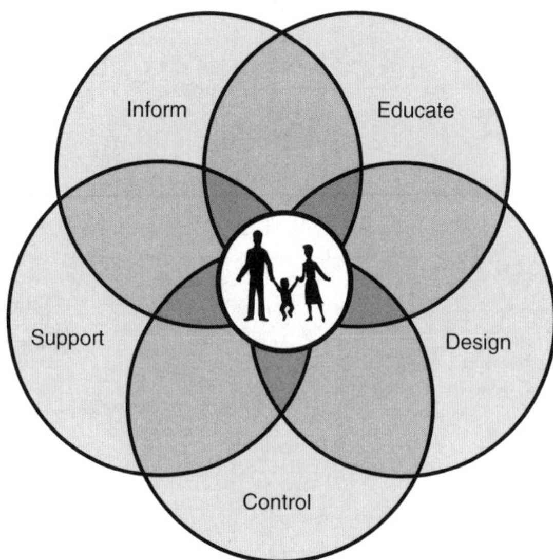

Fig. 4.2 Influencing behaviour: DICES interventions framework. Blair-Stevens and French (2009).
Source: NSMC website paper.

4. **Educate:** Informs and empowers critical reasoning, creates awareness about benefits and develops skills for change and personal development.
5. **Service:** State and other collectively funded products and services provided to support mutually agreed social priorities.

Applying the intervention framework

Each element of the DICES intervention framework links and overlaps, but understanding them and looking at ways to harness each in trying to achieve a particular behavioural goal is important. Reliance on any one in isolation can create problems and, in some cases, counter-consequences. For example, just using 'control' approaches can generate negative impacts and reactions that may achieve something in the short term but be undermined in the longer term.

Voluntary choice

In the development of social marketing, there has been a lively debate about the principle of voluntary choice, and indeed, many key social marketing writers have included voluntary choice as a defining principle of social marketing. This links into a similarly long-standing debate in public health and health promotion about the balance between the needs of the individual versus the needs of communities and society as a whole, and the role of governments or authorities to require and regulate behaviour alongside encouraging and promoting it. Although we do not hold the view that social marketing only deals with voluntary propositions, we do nevertheless hold to the ethical principle that before non-voluntary options are considered we need to ensure that we have properly assessed whether interventions to build voluntary engagement and ownership have been properly explored and ruled out for legitimate and therefore ethical reasons.

Models of individual and wider influences

In the past, there has been somewhat of an artificial debate about the merits of a focus on individual factors (e.g. lifestyle options and choices) versus wider influences or determinants (e.g. environment, education, housing, and employment). This was fuelled by genuine concern that some decision makers and politicians have tried to sidestep addressing the often more challenging and complex wider influences by shifting the focus of attention, and therefore

Table 4.1 Example of the application of the intervention framework

The parents seeking to protect their children from the danger of an open fire	The government seeking to protect and improve health from the harms of tobacco smoking
◆ *Inform* the child that the flame can burn and that burns hurt. ◆ *Educate* from an early age to explain to the child the need for protection from fire and build awareness. ◆ *Support* to monitor and oversee the child and steer them away from any dangers. ◆ *Design* to use a physical barrier such as a fireguard to reduced the risk. ◆ *Control* to set rules, enforce these, and where necessary punish	◆ *Inform* regarding the dangers of smoking and how to get help to stop. ◆ *Educate* by inclusion in schoolwork. ◆ *Support* by providing community and smoking cessation services. ◆ *Design* by limiting physical places where people can smoke. ◆ *Control* by regulating advertising, enacting smoke-free legislation, and enforcing an underage rule.

responsibility (or 'blame'), onto the actions or choices of individuals. Conversely, some have countered this by focusing so much on the wider determinants that there has been a tendency to lose sight of the individual or to infantilize them. This has occurred to such an extent that it has become less important to seek to understand the individual, and develop insights into their everyday lives and experiences (and from this to find ways to motivate and empower them), than it has to tackle the wider political decisions and determinants.

Clearly, both aspects are key to any systematic and coordinated effort to improve people's lives. Thankfully, academics, practitioners, policymakers, and politicians of different persuasions now generally acknowledge that any attempt to seek to positively influence the behaviour of individuals and communities will fail unless it systematically integrates a focus on both the individual options people have and the factors that lie outside of their immediate control but which can be powerful influences on them.

Two wider influences/determinants models

The two models described in the following are examples of ways to understand the range of wider influences on people (beyond the choices individuals might make for themselves) and can help intervention planners and developers consider and adopt a more comprehensive and systematic approach in their work.

The first (see Fig. 4.3) clearly shows that lifestyle factors and choices can have important direct impacts on people's lives. In the example shown, we have used 'health and well-being' as the theme, but the same principle and approach can be used to highlight the impacts on the environment and sustainable resourcing issues. The model also shows clearly that the wider influences around these lifestyle issues have a critical impact on the options people have and, therefore, the choices they personally make. Choice is not neutral and equally distributed. Some people have many more options than others in a given situation, and this will clearly impact on

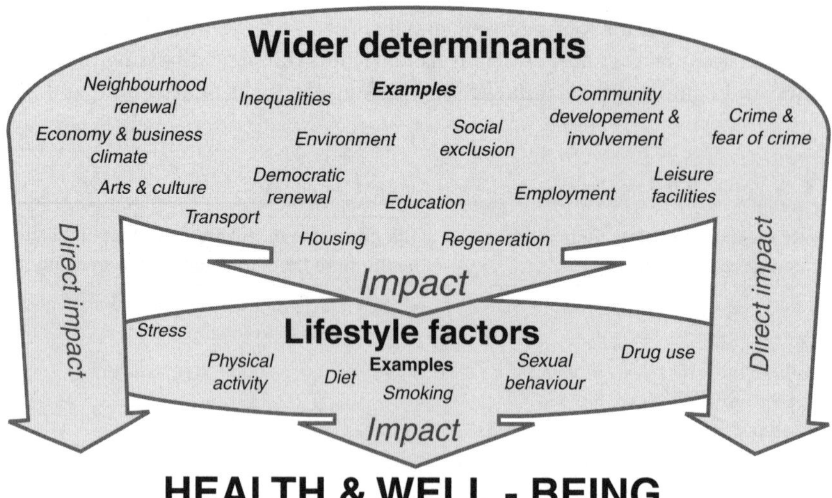

Fig. 4.3 Direct and indirect impact of wider determinants on health and well-being.
Source: French and Blair-Stevens (2007), adapted with permission from *Our Healthier Nation*, Department of Health ©1999.

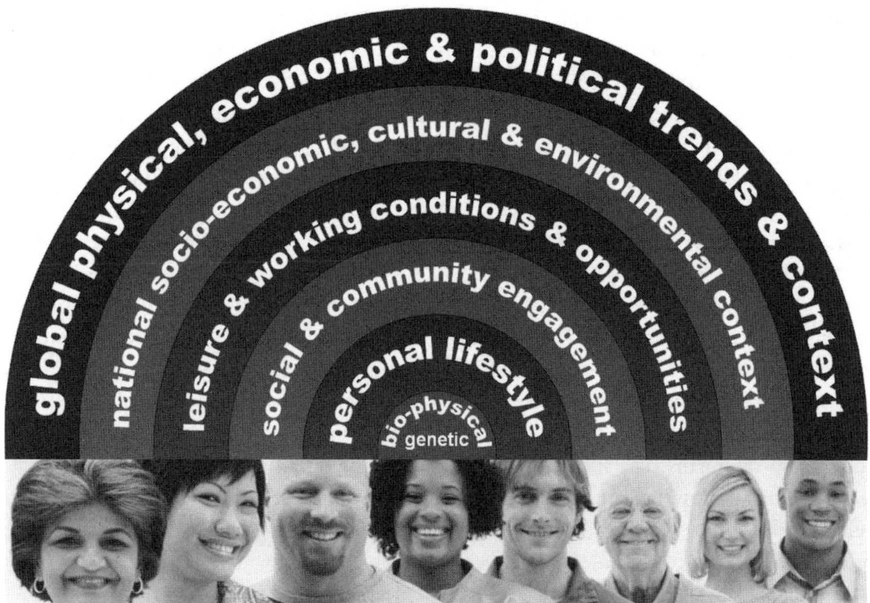
global physical, economic & political trends & context
national socio-economic, cultural & environmental context
leisure & working conditions & opportunities
social & community engagement
personal lifestyle
bio-physical
genetic

Fig. 4.4 Individual and wider determinants of the behaviour model.
Source: French and Blair-Stevens (2008).

the choices they make. Education and employment opportunities are just two obvious examples that will impact on people's choices and, ultimately, their lives and well-being.

However, the impact of these wider influences and determinants goes beyond simply influencing people's individual lifestyle choices and the determinants also have direct impacts on people in their own right. An obvious example would be housing conditions, where poor housing or even homelessness will clearly have major direct impacts on people's health and well-being, outside of any personal decisions or choices they may make.

The second model (see Fig. 4.4) is an adaptation from the seminal work of Dahlgren and Whitehead (2007) to highlight the layers of influence on people. Their work had a particular focus on the health context, but the adapted model we give shows that this can be used in a much wider context to address the factors influencing people's lives.

Conclusion

Whatever our own academic, professional, or personal background, we all develop ideas and 'theories' about what we think influences individuals and communities. This section has been about helping to put the spotlight on a few of these, and for some, this will be giving a name to the ideas they have had but not necessarily been aware of as a particular published theory.

Attempts in the past to develop a 'single theory' that will explain everything have failed, and although perhaps this is a seductive endeavour, it is far more important to develop an appreciation of how different theories can be utilized in different contexts and situations. When we become truly 'customer-focused', we can only really conclude that what influences a person in a particular situation, cultural context, or time frame (day, week, year, life stage) will vary. Recognizing this is critical to being able to develop and deliver effective interventions.

It is not common to find people specifically examining and selecting behavioural theory and then choosing and developing intervention options based on this. But we know that a more open and transparent consideration of the theoretical underpinnings and assumptions informing intervention selection, development, and design can significantly assist systematic application and planning. As suggested previously, it is not necessarily the particular behavioural theory that matters, but that you have an appreciation of the theories that are available when considering ways to influence behaviour. Using an integrated theory framework enables those considering or planning interventions to appreciate the wider thinking and approaches of different theories. It helps avoid the unquestioned and unconscious adoption of a theoretical approach and a failure to consider the benefits of drawing from different theories in different contexts and situations.

A study funded by the Economic and Social Research Council (Sheerin, 2006) looked at the effects of an intervention in 214 published and unpublished studies, asking the question 'Does changing attitudes, norms and self-efficacy change intentions and behaviour?' Interestingly, the report found that interventions aimed at increasing an individual's level of self-efficacy had a much larger impact on intention and behaviour than interventions that aimed to change attitudes or social norms. The study found that 44% of the interventions it looked at did not state a theoretical basis. However, by coding the different elements of intervention strategies (such as agreeing a behavioural contract), it was able to examine those characteristics of more successful interventions. It revealed that the most effective strategies were to

- Prompt practice;
- Prompt specific goal setting;
- Generate self-talk;
- Agree on a behavioural contract;
- Prompt a review of behavioural goals; and
- Discuss relapse prevention.

The strategies it found least effective were those that prompted anticipated regret and fear arousal. This study is a good example of using an integrated theory approach, with which a social marketer can learn from the most effective elements of different theories.

References

Dahlgren, G. and Whitehead, M. (2007). *European Strategies for Tackling Social Inequities in Health: Levelling Up Part 2.* Copenhagen, Denmark: World Health Organization.

DH (1999). *Our Healthier Nation.* London: Department of Health.

French, J. and Blair-Stevens, C. (2007). *Big Pocket Guide: Social Marketing.* London: National Social Marketing Centre.

Sheerin, P. (2006). *Does Changing Attitudes, Norms or Self-efficacy Change Intentions and Behaviour?* Swindon: The Economic and Social Research Council.

Appendix: Behavioural theory snapshots

The following section covers an illustrative selection of potentially useful behavioural theories. It is inevitably selective and only seeks to provide a short overview and 'snapshot' of the basics of the particular theory. This means that it is not possible here to do full justice to the nuances and complexities of each theory. However, for those who may have never specifically studied behavioural theory, we hope that it provides a useful overview. References are included at the end for those wanting to explore these in more detail. For others who may have some familiarity with behavioural theory, we hope that the section provides a useful reminder of the ideas that underpin the different theories, and helps them to reconsider their potential value and utility in their current work.

The integrated theory framework explained previously provides a simple way to consider what areas of theory we may be drawing from and a useful check and balance to just automatically relying on a set of ideas or theories that we may be familiar with. Each of the theories highlighted in the following can offer something to the policymaker and practitioner. Some may be judged as more useful than others; however, avoiding the unquestioning use of a theory is what we hope this section will help to achieve, so that a more conscious and active consideration of the potential benefits of theory can be gained.

- Attribution theory
- Cognitive dissonance theory
- Diffusion of innovations theory
- Goal-setting theory
- Health action process approach
- Health belief model
- Protection motivation theory
- Prototype-willingness model
- Social capital theory
- Social cognitive theory
- Social learning theory
- Theory of group relations
- Theory of interpersonal behaviour
- Theory of reasoned action/Theory of planned behaviour
- Theory of trying
- Transtheoretical (stages of change) model

Attribution theory

Summary

The attribution theory considers how people explain or attribute their own behaviour or that of others. It helps to reveal why people act as they do and further clarify the complexity of behaviour. This theory also looks at how levels of motivation may be affected by the process of attribution.

The attribution theory looks at two different ways in which people explain how their behaviour is determined:

- 'External' attribution: This looks at behaviour as a consequence of outside factors, which are elements that you feel you have little control over. For example, you could blame your poor presentation on the terrible heat of the conference room.
- 'Internal' attribution: This happens when an individual explains their behaviour as being due to factors within themselves, where they feel responsible for a particular occurrence. For example, you may explain that your presentation went well due to the preparation you had done and your ability to cope well under pressure.

This theory suggests that we are more likely to cite external than internal factors when we have made a mistake or done something wrong; however, if it is someone else, we attribute it to internal factors. Conversely, when we have done something right, we are more likely to say that this is due to internal factors such as our intelligence, but when others succeed, we are more likely to put it down to external factors.

For example, if ten children are asked to carry a brimful bowl of water over a certain distance without spilling any, all children will spill some water. Some will blame the spillage on the bowl or the terrain—'it was too full,' 'it was too bumpy' (external attribution); others will blame the spillage on themselves—'I walked too fast,' 'I wasn't careful enough' (internal attribution). Where these children attribute blame will directly correlate with their motivation to try again, and their own sense of self-efficacy and potential.

However, the attribution theory does not always assume that good things are attributed internally and bad externally. Attribution can be influenced by self-efficacy—how capable people perceive they are at doing certain behaviours. Therefore, improving people's self-efficacy has the potential to empower them towards responsibility for certain behaviours and consequently increases their potential for achieving and sustaining behaviours.

Application

This theory is useful in understanding individuals' responses to different behavioural challenges, as well as how people cope with or rationalize behavioural outcomes. Consideration of the attribution theory gives social marketers the opportunity to look at internal and external attribution in their research to better appreciate how an intervention may fit with an individual's perception of their action. For example, a campaign highlighting that it is an individual's responsibility to save the environment may not resonate with them if they feel that damage is caused by big businesses.

Cognitive dissonance theory

Summary

Cognitive dissonance is the uncomfortable tension that arises from having two conflicting thoughts at the same time, or from behaving in a way that conflicts with one's own beliefs. This conflict within an individual's belief system can compel the mind to invent or acquire new thoughts or beliefs, or to alter existing beliefs, in order to reduce the amount of dissonance (conflict) between cognitions.

Application

This theory can be used to understand how, when beliefs and behaviour are in conflict, people often change their beliefs in order to match their behaviour. It can also be used to understand people's tendency to resist information that they do not want to consider. For example, if you present people with information that requires them to break comfortable habits and act in new ways, they may resist or ignore it, in order to avoid cognitive dissonance. This is known as a state of denial as individuals have partial awareness of information and yet choose not to move towards full acceptance of it or any resultant behavioural change.

Diffusion of innovations theory

Summary

This theory considers how new inventions or ideas spread through a given society, being adopted first by one social group and then successively by others. An innovation is something that is new to a particular group or area, but not necessarily to the world (e.g. broadband television, a progressive type of surgery, a redesigned bank service, etc.) This theory recognizes that people will not embrace something new just *because* it is new, or because a mass media campaign promotes it to them. Instead, people are influenced by the actions of those around them, and take varying amounts of time to adopt a new innovation.

Adopters are classed under five headings:

1. **Innovators:** Risk takers who serve as opinion leaders and willingly try new things
2. **Early adopters:** Well educated and wealthy, like the innovators, but more influential with their peers and so key influencers of the time it takes for an innovation to be adopted by others
3. **Early majority:** Do not risk being the first to adopt, but do accept an innovation more quickly than average; followers in their social groups, but above average in education and income
4. **Late majority:** Embrace an innovation just after the average person has; limited education and income and reluctant to take a risk unless the majority has already embraced the innovation
5. **Laggards:** The last group to adopt; typically sceptical about innovations

Each of these levels is influenced by the others (e.g. innovators can influence early adopters, who can then influence the early majority, etc.) Media messages might reinforce the spread of opinion from one adopter level down to the next, but it is recognized that lower levels are unlikely to respond until the level above them has fully adopted.

There are four key elements that are considered through the diffusion of innovations theory:

- **Innovation:** The thing, idea, product, or service that is conceived as 'new' by the consumer
- **Communication:** The process by which this new idea travels from one person to another
- **Social System:** The group of individuals who together adopt an innovation
- **Time:** The duration it takes for the group to adopt an innovation

Application

This theory emphasizes peer pressure and social imitation as crucial factors in the diffusion of a new idea, product, or service. People are more likely to adopt something new if the people they know or respect are seen to have adopted it. This has important implications for those developing interventions suggesting that an effective strategy can be to target a behavioural message or service to the innovators and early adopters, and then to reinforce its diffusion through each successive level. It also suggests that resources should not be invested in trying to reach a given level if the level above has not already adopted.

Goal-setting theory

Summary

The goal-setting theory came out of research looking at how goals can influence performance. The main premise of this theory is that people are influenced by setting goals. Goal setting can help to motivate or stimulate an individual into action. It is argued that setting a goal helps individuals to focus their activities onto one particular target. This focus on the exact goal means that individuals can adapt performance as needed to achieve their goals—for example, trying harder at certain points because they know how far they need to travel to satisfy their objective.

However, the relationship is not as simple as 'goal setting = performance'. There are many different ways in which goals can be framed and this can impact on the resultant level of performance. Locke's (1968) research found that specific, clear goals that are realistically achievable are more effective than ambiguous and easy ones. An element of challenge is important in motivating an individual to try to achieve their goal. Without it, the activity can feel boring or tedious. However, although a degree of challenge is important, it is vital to ensure that goals are actually achievable—expectations that are too high are likely to demotivate individuals from undertaking an activity.

Studies into the goal-setting theory also found that empowerment is important when setting goals. An individual is more likely to be motivated to work hard if they have set the goals or been involved in their development. The importance of goal setting is underlined when we consider the sense of satisfaction, capability, and accomplishment we have when a goal has been achieved. However, the converse is also true: if we do not achieve our goals, we may be dissatisfied and demotivated, which may then act as a barrier to trying to achieve the goal again.

This theory also stresses the importance of feedback as long as it is done constructively and understandingly. This can encourage individuals, letting them know if they are on track to achieving their goal or, if not, what adaptations they may need to make. This feedback does not necessarily need to be from others: it can also be internal feedback.

Application

The goal-setting theory gives the social marketer an appreciation of how the type of behavioural goal individuals set can influence the likelihood of its adoption. It underlines the importance of setting SMART (i.e. specific, measurable, achievable, realistic, and timely) objectives, as highlighted later on in this book. In addition, this theory stresses the importance of involving people when setting goals, which should be an important consideration in the scoping stage of an intervention.

Health action process approach

Summary

The health action process approach suggests that certain elements need be in place for an individual to initiate, adopt, or maintain a certain behaviour. The theory proposes that an individual needs to have an intention to change their behaviour—the 'motivation' phase. In addition, individuals need to have the 'volition' or will to undertake the behaviour. The motivation phase involves the intent to undertake an action and the volition phase the extent to which they attempt to initiate the behaviour. The type of decisions involved in the volition phase include factors such as how long an individual is willing to try a particular activity, the level of effort they devote to it, or how hard they try.

However, the health action process approach does not assume that the two phases operate in isolation to other cognitive process that impact on the levels of motivation and volition to action. For example, the level of perceived self-efficacy impacts on both stages: that is, how capable do you feel you are at undertaking a particular action. It is likely that if an individual does not feel capable of undertaking an action, they will not feel motivated to do it. Perception of the level of risk attached to a behaviour also impacts on motivation towards an action.

Application

The health action process approach is a useful model to take into account when designing behavioural interventions. By considering the impact of self-efficacy and outcome expectancies on behavioural intentions, a social marketer can better understand levels of motivation and will towards an action. For example, if research shows that people have low levels of motivation towards undertaking an action, further investigations can explore whether this might be because they feel they cannot do it, fear the risks of doing it, or do not see the value of the outcome. This information is important when designing interventions.

Health belief model

Summary

This model seeks to explain why individuals do or do not carry out certain health-related behaviours, such as attending for screening, exercising regularly, or using smoking-cessation services.

It suggests that a person's willingness to change their health behaviour is based on the following factors:

- **Perceived susceptibility:** How likely an individual thinks they are to develop a certain condition. Unless they believe that they are at risk, an individual is unlikely to change their health behaviours.
- **Perceived severity:** How serious the individual thinks the condition and its consequences are.
- **Perceived benefits:** What benefits the individual sees in terms of the positive effects of adopting the behaviour (i.e. what is in it for them).
- **Perceived barriers:** How 'hard' the individual thinks it will be to change their behaviour, and the costs that are involved—money, but also effort, time, inconvenience, disruption of regular routines, and so on.

Two further factors were added to the model in the 1980s:

- **Perceived efficacy:** A person's belief in his or her actual ability to make a health-related change (belief in your own ability to achieve something is key—thinking that you will fail means you often will.)
- **Cues to action:** The external influences that might prompt an individual to adopt the desired behaviour (e.g. seeing a poster, walking past a service, losing a relative to a certain condition, being persuaded by a partner, etc.)

Application

The health belief model can be used to predict and prompt health behaviours, and to understand the reasons why individuals do or do not use the available services. It recognizes that it is not enough simply to encourage individuals to *want* to change a health behaviour—there are a range of other factors that affect their intention and ability to change.

Protection motivation theory

Summary

The protection motivation theory looks at how people can be persuaded to adopt risk-reduction behaviours. It considers the influence of fear or persuasion campaigns on individuals' thought processes and the resultant behaviours. It states that, when faced with a health threat, individuals react by either

- Adopting adaptive behaviours to minimize risk, such as taking up regular exercise or stopping smoking (i.e. they are motivated to protect themselves); or
- Carrying out maladaptive behaviours, which place them at health risk either because they continue a harmful behaviour, such as heavy drinking, or because they fail to take a positive step that may reduce health risks, such as having a blood pressure check.

Whether an individual chooses an adaptive or maladaptive behaviour depends on their personal evaluation of four factors:

1. The perceived severity of the threat
2. Their own vulnerability to this risk
3. How effective the recommended preventive behaviour might be
4. How confident they are that they will be able to carry out the preventive behaviour

Application

This theory helps to predict various health-related behaviours and whether individuals will engage in these behaviours. In particular, it can be used when working on topics such as smoking cessation, alcohol reduction, and healthy lifestyle programmes. It allows practitioners to understand what will (or will not) prompt an individual to behave healthily, and to design interventions that maximize the chances of positive adaptive behaviour.

Prototype-willingness model

Summary

This model considers the concept of social 'prototypes', and the ways in which they influence adolescents' engagement in risk behaviours. Perceptions about the type of person who carries out a behaviour are known as 'prototypes'. People associate certain attributes (e.g. coolness, maturity, rebelliousness) with the type of person who typically performs a given behaviour (e.g. drinking or smoking). If the attributes the prototype represents are desirable, individuals will adopt that behaviour in order to become associated with them (i.e. if I smoke, it will make me look cool, because person A smokes and he is cool.)

Application

This model stresses the extent to which social influence affects behaviour, especially among adolescents. Lots of studies have shown that substance-related prototypes influence substance use among teens. However, the model can also be applied to broader health and behavioural issues, and can help to inform understanding about young people's attitudes to their peers and to risk behaviours.

Social capital theory

Summary

Social capital can be defined as the links, resources, and assets that are built both *between* and *within* social networks, which can enable collective action. Such links, resources, and assets can include social norms (such as believing in equal rights), trust, social networks, and social groups.

High levels of social capital can benefit both a community and an individual. For example, being linked and connected within the community can help people at an individual level, such as maybe giving them access to more opportunities for employment. Also, the community may benefit through safer neighbourhoods or getting a better deal from the local government due to a more empowered and connected community.

Application

Considering the levels of social capital can help to give a better perspective of the uniqueness of different communities and the opportunities or challenges that this can bring. Often, interventions may be thought of at an individual, group, or community level; however, the social capital theory gives a stronger focus on the connections *within* the community and helps us to better appreciate that not all are the same.

The social capital theory can be used to understand the ways in which different communities might respond to government interventions or policies. For example, an intervention seeking to change the behaviour of a community, such as increasing their recycling rates, may need to use different approaches depending on the level of social capital within the community. If social capital is high, the intervention may seek to use existing strong social networks to address behaviour; however, with low capital, interventions may need to focus on a more individual level.

Social cognitive theory

Summary

The social cognitive theory (SCT) looks at how people learn certain behaviours. It proposes that learning, or the development of behaviour, is achieved through the interaction of three different factors: personal, environmental, and behavioural. The SCT looks at how these factors interact with each other to influence changes in behaviour.

A broad range of influences can be included in environmental factors. For example, you could be influenced by the *social* environment, which might be your peers or family, or the *physical* environment, which might be the design or location of your building. The *situation* determines the way in which we interpret the environment. For example, depending on the situation, sometimes the views of your peers matter strongly whereas at other times they do not.

The three factors are interrelated and constantly affect each other—one aspect is not simply the consequence of another. Therefore, it is not just how you interact with the environment but also how your internal processes influence how you interpret this. The nature of the interaction between the three factors involves our personal factors (e.g. beliefs and values) as well as the environment and wider social influences. Our cognitions constantly encode and construct structure in situations, which is why we sometimes act differently in similar situations. This is illustrated by the fact that experience and feedback can influence our behaviour.

Bandura (1997) discusses how the environment gives us different models that can help to impact on our own behaviour through observation. How we see things affects our own cognitions. How we react to models depends on whether we see them as believable or credible.

The SCT also stresses that it is important for individuals to believe that the benefits of undertaking a behaviour outweigh the costs. Self-efficacy also plays a key role in the SCT—individuals need to believe that they can actually undertake an action.

Application

The SCT can help provide an appreciation of the way in which different factors interact to influence behaviour. It helps to stress that simply looking at one of the factors in isolation may not yield a large impact because of the influence of wider factors. This theory also provides a good background to the way in which an individual constructs their world and how observations can affect their behaviour.

Social learning theory

Summary

This theory looks at how people learn behaviour. Although people do learn from their own trial and error, they also learn by watching other people—letting someone else try out the behaviour, seeing if it looks sensible, rehearsing it in their own minds, and then trying it for themselves. In addition, people are most likely to imitate behaviour if they see it leading to positive outcomes in another person.

Based on these observations, the theory suggests that learning results from a combination of watching, thinking, and trying. The theory also links attempts at learning with self-efficacy. Most individuals get an initial 'buzz' from learning something new. However, this inevitably reduces as the individual becomes more competent at the new behaviour. In order to get this buzz again, individuals will set themselves higher and higher performance objectives every time they successfully learn something new. By contrast, if an individual fails at a learning attempt, they will set their sights lower to avoid repeated failure.

Application

Individuals can learn from the people they identify with, such as parents, peers, and celebrities. Based on this, it is possible to better understand who will have the most influence over an individual's learning behaviour, and how champions or role models can be used to encourage imitation of positive learnt behaviour. For instance, in a campaign to increase healthy eating, children might be shown how a certain celebrity eats a healthy diet, how this has led to sports success, and how this is a positive behaviour that they are able to imitate.

Theory of group relations

Summary

The theory of group relations looks at how people perform different roles within groups. A group can be defined as two or more people interacting to achieve a common task, and can therefore include work groups, teams, organizations, or social groups. The basis of this theory is that groups move in and out of focusing on their task and a number of different defensive positions based on unarticulated group phantasy (unconscious desires, fears, drives, etc.)

The key conclusions are as follows:

- Individuals lose some of their individuality when joining a group, and might be more easily influenced as a result (Gustave le Bon, 1896).
- The behaviour of organized groups is different from that of unorganized groups (William McDougall, 1921).
- Workers are more committed to work when they are involved in the development of a solution to a problem (Mary Parker Follett, 1941).
- Groups have properties that are different from their subgroups or their individual members (Kurt Lewin, 1948).
- Groups operate on two levels: the work level, where concern is for completing the task, and the unconscious level, where group members act as if they had made assumptions about the purpose of the group which may be different from its conscious level (Wilfred Bion, 1961/1989).

Application

This theory marks an important development in how people think about work and organizations. It can be applied to help shift a focus towards the human elements of work and organizational life.

Theory of interpersonal behaviour

Summary

This theory (Triandis, 1977) seeks to explain people's interpersonal behaviour by looking at variables such as attitudes, values, social factors, and behavioural dispositions. It considers two core factors behind specific behaviours: intention and habit.

The model posits two key equations for behaviour:

- Equation 1 suggests that individuals behave in a certain way as a combined result of their habits and their intentions, and that these two balance each other out. If a behaviour is easy to perform and familiar, it is likely to become a habit. This means the individual requires little intention in order to perform it. On the other hand, if a behaviour is difficult or unfamiliar, the individual will need a high level of intention to perform it. However, external environmental factors also influence behaviour—even if both habit and intention exist, individuals will not be able to behave in a certain way if their social or environmental surroundings prevent them.
- Equation 2 considers the influences that determine behavioural intention itself. It suggests that an individual's intention to behave in a certain way is influenced by how that person feels about the behaviour, the consequences they see the behaviour to have, and the subjective norms and values they have absorbed from their social group.

Application

This theory can help programme planners to understand the relationship between people's attitudes and their behaviour. It can also help to explain the differences between intention-based behaviour and habit-based behaviour. For a health behaviour intervention to work, it will require individuals' voluntary cooperation: that is, they will need to shift away from habit behaviour, and be supported to develop intention-based behaviours.

Theory of reasoned action/Theory of planned behaviour

Summary

The theory of reasoned action was developed by Ajzen and Fishbein (1980) when they were looking at the relationship between attitudes and behaviour. This theory proposes that behaviour can be determined by the intention to perform the behaviour. While intention can be determined by attitudes towards the behaviour and wider social norms.

In this context, social norms can be seen as the way individuals believe their significant others will feel about them undertaking a certain behaviour. Attitudes are defined as the way in which individuals view or evaluate the given behaviour: for example, is it positive or negative? Finally, intention is the individual's readiness to perform the behaviour.

According to this theory, if an individual thinks that a behaviour is positive (their *attitude* towards it) and feels that others will accept their undertaking it (the *social norm*), their *intention* to embark will increase. However, some studies have shown that intention does not always lead to behaviour and that there are other circumstantial factors that can influence this relationship. Ajzen (1991) felt that intention cannot be the sole determinant of behaviour where an individual's control over their behaviour is not complete.

In response to this observation, the theory of planned behaviour was developed. This adds 'perceived behavioural control' as an influencer of intention and therefore further explains the relationship between intention and actual behaviour. This theory focuses on attitudes, social norms, and perceived behavioural control, which collectively affect an individual's level of intention and therefore influence behaviour.

A number of different factors impact on the level of perceived behavioural control, such as the level of skills, opportunities, and the perception of the importance of achieving results. This theory also highlights the influence of self-efficacy over behaviour. For example, if two friends are running a marathon where one feels they can do it and the other does not, it may be that the one more confident in their capabilities tries harder and achieves the behaviour.

Application

A consideration of these theories will give the reader the opportunity to reflect on the complexities involved in generating intention to behave in a particular way. It is important to look at social norms and attitudes and also the level of perceived behavioural control, which the theory of planned behaviour highlights. Those developing interventions may wish to explore these areas in their research, the findings of which may be used to predict behaviour or to highlight the challenges apparent when looking to increase intention.

Theory of trying

Summary

The theory of trying views action or behaviour as a series of attempts and reattempts to realize a dynamic goal, rather than as a single intention towards an inactive behavioural target. Therefore, measures of past behaviour (such as the frequency and recency with which an individual has attempted to achieve a certain action) are valued as indicators of predicted future behaviour.

In addition, an individual's views on the consequences of trying and their perception of these consequences will also affect their attitude of whether to try. So that understanding how people process failures, because a key consideration.

Application

This theory allows those planning interventions to consider recent past behaviour when predicting current and future behaviour and to see how the experience of trying affects the likelihood to do it again. For example, if an individual has tried a number of times to give up smoking through nicotine patches unsuccessfully and has also felt drowsy through them, this may impact on their likelihood to do so again.

Transtheoretical (stages of change) model

Summary

Stages of change is one of the most commonly mentioned behavioural theories and identifies some key stages that people can (in particular contexts) go through when adopting different behaviours. This theory sees behaviour as a process rather than an event; it also recognizes that there are different levels of motivation and readiness to change.

The theory outlines five main stages that individuals go through when adopting a behaviour:

1. **Pre-contemplation:** The person is unaware, and not currently considering or intending to adopt a particular behaviour.
2. **Contemplation:** The person has become aware and is beginning to understand and consider adopting a behaviour, and may be prepared to seek more information
3. **Preparation:** The person is actively considering and beginning to make a commitment to adopting a given behaviour.
4. **Action:** The person undertakes or starts to undertake a given behaviour.
5. **Maintenance:** The person sustains and consolidates the behaviour, although potential for 'relapse' or return to previous behaviour exists.

The theory suggests that people do not always move through these stages at the same rate, and sometimes might remain at a stage for a long time. Therefore, it is valuable to look into the reasons why some people stay at particular stages and why others move on. It discusses the factors that might help people go through these changes, including the following:

- Decisional balance: This is the balance of the positives and negatives of a behaviour, depending on the consequence; this can affect levels of motivation.
- Self-efficacy: This is the level of confidence in the ability and capabilities to undertake the behaviour.

Application

This theory can be useful when segmenting an audience and tailoring interventions to different needs. By seeing behaviour more as a process it is possible to appreciate how different people may respond. It is important however not to consider the stages as rigid or deterministic, since people can move back and forth between stages in dynamic ways.

This understanding of potential stages can help those planning interventions to consider tailoring work to different clusters or groups of people. For example, an awareness raising campaign could be targeted at the precontemplation stage to let the target audience know about the positive aspects of the behaviour, whereas a service might be adapted slightly to help those in the maintenance stage to sustain their positive behaviour.

Behavioural theory references

Attribution theory

Heider, F. (1958). *The Psychology of Interpersonal Relations.* New York, NY: John Wiley & Sons.

Cognitive dissonance theory

Festinger, L. (1957). *A Theory of Cognitive Dissonance.* Stanford, CA: Stanford University Press.

Diffusion of innovations

Rogers, E.M. (1962). *Diffusion of Innovations.* New York, NY: Free Press.

Rogers, E.M. (1983). *Diffusion of Innovations*, 3rd ed. New York, NY: Free Press.

Goal-setting theory

Latham, G. and Locke, E.A. (2002). Building a practically useful theory of goal setting and task motivation. *American Psychologist*, 9(57): 705–717.

Locke, E.A. (1968). Toward a theory of task motivation and incentives. *Organizational Behavior and Human Performance*, 2(3): 157–189.

Health action process approach

Schwarzer, R. (1992). *Psychologie des Gesundheitsverhaltens.* Göttingen, Germany: Hogrefe.

Schwarzer, R. and Fuchs, R. (1996). Self-efficacy and health behaviors. In M. Conner and P. Norman (eds.) *Predicting Health Behaviour: Research and Practice with Social-Cognitive Models*, pp. 163–196. Buckingham: Open University Press.

Health belief model

Rosenstock, I. (1974). Historical origins of the health belief model. *Health Education Monographs*, 2(4).

Rosenstock, I.M., Strecher, V.J. and Becker, M.H. (1988). Social learning theory and the health belief model. *Health Education Quarterly*, 15(2):175–183.

Protection motivation theory

Rogers, R.W. (1975). A protection motivation theory of fear appeals and attitude change. *Journal of Psychology*, 91: 93–114.

Rogers, R.W. (1983). Cognitive and physiological processes in fear appeals and attitude change: a revised theory of protection motivation. In J. Cacioppo and R. Petty (eds.) *Social Psychophysiology.* New York, NY: Guilford Press.

Prototype-willingness model

Gibbons, F.X. and Gerrard, M. (1995). Predicting young adults' health risk behavior. *Journal of Personality and Social Psychology*, 69: 505–517.

Gibbons, F.X., Gerrard, M., Blanton, H. and Russel, D.W. (1998). Reasoned action and social reaction: willingness and intention as independent predictors of health risk. *Journal of Personality and Social Psychology*, 74(5): 1165–1180.

Social capital theory

Brehm, J. and Rahn, W. (1997). Individual-level evidence for the causes and consequences of social capital. *American Journal of Political Science*, 41(3): 999–1024.

Putnam, R.D. (1995). Bowling alone: America's declining social capital. *Journal of Democracy*, 6: 65–78.

Social cognitive theory

Bandura, A. (1986). *Social Foundations of Thought and Action: A Social Cognitive Approach.* Englewood Cliffs, NJ: Prentice-Hall.

Bandura, A. (1997). *Self-efficacy: The Exercise of Control.* New York, NY: Freeman.

Social learning theory

Akers, R.L. (1973). *Deviant Behavior: A Social Learning Approach.* Belmont, CA: Wadsworth Publishing Co.

Theory of group relations

Bion, W.R. (1961/1989). *Experiences in Groups, and Other Papers.* London: Tavistock (reprinted by Routledge).

Follett, M.P. (1941). In H. Metcalf and L. Urwick (eds.) *Dynamic Administration: The Collected Papers of Mary Parker Follett.* London: Pitman.

Le Bon, G. (1896). *The Crowd: A Study of the Popular Mind.* London: Ernest Benn Limited.

Lewin, K (1948). *Resolving Social Conflicts: Selected Papers on Group Dynamics.* New York, NY: Harper & Row.

McDougall, W. (1921). *The Group Mind.* Cambridge, MA: Cambridge University Press.

Theory of interpersonal behaviour

Triandis, H.C. (1977). *Interpersonal Behavior.* Monterey, CA: Brooks/Cole.

Theory of reasoned action/Theory of planned behaviour

Ajzen, J. (1991). The theory of planned behaviour. *Organizational Behaviour and Human Decision Processes,* 50(2): 179–211.

Ajzen, I. and Fishbein, M. (1980). *Understanding Attitudes and Predicting Social Behavior.* Englewood Cliffs, NJ: Prentice-Hall.

Fishbein, M. and Ajzen, I. (1975). *Belief, Attitude, Intention, and Behavior: An Introduction to Theory and Research.* Reading, MA: Addison-Wesley.

Theory of trying

Bagozzi, R.P. and Warshaw, P.R. (1990). Trying to consume. *Journal of Consumer Research,* 17: 127–140.

Transtheoretical (stages of change) model

Prochaska, J.O. and DiClemente, C.C. (1983). Stages and processes of self-change of smoking: towards an integrated model of change. *Journal of Consulting and Clinical Psychology,* 51(3): 390–395.

Prochaska, J.O. and Velicer, W.F. (1997). The transtheoretical model of health behavior change. *American Journal of Health Promotion,* 12(1): 38–48.

Prochaska, J.O., DiClemente, C.C. and Norcross, J.C. (1992). In search of how people change. *American Psychologist,* 47: 1102–1114.

Chapter 5

Using social marketing to develop policy, strategy, and operational synergy

Jeff French and Clive Blair-Stevens

When it shall be said in any country in the world, my poor are happy, neither ignorance nor distress is to be found among them; my jails are empty of prisoners, my streets of beggars; the aged are not in want; the taxes are not oppressive; the rational world is my friend, because I am the friend of its happiness. When these things can be said, then may that country boast its constitution and its government.
Thomas Paine

Learning points

This chapter helps

- To develop an understanding of the differences between operational and strategic application of social marketing;
- To understand how social marketing can be used to inform the strategic development of social programmes;
- To understand how social marketing can and should be integrated into the policy and strategy development within the public sector.

Chapter overview

This chapter covers the application of strategic thinking in social marketing and the difference between policy, strategy, and operational social marketing. The concepts of the policy intervention mix and the marketing mix in the public sector are compared and contrasted. The chapter explores the challenges of influencing public policy and approaches to using social marketing principles to inform policy and strategy development. Developing a strategic approach to social marketing is covered, including a description of what constitutes a strategic social marketing approach and how it can be analysed and evaluated. The implications for the delivery of operational social marketing, including the need for programmes of action and vertical and horizontal integration, are also included. The chapter concludes with a call for social marketing to be embedded as an integral part of public sector policymaking and strategy development as well as improved operational implementation.

Introduction

Policymakers today face a very different environment and set of challenges to those which taxed previous generations, as discussed in the first chapter. Today, in developed countries at least, we live in an increasingly complex social and cultural environment, with increasingly articulate, educated, and ethnically and culturally diverse populations. Citizens, who through mass consumption, mass media, and globalization, have become accustomed to accessing increasingly individualized solutions that fit with their own lifestyles and aspirations. Changing attitudes, interrelationships with authority figures, and mass literacy mean that the demands on, and expectations of, the state have changed greatly, with a renewed focus on the citizen and consumer power driving policy.

As discussed in the previous chapter, behavioural change is high on the political agenda of many governments, with books such as *Nudge* (Thaler and Sunstein, 2008) becoming must-read texts for many politicians and public officials. This growing interest in the application of what is known about influencing behaviour is helpful; however, there is a danger of developing a new naivety. This naivety gives the impression that the science and art of influencing behaviour can replace the science and art of public policymaking. Even if we were ever to get to a situation where we could precisely predict and influence behaviour, there would still be a need for political and broader civic debate about what to do and how to do it.

For example, long-running educational programmes have done much to create a climate in which a ban on smoking in the workplace has become acceptable. However, in the end, governments have to legislate to ensure smoke-free working environments. In this sense, some public health interventions cannot simply be 'nudged' onto the statute book. What is required is a decision to legislate to restrict some freedoms in order to promote others. This judgement call is rightly increasingly being influenced by the views of citizens and by expert opinion. However, although most policy is developed through the political process of interaction with citizens, most strategy is still driven by policy advisers who view 'policymaking by focus group' as a sign of sloppy thinking and a lack of political will. This view is often characterized by a belief that the attitudes, beliefs, and views of citizens are less important in delivering on policy commitments than an often simplistic notion of 'hard evidence' about what works, or self-evident requirements to educate or legislate for change. This mindset often results in a culture of professional policymaking that favours professionally defined solutions over those derived from citizen-focused research. This product or service focus stands in contrast with the consumer orientation of successful social and commercial enterprises. Such enterprises are not only driven by expert opinion or expert-interpreted evidence but also by an obsession with listening to the people they serve and using that intelligence to create services and products that people actually want and will help them. Fig. 5.1 illustrates how people's views, beliefs, and needs can and should be factored into the development of policy, strategy, and operational delivery of social programmes. The rest of this chapter illustrates how social marketing principles can also be used to inform these three levels of public policymaking and delivery.

Applying strategic thinking in social marketing

Avoiding social marketing myopia

One of the most famous marketing papers was written by Theodore Levitt in 1960, called 'Marketing myopia'. Levitt argued that marketing strategy is not about starting from an analysis

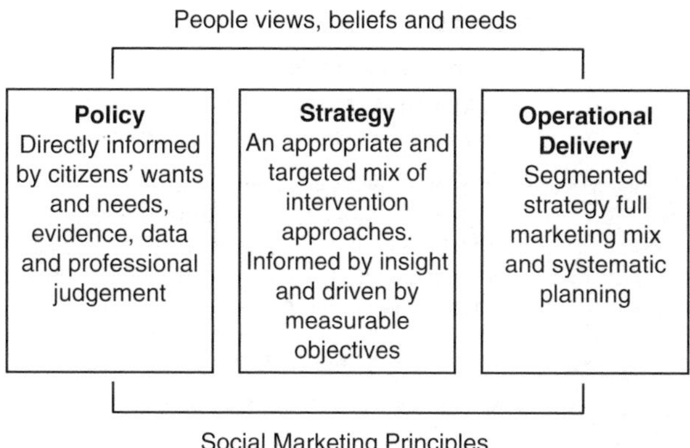
People views, beliefs and needs
Policy
Directly informed by citizens' wants and needs, evidence, data and professional judgement
Strategy
An appropriate and targeted mix of intervention approaches. Informed by insight and driven by measurable objectives
Operational Delivery
Segmented strategy full marketing mix and systematic planning
Social Marketing Principles

Fig. 5.1 Factoring people into policy.

of your products and services and how they can be improved and sold to the public; instead, the key is to focus on understanding what business you are in and what the needs of your customers are. Levitt uses the example of the American railroad operators to illustrate the mistake they made of assuming they were in the railroad business rather than the transportation business.

In social marketing, the mistake of viewing a social marketing strategy as being about fixing a social problem rather than providing a solution to people's needs is the equivalent of Levitt's myopia analysis. Social marketing is a powerful process for tackling social issues, but in strategic terms it needs to keep a clear focus on meeting the needs of the citizens it is seeking to serve rather than on just meeting the policy goals of politicians. Fortunately, in free democratic societies, there is often a great deal of overlap in policy goals, which have usually been developed by governments through a process of dialogue with the electorate. In this situation, the political process is based on the views of citizens served by governments; however, it is possible for governments to lose touch with the electorate. Social marketing, with its prime focus on developing deep understanding of people's needs and wants, can help maintain this link between the development of policy and people's preferences.

When considering how social marketing might be able to make its contribution to the achievement of positive social goals, it is useful to make the distinction between using social marketing strategically and operationally. Social marketing can be used to inform and assist policy formulation, strategy development, and to guide and plan the implementation and delivery of specific interventions.

Fig. 5.2 illustrates the differences between strategic and operational social marketing. Social marketing can be used to inform all three levels and is most effective when it works at all three levels simultaneously to ensure that social programmes are based on common understanding of evidence, citizens' views, and a common and mutually reinforcing hierarchy of objectives and programmes of action.

What are we talking about?

Many terms are used to describe different levels of strategic planning, and it is important to distinguish between policy, strategy, and operational goals, objectives, and processes. In social marketing, it is possible to distinguish between a hierarchy of goals and processes that together make up the range of processes required to ensure a consistent and planned approach to tackling social issues. Box 5.1 lists the three levels of policy, strategy, and operational planning with their attendant objectives and processes.

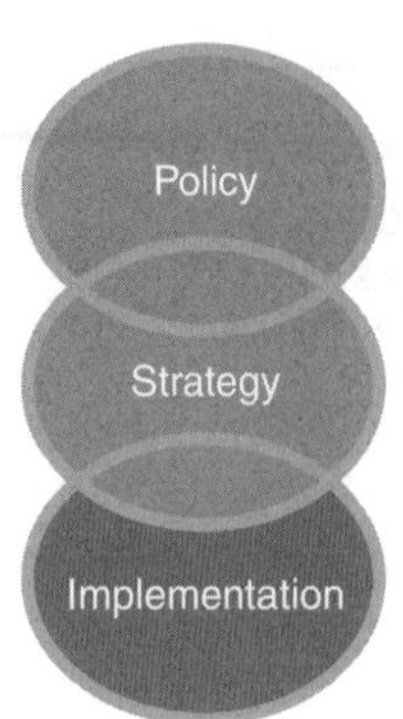

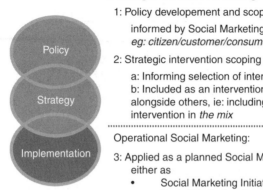

Strategic Social Marketing:

1: Policy developement and scoping

informed by Social Marketing
eg: citizen/customer/consumer insight

2: Strategic intervention scoping

a: Informing selection of interventions to achieve goals
b: Included as an intervention option in its own right, alongside others, ie: including a Social Marketing intervention in *the mix*

Operational Social Marketing:

3: Applied as a planned Social Marketing process either as

- Social Marketing Initiative
- Social Marketing Campaign
- Social Marketing Programme

4: Also able to directly inform developement of:
– other interventions and/or
– service developement and delivery

Fig. 5.2 Strategic and operational social marketing.

Box 5.1 Policy, strategy, and operational planning

1 Policy

1.1 Policy objectives/goals

- Statement of the broad improvements required

1.2 Policy process

- Ideological and political vision
- Understanding the problem
- Identifying stakeholders and responsibilities
- Processes based on evidence reviews for achieving goals
- Time frame for achievement

2 Strategy

2.1 **Strategic mission statement** that summarizes intent, philosophy, and expected outcome; **Strategic objectives** more detailed and related to all policy objectives and goals

2.2 Strategic process

- What intervention mix will be applied
- What will be invested
- Specific responsibilities of each organization and/or sector
- The expected time frame

3 Operational planning

3.1 Operational objectives

- Impact objectives—short-term targets
- Outcome objectives—ultimate success criteria

3.2 **Operational process**
- What will be done
- What will be invested
- How it will be done
- Who will do it
- The expected time frame
- Evaluation and learning systems
- Projects: one year or less
- Campaigns: two–three years
- Programmes: over three years

The DICES intervention mix and social marketing mix

Applying a social marketing approach means recognizing that in any given situation there are a range of interventional options that could be used to achieve a particular goal with different groups of people. As discussed in Chapter 4, single interventions are generally less effective than multilevel interventions. The point is to make reasoned judgements about the relative balance or mix between the interventions selected. Where this is done at the strategic level, it can be described as the 'strategic intervention mix', which is different from the social marketing mix described in Chapter 3. The marketing mix, commonly known as the 4Ps (i.e. price, place, product, and promotion), is a useful mnemonic for some of the key principles used to develop and deliver social marketing interventions. The strategic intervention mix refers to the mix of five key public sector tools that governments and organizations can use to improve people's lives. All liberal democratic societies have five basic tools that can be used to deliver a better life experience for citizens (see Fig. 5.3) which we have called the DICES strategic intervention mix.

Each domain in isolation has the potential to influence behaviour, and each has it associated strengths and weaknesses. However, the evidence is increasingly showing that orchestrating a coordinated response drawing from approaches across all of the five domains has the greatest potential not only to influence behaviour but also, importantly, to help sustain this influence over time. Using isolated approaches can sometimes achieve short-term 'behavioural change', but the greatest challenges we face require us not simply to focus on 'changing behaviour' but on maintaining and sustaining this over time.

A good example of such an approach is the national tobacco control campaign in England. *Go Smokefree* uses a sustained approach and a wide range of interventions to reduce smoking (www.gosmokefree.co.uk). These include cessation services run alongside a national ban on smoking in public combined with educational programmes and tax disincentives on the purchase of tobacco products. The *Go Smokefree* strategy also makes use of the marketing mix, by offering different 'products', at the right 'price' (addressing costs and sacrifices as well as savings), in different 'places' (online, by telephone, through primary care facilities), which are promoted appropriately (through integrated marketing and media programmes).

Using social marketing to inform policy

The policy challenge

The fifth 'P' in social marketing is policy. Many of the challenges faced by governments are reflected in transnational and global trends. As discussed in Chapter 1, the connections between

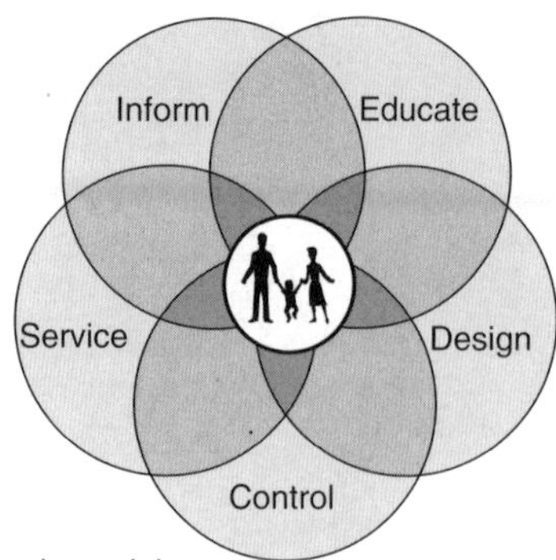

The DICES intervention mix model

1. **Design:** Creates the environment and procedures that support self and community development, and safety.
2. **Inform:** Informs and communicates facts and attitudes, and may seek to persuade and suggested behaviours.
3. **Control:** Using the power of the law and regulation as a body of rules and having binding force to incentivise and penalize the behaviour of individuals, organizations and markets for social good.
4. **Educate:** Informs and empowers critical reasoning, creates awareness about benefits and develops skills for change and personal development.
5. **Service:** State and other collectively funded products and services provided to support mutually agreed social priorities.

Fig. 5.3 The DICES strategic intervention mix—five primary domains for influencing behaviour.

people, government, and the wider global economy are evolving rapidly, reflecting new challenges in the development of policy. The influences on political policy are many (see Box 5.2).

When we look at policy as it relates to the health and well-being agenda, we increasingly see a wider, more holistic approach being adopted. In most health policy over the last twenty years, the word 'health' is used broadly to refer not merely to the absence of disease or even simply the provision of health 'services'. Rather, it refers to a much fuller concept focusing on the promotion of well-being and social justice. Health has also been promoted as a fundamental 'human right' at least since the 1974 World Health Organization (WHO) Alma Ata declaration. The WHO has argued that this 'right to health' can only be realized through the combined and coordinated action using all policy tools and across all sectors. This is a reasonable proposition supported by a wealth of insights and evidence from many academic and practice fields. Health can be understood as an emergent capacity arising from the integrated effects of somatic, social, economic, and cultural activity. It is not something that can be attained solely from heath sector-directed expenditure, or attempts to get people to live healthy lives. If we accept that health is determined by a broad range of factors, we also accept that the development of better health will require whole systems solutions driven by coherent and consistent policymaking and joined-up delivery. Whole systems solutions however depend on how the system is conceived and the role of state-sponsored efforts within this concept.

The WHO and many public health practitioners have, for over thirty years, argued that the promotion of health and prevention and treatment of disease should be viewed by all governments as a primary duty. Smith et al. (2003) have advocated that health actually constitutes the most important form of 'global health good'. Conceived in this way, public health has

Box 5.2 Key influences on policy

Political ideology and opinion
Evidence about plausible interventions
Evidence about the effectiveness of current interventions
Public opinion
Expert opinion
Observational data
Technological breakthroughs
Financial and budgetary opportunities and constraints
Macro-economic influences
Demographic changes
Global, national, and local cultural and social influences
Systems failures
Environmental changes, threats, and opportunities

increasingly called for no less than a global, political, and economic reorientation, something that is not uncommonly associated with a more radical socialist position. Governments, however, do not always accept this proposition and citizens are often seen as holding views and undertaking behaviour that is not, from a narrow professional public health perspective, perceived as logical. Against this background, achieving the right policy and strategic frameworks to promote the population's well-being is not a simple or linear process but one that will require deep insights into why people do what they do belief in what they do and an understanding of what they say will help them to change together with systematic and coordinated planning, delivery, and evaluation. Which is where adoption and integration of a strategic social marketing approach—based as it is on developing a deeper contextual understanding and insight into people's lives—has much to offer, in terms of effective policy formation and in guiding the strategies that flow from policies.

Social marketing: informing policy

The social marketing concepts set out in Chapters 2 and 3 can be used strategically to ensure that understanding about target audience behaviour and presences directly informs the identification and selection of appropriate policy and interventions. For example, the 2000 *Road Crew* social marketing programme run by the State of Wisconsin in the United States demonstrated that taking a customer-focused approach can lead to highly effective forms of intervention (Wisconsin Department of Transportation, 2000; see also Chapter 9). It should also be remembered that social marketing principles can be applied to influence the decisions and actions of political decision makers and service planners. Social marketing has the potential to be a key tool for convincing decision makers and individuals who are in a position to influence overall health determinants and risk conditions to make significant changes.

Much of the social marketing literature and examples of practice currently lie at the 'operational social marketing' end of the spectrum, where social marketing programmes or campaigns are developed to address specific topic areas and audiences. In contrast, a 'strategic social marketing' approach is increasingly being developed to take a broader viewpoint. Strategic social marketing looks at ways in which a stronger customer understanding and insight approach, aligned with more strategic audience segmentation work, and whole systems planning can inform policy development and strategic planning. As Craig Lefebvre, a professor of Social Marketing at George Washington University suggested whilst being interviewed for the last chapter of this book:

> We need social marketers to be at the policy table when options are being discussed and presented, not just sat at the sidelines. There are glimmers visible of people in policy areas asking for social marketing viewpoints for policy analysis and creation stages. We need to ensure they know and understand the social marketing viewpoint—be part of the discussions. This is about having an upstream focus, not just advising for the policy status. Change needs to be part of the discussion.
>
> Excerpt from an interview, 27 Feb 2008

A key challenge for social marketing then is to focus 'upstream' for example to influence fiscal, food, and transport policy that can in turn impact on factors that affect people's behaviour.

The challenge for social marketers is ensuring that the benefits of adopting a social marketing approach are fully understood. This is not, in many respects, about selling empirical evidence of the effectiveness of social marketing. It is about constructing a narrative that helps policy and planners understand the rationale for social marketing and the value of its application across policy formulation, strategy development, and implementation. The first duty and task for many social marketers is to market social marketing to policymakers and planners. Examples of how this has been done at a national policy level can be found in Kotler and Lee (2008) and French and Blair-Stevens (2006). There are a number of tasks that social marketers need to consider when seeking to influence policymakers and planners. These tasks include asking and answering the following two questions:

- What are the policymakers' and planners' needs?
- What will convince them that applying a social marketing approach will enhance the impact of their programme?

Having ascertained the answers to these questions, the experience in England and elsewhere is that a number of other tactics can help develop policy support for social marketing and embed it in the policy and planning process. These tactics include the following:

- Build a compelling story about the power of social marketing and promoting it.
- Build a network of champions and advocates and support them with examples and evidence.
- Provide champions and advocates with opportunities to experience first hand the power of applying a social marketing approach.
- Be constructively critical of current practice if it can be shown to be ineffective.
- Walk the corridors of power and influence, and take part in face-to-face selling of a strong customer-focused social marketing-informed approach.
- Celebrate and promote success.

A key lesson from the English experience has also been that if the term 'social marketing' is getting in the way due to misunderstanding or confusion, then do not start there. Start with the language and values of the policymakers and planners, and then connect the key social marketing principles to what they care about. The chances of achieving a fuller appreciation of the benefits of social marketing are much greater if you are not written off simply as 'selling social marketing'. Focusing on the benefits to the policymakers and planners and what they care about is, as with any social marketing proposition, the right place to start.

There is, in effect, an 'exchange' (see Chapter 3) for policymakers when considering the application of a social marketing approach. The costs for policymakers are focused on the need to invest time in research and gathering users' views. The increased time and cost is a result of developing and synthesizing a more comprehensive array of different forms of evidence and influence on the policymaking process. This can also result in a delay in being able to deliver high-profile visible action, often in the form of a social advertising programme, if it is not supported by the evidence gathered. However, politicians get a more defendable programme of action based on sound evidence and support from the intended audience. An end programme of action is more likely to be effective due to its explicit measurable objectives that can be used to inform the development of future interventions. Finally, politicians and planners get a programme of action that is not only fit for purpose but also one that can be tested for its utility because it has clear aims and objectives, and known input costs and outcome measures. Box 5.3 provides examples about how social marketing can assist the policymaking process.

The main policy building blocks

We know that in any area of policy where there is a strong knowledge base, and broad consensus about what to do, a high degree of central policy specification can work, so long as it focuses on a few key priorities. Where there is less knowledge about what works, management by setting out broad policy objectives is more likely to succeed. This approach leaves more freedom for frontline managers and staff to develop and test new approaches (Performance and Innovation Unit, 2001; Prime Minister's Strategy Unit, 2006). We also know that involving practitioners in policymaking and ensuring that their knowledge is used early in the policy process improves effectiveness.

Box 5.3 Examples of how social marketing can assist in the policy and strategic selection process

- Input into policy development
  - *Collection and analysis of user and citizen understanding; support for views and needs to inform policy selection and development*
  - *Setting up of clear, measurable policy objectives, targets, and behavioural objectives (individual and organizational)*
  - *Review of evidence and experience regarding the intended policy*
  - *Systems audit and analysis*
  - *Behavioural modelling based on theory,evidence, and practice*
- Input into strategy analysis, development, and evaluation
  - *Audience and stakeholder segmentation*
  - *Understanding and formulation of targeted strategies*
  - *Development and pretesting of services, products, campaigns, and other interventions*
  - *Modelling and projection of impact, outcomes, and potential gains*
  - *Budget development and modelling of return on investment*
  - *Identification of stakeholders and partners and other asset analysis and development that contribute to delivery*

Both of these areas of policy understanding lend themselves to the application of social marketing to help with setting agreed behavioural objectives and engaging people and service delivery workers in the development of programmes. We know that effective policymaking results when horizontal networks are developed to assist in the capture and sharing of best practices (Strategic Policy Making Team, 1999; Prime Minister's Strategy Unit, 2007).

In essence, modern and effective policymaking should involve the following (Bullock et al., 2001):

1. Designing policies around outcomes.
2. Policy should be informed by end-user wants and needs.
3. Policies should be and be seen to be inclusive and fair.
4. Policy should be based on evidence.
5. Policy should avoiding unnecessary burdens on delivery agencies or other sectors.
6. All relevant stakeholders should be involved in policymaking.
7. Policymaking should be forward and outward-looking.
8. Policy should have systems in place to learn from experience.

The core policymaking process is essentially about understand the problem, the context, and the stakeholders who are affected by the issue and who might be part of the solution, and then going on to develop solutions based on a deep understanding of people's lives in turn based on the existing evidence and experience. On the basis of this knowledge, the next phase of the policy-making process is to formulate and test possible interventions and combinations against the agreed criteria and risks, followed by the selection of strategies and agreed achievable objectives and how they will be measured. As previously discussed, social marketing concepts and principles may be used strategically to ensure that a strong customer focus directly informs the identification and selection of appropriate interventions. An example of this is the Department of Health's Change4Life programme, which consists of multiple projects and programmes of action (http://www.nhs.uk/Change4Life/Pages/default.aspx)

Developing a strategic approach to social marketing

Strategy is the coordinated application of all of an organization's resources to achieve its goals. Strategy is not the same as operational social marketing planning, as it involves strategic analysis, strategic choice, and strategic implementation, and these three tasks are iterative in nature. Strategy is focused on how an organization, service, or department is structured and operates as well as develops specific plans and applies its resources to achieve specific goals. The development of strategy involves the following seven steps:

1. Determine and codify explicitly the current mission, goals, and objectives.
2. Agree on the criteria for selecting the new strategy.
3. Describe the current strategy and assess its strengths and weaknesses.
4. Assess the current and future external opportunities and threats.
5. Summarize the results of the analyses and conclusions.
6. Generate new options and analyse each against the results and conclusions of the internal and external analyses.
7. Select the new strategy.

When analysing each possible new strategy, a number of issues need to be considered. These issues should be used to assess and filter strategic options. It can help to think of two kinds of criteria when assessing strategic options. The first set of criteria can be described as essential or critical criteria. Such criteria will always be specific to the issue and context but might include the need for the strategy to be, in the first instance, ethical, non-discriminatory, and deliverable. Strategic options that meet the first set of essential criteria can then be subject to secondary criteria that might include issues such as comparative costs and sustainability. Fig. 5.4 sets out the criteria that are often used to assess strategic options.

The need for programmes of action

As discussed in Chapter 1 and throughout this book, many social marketing programmes need to be sustained over time to bring about measurable change. The term 'programme' is significant in that it indicates the need for sustained action over time rather than short-term interventions, projects, or even campaigns. Realistic time frames and sufficient budgets facilitate both the possibility of achieving programme goals and allowing for appropriate evaluation to be completed. This in turn facilitates the possibility that the learning that flows from the evaluation can be used to develop more effective subsequent programs of action. Social marketing programmes should reflect the 16 characteristics of effective practice summarized in Chapter 1. In addition to long-term programmes of action, we also know that significant investment is often required not just to sustain a programme over time but also to fund it to a level at which it can have a measurable effect. Many behavioural programmes are ineffective, not because they are poorly researched designed or executed but because they are simply not funded to a level that allows them to have an impact. The scale of investment required is dependant on the issue and what other assets can be mobilized to address the issue. Any examination of commercial sector marketing programmes reveals that they have far greater budgets than most public sector interventions. Yet the commercial sector is often working to achieve small percentage shifts

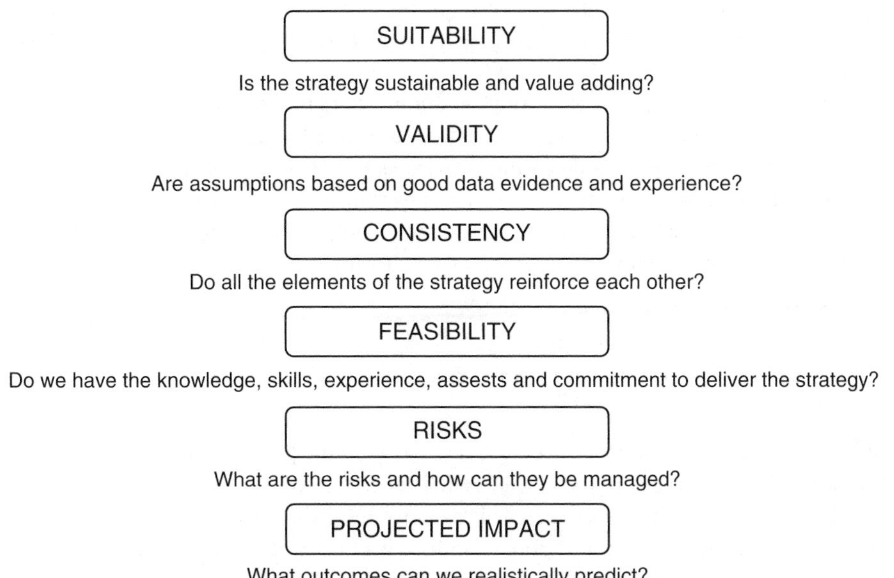
SUITABILITY
Is the strategy sustainable and value adding?
VALIDITY
Are assumptions based on good data evidence and experience?
CONSISTENCY
Do all the elements of the strategy reinforce each other?
FEASIBILITY
Do we have the knowledge, skills, experience, assests and commitment to deliver the strategy?
RISKS
What are the risks and how can they be managed?
PROJECTED IMPACT
What outcomes can we realistically predict?

Fig. 5.4 Criteria for the evaluation of strategic options.

in customer behaviour. In comparison, public sector interventions have often highly ambitious behavioural targets to address issues such as smoking or obesity, with much smaller budgets.

The need for vertical and horizontal integrated programmes

In addition to sustained social marketing programmes, there is also a need for vertical and horizontal integration of specific interventions. Social marketing programmes, like many other public sector, private sector, and non-governmental organization (NGO) sector interventions, tend to have a bigger impact when national, regional, and local action is coordinated. Coordinated action across different sectors such as government, private sector, and NGO sector can also improve the impact. Operational delivery responsibilities undertaken by different sectors or organizations can be clustered and related back to specific strategic areas of action to ensure that a consistent approach is maintained. In order for such a coordinated approach to work, there is always a need to develop clear systems for ensuring that all organizations know their and the other organization's responsibilities. Strong internal communication strategies together with clear performance management and feedback systems can help to ensure that social marketing strategies are effectively delivered.

Conclusion

In this chapter, we have argued for the need to move beyond the more traditional 'operational social marketing' approach (albeit important in its own right) towards a much more 'strategic social marketing' application and adoption, where the principles of social marketing can directly inform and drive both policy and strategy developments.

What the history of different types of social reform and public health in particular teaches us is that attempts to bring about improvement across populations usually requires coordinated multiple interventions as part of wider programmes sustained over time. Interventional approaches must be based on deeper contextual understanding of people's lives and what will move and motivate them, and in the process, work to achieve the popular consent and engagement of citizens. There is now growing recognition that social marketing as both a mindset and process must actively involve all sectors, all levels of government, and a wide range of professionals and activists.

What is required is a shift away from single monolithic organizational solutions towards solutions that also include and encourage contributions from all sectors of society. Despite good intentions, there is a persistent tendency for knowledge, power, authority, learning, and information flows to be top-down from the 'experts'. This phenomenon has been documented in reviews across many areas of social development. For example, in the field of international development over the last forty years, initiatives have largely failed because they ...

- Were wrongly conceived, often doing harm rather than good;
- Created a further burden of debt on the recipients of help; and
- Failed to learn from knowledge that was already available.

(Chambers, 1997)

Chambers sites the main problem as being focused around the problem of distance and believes that *Distance blocks, blurs, and distorts vision*. A division is created between the 'experts' at the top level and the deliverers at the front line. This distance results in those at the top being isolated from the deliverers' knowledge and understanding, and instead relying on secondary data to formulate strategy. The distance is also elongated through a whole professional and technological top-level community, which reiterates the belief that expert thinking is more likely to be driven from lateral sources than from filed level understanding. Consequently, those at the top are more likely to follow current ideologies and academic stimulus than the unfolding experience on the ground.

One solution to this problem is to develop social marketing as an 'embedded capacity' and capability within public sector institutions. Practically, this means not just developing social marketing centres and social marketing specialists but also supporting all agencies, groups, and communities to apply social marketing principles when developing their interventions, services, or other 'products'. Such action needs to be facilitated by strategies that encourage diversity of response, and pay great attention to capturing and spreading the learning from these initiatives as they unfold. This analysis represents a sophisticated system of action research, which can help to inform and shape future initiatives. The support for diversity of response does not negate the need for the establishment of clear central strategy and systems of support but in fact requires a synthesis of approach between the centre and periphery. In summary, the two big policy challenges for social marketing are to move beyond just being a specialist technical function and embed social marketing across the public sector. Social marketing must therefore be at the heart of shaping policy and strategy, and not just informing the implementation of specific operational interventions.

References

Bullock, H., Mountford, J., Stanley, R. et al. (2001). *Better Policy Making*. London: Centre for Management and Policy Studies.

Chambers, R. (1997). *Whose Reality Counts? Putting the First Last*. London: Intermediate Technology Development Group.

French, J. and Blair-Stevens, C. (2006). From snake oil salesmen to trusted policy advisors: the development of a strategic approach to the application of social marketing in England. *Social Marketing Quarterly*, XII(3): 29–40.

Kotler, P. and Lee, N. (2008). *Social Marketing: Influencing Behaviors for Good*, 3rd ed. Thousand Oaks, CA: Sage Publications.

Levitt, T. (1960). Marketing myopia. *Harvard Business Review*, 38(July–Aug): 29–47.

Performance and Innovation Unit (2001). *Better Policy Delivery and Design*. London: Cabinet Office.

Prime Ministers Strategy Unit (2006). *The UK Government's Approach to Public Service Reform*. London: Cabinet Office.

Prime Ministers Strategy Unit (2007). *Building on Progress: Public Services: HM Government Policy Review*. London: Cabinet Office.

Smith, R., Beaglehole, R., Woodward, D., and Drager, N. (eds.) (2003). *Global Public Goods for Health*. Oxford: Oxford University Press.

Strategic Policy Making Team (1999). *Professional Policy Making for the Twenty First Century*. London: Cabinet Office.

Thaler, R. and Sunstein, C. (2008). *Nudge. Improving Decisions about Health, Wealth and Happiness*. New Haven and London: Yale University Press.

WHO (1974). *Declaration of Alma Ata*. Geneva: World Health Organization. Available at: http://www.who.int/publications/almaata_declaration_en.pdf [accessed 19 January 2009].

Wisconsin Department of Transportation (2000). *Statistical and Technical Reports: Road Crew*. Available at: http://www.dot.wisconsin.gov/library/publications/format/reports.htm [accessed 3 October 2007].

Chapter 6

Providing evidence for social marketing's effectiveness

Martine Stead and Ross Gordon

If you can't measure it you can't manage it.
Anon

Learning points

This chapter

- Sets out the challenges social marketers face when seeking evidence of their initiatives' effectiveness;
- Calls for a broader vision of evidence-based practice that reflects the complexity of the challenges faced; and
- Provides an overview of the evidence for social marketing within four health-related areas.

Chapter overview

This chapter sets out the need for providing evidence of effectiveness and examines the challenges this poses to social marketing. It focuses primarily on reviewing evidence of social marketing's effectiveness in four areas:

- Nutrition
- Substance misuse
- Physical activity
- The workplace.

It concludes that although definitive proof of effectiveness is often unobtainable, efforts to develop and refine evidence of the impact of social marketing initiatives should, and indeed must, continue. In the pursuit of more comprehensive and meaningful evidence, social marketers must acknowledge the wider and more complex factors that influence change.

Introduction

Social marketing increasingly faces calls to demonstrate its effectiveness. As funders become more interested in the discipline's ideas and are more prepared to invest money in social marketing initiatives, these calls have become more pressing. Equally, those involved in conducting social marketing feel the need for concrete proof that what they are doing works, as reassurance to themselves and to their managers, collaborators, and target groups.

These demands for rigorous proof of effectiveness reflect wider trends in social and health policy. Increasingly, funders and policymakers rightly demand evidence that programmes are worthy of investment. In the case of medicine, for example, the demand for evidence-based practice perhaps appears a self-evident requirement. But the reality is that this demand is a relatively recent development, and there remain many therapies that lack a sound evidence base.

Doctors have to make decisions about what works and what side effects are acceptable; they also have to liaise with policymakers to manage their interface with society. The concept of evidence-based decision making, with its emphasis on rigorous methodologies for sifting, prioritizing, and interpreting evidence, has arisen in response to this need (Mulrow, 1994). It is defined as *the conscientious, explicit, and judicious use of current best evidence in making decisions about the care of individual patients* (Sackett et al., 1996, p. 71).

The challenge of being evidence-based

The concept of evidence-based decision making, often based on systematic review evidence, is now well established in the United Kingdom (Solesbury, 2001). In turn, the experience of the evidence-based medicine movement has encouraged the expansion of the concept into areas further afield, such as health promotion and social policy (Victora et al., 2004).

However, there are problems in transferring the evidence-based approach, which originated in clinical intervention, to non-clinical forms of intervention. Comparing alternative treatments for a heart condition lends itself to clear-cut and rigorous experimental studies—typically gold standard randomized controlled trials (RCTs)—whose findings meet exacting standards and can be combined through systematic review and meta-analytical procedures to produce clear evidence of the most effective approaches to achieve a desired outcome(s). In contrast, public health and health promotion initiatives tend to have longer and more complex causal pathways than clinical interventions (Victora et al., 2004). Even a relatively simple intervention such as advising general practice patients who smoke to quit relies on several steps: large numbers of general practitioners (GPs) must be informed that they should give advice; large numbers of GPs must give this advice; the advice must be given to a large number of patients; the advice must be given correctly; patients must be receptive to the information and understand it, and so on. A universal and consistent response to interventions cannot be assumed, because so many factors, some of which are likely to be out of the control of the intervention, can affect its delivery and outcomes (ibid.) The problems are intensified when the intervention is one which seeks not to impact on individual knowledge, attitudes, and behaviour but to tackle social and environmental determinants of health by impacting on communities, structures, and policies (Jackson and Waters, 2005).

McKinlay (1993) suggests that traditional experimental designs intended for measuring change in individual subjects are 'suboptimal or even inappropriate' when the mechanisms and settings under investigation are organizations, communities, and social policy. RCTs are unable to accommodate the complexity and flexibility that characterize such programmes (Rychetnik et al., 2002). In addition, even if resources were available, the experimental design would be inappropriate for initiatives that are unpredictable, which take place over a long, and perhaps unforeseen, timescale—with changes potentially occurring after the evaluation period has lapsed (Jackson and Waters, 2005)—or which involve changes in tactics and actions in response to environmental factors (such as statements by government or the tobacco industry; e.g. see Samuels and Glantz, 1991; Heiser and Begay, 1997).

The same challenges apply to social marketing:

- No two social marketing programmes are exactly the same, or at least they should not be. Social marketing puts the consumer at the centre of every intervention and initiative, and this means that messages, services, products, and activities should be designed with the needs of the particular target consumer group in mind. Although the *principles* behind a social marketing programme are transferable, programmes should always be adapted for local needs and contexts. This makes it difficult to prove effectiveness, because conventional procedures for establishing evidence require the comparison and synthesis of results from interventions that are essentially the same.
- Social marketing often requires a multifaceted, multicomponent approach. Initiatives typically involve multiple actions and channels: products, promotional materials, services, publicity, and so on. Such complex interventions do not lend themselves to a precise statement of independent variables whose effects can be measured and easily replicated. McQueen (2001, p. 266) argues, while discussing the challenge of assessing the effectiveness of complex health promotion interventions, that complexity affects evaluation, measurement, and design:

  > The methods one needs to use and develop are tied to the complexity. As the complexity of an intervention increases we need more complicated methods of assessment [and] answers provided by the assessment may be less certain. It is also clear that the most rigorous method of assessment that many propose for evaluation, namely an RCT, is best suited to a simple intervention.

- Social marketing programmes are, by their nature, designed to reflect, and be implemented in, real-world conditions: schools, neighbourhoods, people's homes, and workplaces. This means that it is very difficult to control the context in which an intervention is implemented. As Livingstone (2005) points out, it is difficult in naturalistic settings to eliminate possible confounding variables. In social science, the 'perfect study' often simply cannot exist, for technical, ethical, or other reasons.
- Social marketing programmes are not always predictable. A social marketing programme may evolve flexibly in response to changing needs and circumstances, or in response to research findings suggesting that a certain strategy needs modifying. This inability to specify in advance and then to control the 'active ingredient' in the intervention is incompatible with the typical approach to establishing effectiveness, which requires a treatment or procedure to be tightly specified, implemented consistently, and compared across different cases. Where interventions are by necessity opportunistic and flexible, such as where the intervention is focused on changing policy (Clark and McLeroy, 1998), it is difficult to 'keep the intervention stable', as is required in the conventional controlled design.
- Social marketing is multidisciplinary and draws inspiration from a range of academic and practical domains. One of its strengths is that it does not adhere tightly to any single discipline, approach, or sector, but cuts across these, drawing on tools and theories as appropriate. Although this flexibility is a key strength of social marketing, it poses particular challenges for establishing effectiveness. Strategies that are appropriate for measuring social marketing programme elements and which draw on psychology or education may, for example, be completely inappropriate for assessing the success of features informed by anthropology or sociology.

All of the above contribute to the increasingly accepted argument that, for intervention approaches that seek to bring about behavioural, social, and policy change (including social marketing), the traditional biomedical approach to evaluation has limited relevance (e.g. see McKinlay, 1993; Davies and MacDonald, 1998; Learmonth and Mackie, 2000; Tones, 2000; Stead et al., 2002).

Rigid adherence to a hierarchical view of evidence that values methodological purity as the most important factor may be unhelpful to public health and health promotion (Ogilvie et al., 2005). Many interventions of interest within public health simply cannot be studied using RCTs for scientific, political, ethical, or practical reasons (ibid.) Reliance on levels of evidence alone will favour interventions with a medical rather than social focus, and those that target individuals rather than communities or 'upstream' determinants. This can result in flawed, narrow, or even no decisions about how to proceed (Rychetnik et al., 2002). Furthermore, certain types of intervention are more likely to be subject to high-quality evaluation because there are strong financial interests behind them, resulting in more resources to conduct studies (e.g. pharmaceutical interventions; Rychetnik et al., 2002). 'Best' evidence is often gathered on simple interventions conducted on groups that are the easiest to reach. Social marketing, like public health in general, is often more concerned with complex interventions conducted with disadvantaged groups (Rychetnik et al., 2002). Therefore, considerations of equity should also inform decision making in formulating recommendations (ibid.)

The RCT design also leaves many important questions unanswered or uninvestigated: it fails to capture the detail and complexity of intervention inputs and tactics; it reveals little, if anything, about the processes by which interventions exert an influence; and it neglects events and factors outside the scope of the experiment. Fawcett et al. (1997, p. 826) argue that *the usual research goal of establishing links between project activities ... and particular outcomes* is particularly challenging when interventions use an array of actions, aimed at different targets, over varying periods of time, the effects of which are often delayed. Furthermore, less easily measurable effects, which may in themselves be deemed worthwhile (such as increases in community participation in improving their own health or their neighbourhood, or gradual shifts in community attitudes towards a health problem), are unlikely to be captured. Allison and Rootman (1996) note that the very processes used and valued in many interventions, such as community participation, tend to make randomized designs impossible. Similarly, in social marketing, some of the aspects that make social marketing an ideal interventional approach in many contexts (e.g. its flexibility and pragmatism) are also the ones which cause the most difficulties when trying to measure effectiveness.

The way forward: a broader view of evidence

Gathering evidence for the value of approaches such as social marketing is a challenging task. What is required is a broad vision of evidence-based practice—one that embraces the inherent complexity of the approach. Rather than retreating to limited rules regarding what constitutes evidence, there is a need to develop analytic frameworks that recognize the complexity of the field.

This is by no means a counsel of despair. Efforts to assess effectiveness in social interventions continue, using both traditional biomedical models and expanding and modifying these models to incorporate more complex dimensions (see Kennedy and Abbatangelo, 2005; NICE, 2007). Assisted by this sort of thinking, the principles of evidence-based decision making are now increasingly being taken beyond medicine into fields such as crime and criminal justice, social welfare, and health education, where practice and policy options are also actively debated and the balance between professional and public interest has to be determined. For example, a recent study funded by the Economic and Social Research Council (ESRC) used systematic review methods to assess the effectiveness of financial 'safety net' products designed to protect mortgagors against the risk of arrears and repossession (Baldwin et al., 2002).

As with medical research, institutions have been established to guide and progress the preparation and dissemination of research used to inform social policy. In 2002, the Campbell Collaboration (http://www.campbellcollaboration.org) was established to build on the experience of the Cochrane Collaboration and carry out evidence reviews of initiatives in the fields of education, criminal justice, and social work. Similarly, the Centre for Evidence Based Policy and Practice (http://www.kcl.ac.uk/schools/sspp/interdisciplinary/evidence) was established to produce and disseminate social science research and publications relevant to policy and practice among a variety of stakeholders, including the research community, central and local government, and industry. Reviews now exist on a disparate range of topics, including teaching approaches (Higgins et al., 2005), social care (Turner et al., 2005), and crime reduction (Petrosino et al., 2002). In the United Kingdom, this growing interest in evidence-based decision making is reflected at the highest levels of government (Cabinet Office, 1999), where commitments have been made to use research evidence to inform policy and practice, and great emphasis is put on establishing 'what works' (Boaz et al., 2002) to ensure efficient use of taxpayers' money.

The new evaluation agenda is informed by an acknowledgement that there is a need to develop a broader view of evidence, one which acknowledges the utility of alternative types of study and other forms of knowledge, such as practitioner and target group perspectives. Systematic reviews of evidence are likely to be more relevant to the end user if they are informed by the perspectives of people with experience of the topic and practice issues (Jackson and Waters, 2005). Importantly, there is recognition that the desire for 'best' evidence should not stand in the way of using the 'best available' evidence (Ogilvie et al., 2005). Learning in public health and social marketing is best promoted by critical sharing of all types of evidence, and not by suppressing some sorts of evidence because they are deemed suboptimal (Ogilvie et al., 2005).

Importantly, it is essential to recognize the limits of so-called 'gold standard' research designs when applied to social interventions. Even where a social intervention has been subjected to an RCT-type evaluation and been proven effective, this does not mean it will be acceptable or appropriate in every context or with every target group.

Assessing social marketing effectiveness

Although many primary studies have examined the effectiveness of individual social marketing programmes, there have been only a small number of reviews of its effectiveness in general as a health behavioural-change approach. For example, a recent review of the effectiveness of social marketing initiatives designed to promote condom use among 'poor and vulnerable' groups found that although the initiatives were struggling to reach the poorest groups, they had achieved some success in addressing social and regulatory constraints to access (Price, 2001). Another review, of social marketing nutrition and physical activity initiatives, found that although social marketing had been effective in altering some behaviours, its overall effects were limited (Alcalay and Bell, 2000). However, these reviews have a number of limitations. Methods have not always been systematic, and there is often insufficient information on the search strategy and inclusion criteria. In particular, reviews often fail to state explicitly how social marketing interventions have been defined, and they conceptualize social marketing in widely differing ways. For example, in family planning reviews, social marketing is often taken to mean, primarily, free distribution of condoms. In others, social marketing is misconstrued as simply social advertising or communications (e.g. see Alcalay and Bell, 2000).

One difficulty has been the lack of an agreed and easily operationalized definition of a social marketing initiative (see also Chapter 3 for more discussion on the challenge of defining social marketing). Consider Andreasen's definition (1995, p. 7):

> The application of commercial marketing technologies to the analysis, planning, execution and evaluation of programs designed to influence the voluntary behaviour of target audiences in order to improve their personal welfare and that of society.

Such generic definitions are not precise enough to help decide whether a specific initiative does or does not qualify as social marketing. One solution to the difficulty is simply to select initiatives that are labelled 'social marketing' by their managers or evaluators. However, recent experience of reviewing 'social marketing nutrition initiatives demonstrated that relying solely on the label is a problematic approach (McDermott et al., 2005a, 2005b). Firstly, it excludes many initiatives that are not labelled 'social marketing' but which appear to incorporate social marketing principles. Secondly, it includes initiatives that, despite their label, are poor examples of social marketing or are not social marketing at all. For example, the misperception that social marketing equals advertising means that many initiatives that are essentially media campaigns are erroneously described as social marketing (Stead and Hastings, 1997). The resulting evidence base, if a search is restricted only to initiatives called 'social marketing', is likely to be limited and flawed.

A more useful solution is to ask what essential ingredients should be present in a social marketing initiative. In 2002, Andreasen identified what he termed six essential benchmarks of a 'genuine' social marketing intervention, one which applies social marketing throughout rather than as an add-on (see Table 6.1).

Recent reviews of social marketing effectiveness

In response to the National Social Marketing Strategy and the white paper *Choosing Health* (DoH, 2004), which culminated in the formation of the National Social Marketing Centre (NSMC), and also as part of the work to *help realise the full potential of effective social marketing in contributing to national and local efforts to improve health and reduce health inequalities* (NCC and DoH, 2005, p. 4), a review of social marketing effectiveness was conducted. The Department of Health and National Consumer Council commissioned a series of literature reviews to investigate the effectiveness of social marketing interventions as a health behavioural-change approach. Three separate reviews, which were largely systematic in nature, were conducted on the effectiveness of social marketing interventions tackling substance misuse, physical activity, and nutrition (Gordon et al., 2006a; Stead et al., 2007a). As part of a separate strand of work, funded by the Health and Safety Executive, a review was later conducted on the potential of social marketing as an approach for promoting workplace health and well-being (Stead and Angus, 2007).

For each of the reviews, potential interventions were assessed against Andreasen's six essential benchmarks of a 'genuine' social marketing initiative. If an initiative was judged to have met each of the six benchmark criteria, it was defined as having adopted a social marketing approach, irrespective of the label that the author used to describe the initiative. If it failed to meet any one of the benchmark criteria, the initiative was excluded from the review. These criteria have since been further developed by the NSMC to include use of theory and customer insight (French and Blair-Stevens, 2005).

Table 6.1 Andreasen's benchmark criteria

	Benchmark	Explanation
1	Behavioural change	Intervention seeks to change behaviour and has specific measurable behavioural objectives.
2	Consumer research	Intervention is based on an understanding of consumer experiences, values, and needs. Formative research is conducted to identify these. Intervention elements are pretested with the target group.
3	Segmentation and targeting	Different segmentation variables are considered when selecting the intervention target group. Intervention strategy is tailored for the selected segment(s).
4	Marketing mix	Intervention considers the best strategic application of the 'marketing mix'. This consists of the four Ps: 'product', 'price', 'place', and 'promotion'. Other Ps might include 'policy change' or 'people' (e.g. training is provided to intervention delivery agents). Interventions that use only the promotion P are social advertising, and not social marketing.
5	Exchange	Intervention considers what will motivate people to engage voluntarily with the intervention and offers them something beneficial in return. The offered benefit may be intangible (e.g. personal satisfaction) or tangible (e.g. rewards for participating in the programme and making behavioural changes).
6	Competition	Competing forces to the behavioural change are analysed. Intervention considers the appeal of competing behaviours (including current behaviour) and uses strategies that seek to remove or minimize this competition.

Data adapted from Andreasen (2002).

Different search strategies were used for each of the three reviews. The nutrition review updated a previous review (McDermott et al., 2005b) and was fully systematic in nature. To update the review, eight electronic databases were searched for the relevant literature from 2003 onwards. This resulted in 67 articles that were assessed against the benchmark criteria, of which 31 met all six criteria and were included in the review.

For the physical activity review, eight electronic databases were searched using combinations of the terms 'physical activity', 'exercise', and 'social marketing'. This yielded 110 articles that were reviewed against the benchmarks, with 22 interventions meeting all the criteria and being included in the review.

Due to the large number of substance misuse intervention studies, a search was conducted for good-quality reviews on the topic, and the reference lists from these existing reviews formed the basis of a sampling frame for potentially eligible social marketing initiatives. The search yielded 35 systematic reviews, and from these, 310 individual studies were assessed against the benchmarks. Thirty-five studies met all of Andreasen's six criteria for a social marketing intervention and were included in the review.

A similar approach was adopted for the workplace review. Reference lists of systematic reviews were searched for intervention studies that might have adopted a social marketing approach, and the original studies were retrieved and assessed against the benchmarks. Of these, 14 studies met the criteria and could be described as having used social marketing principles in their design and implementation. In addition, grey literature and company websites were searched for contemporary examples of initiatives that adopted some the social marketing principles. These were included in the review as case studies illustrating what a social marketing approach to workplace health and well-being might look like in practice.

The findings from the reviews demonstrated the applicability of a social marketing approach in each arena (Gordon et al., 2006b; McDermott et al., 2006; Stead and Angus, 2007; Stead et al., 2006, 2007a). A summary of their findings is presented in the following subsections.

Nutrition

In the nutrition review, of the 18 interventions that aimed to increase fruit and vegetable intake, 10 had a positive overall effect, six had mixed or moderate effects, one had no effect, and one was counterproductive. One successful programme reported significant improvements in the fruit and vegetable consumption of primary school children in England and Wales following the implementation of a rewards-based peer modelling intervention (Lowe et al., 2004). Overall, the results provided strong evidence that social marketing can improve fruit and vegetable intake.

Another 18 interventions sought to reduce fat intake, and of these, eight had a positive overall effect, seven had mixed or moderate effects, and three had no effect, demonstrating that social marketing can influence fat intake. An example is the Child and Adolescent Trial for Cardiovascular Health (CATCH), a school-based, extensively implemented programme in the United States that incorporated educational, behavioural, and school environmental components. The trial reported a significant reduction in fat intake among students in schools partaking in the initiative compared with control schools ($p < 0.001$), and also successfully lowered the percentage of calories from total fat in school meals (Luepker et al., 1996).

Of the 11 studies that aimed to improve dietary knowledge, nine reported a positive overall effect and two had no effect. For example, a '5-a-Day' programme with low-income women (comprising nutrition sessions, printed materials, and direct mail) significantly increased their knowledge of the recommendation to eat five or more portions of fruit and vegetables a day (Luepker et al., 1996).

Social marketing initiatives were also successful in influencing psychosocial factors associated with nutrition, such as attitudes towards healthy eating and self-efficacy for eating a better diet. Of 17 studies, 13 had a positive effect on at least one psychosocial variable. One such programme was a church-based intervention that brought about significant improvements in self-efficacy for eating five daily portions of fruit and vegetables among African-American church members (Campbell et al., 2000). However, only three of 13 studies that aimed to influence physiological variables such as blood pressure, cholesterol, or body mass index (BMI) showed an effect.

Overall, the evidence from the nutrition review demonstrated that social marketing is an effective approach to use in nutrition interventions.

Substance misuse

In the review of substance misuse social marketing initiatives, 13 of 18 studies aimed at smoking prevention had a positive effect, four had mixed or moderate effects, and one had no effect, providing strong evidence that social marketing interventions can be successful at preventing smoking. One example, Project SixTeen (designed to reduce both illegal sales of tobacco and youth tobacco use), had a significant effect on smoking prevalence (smoking in the past week) 5 years after the start of a 3-year intervention ($p < 0.05\%$): the prevalence was 3.8% lower in the intervention communities compared with the communities that had received only a school-based programme (Biglan et al., 2000).

Of the substance misuse interventions targeting alcohol prevention and harm minimization, eight of 13 had a positive overall effect, four had mixed or moderate effects, and one had no effect, again demonstrating that social marketing can be an effective approach for tackling drinking. As an example, Project Northland, comprising a 3-year school curriculum, peer and parent activities, and community task forces, found a significant impact on past month and past week alcohol use ($p < 0.05$ for each) in the intervention group compared with the control group at 2.5 years, although the effect dissipated at 4 years (Perry et al., 1996).

Of the 12 substance misuse interventions dealing with illicit drug use, eight had a positive effect, three had mixed or moderate effects, and one had no effect. One effective campaign was Project STAR, which reported significant reductions in last month marijuana use in intervention students compared with controls both in the short term and at 2-year follow-up (Pentz et al., 1989).

For smoking cessation, the evidence was less strong, with only two of nine interventions aimed at influencing cessation rates having a positive effect, five having modest or weak effects, and two having no effect.

Physical activity

In the review of social marketing interventions for physical activity, 21 of 22 studies aimed to influence behavioural outcomes. Of these, eight had a positive overall effect, seven reported mixed results, and six had no effect, demonstrating that social marketing initiatives can have a positive impact—but with more mixed results than in the nutrition review. One of the successful interventions was the Social Marketing for Public Health Employees Interventions (Neiger et al., 2001), a workplace-based initiative comprising communications and promotions, various ongoing activities, one-off events, and environmental changes, which resulted in pretest to post-test increases in the primary interventions group on three measures of physical activity. Similarly, the Wheeling Walks interventions (Reger et al., 2002), a community-based campaign to promote walking among sedentary people aged between 50 and 65 (underpinned by the Theory of Planned Behaviour), had a positive effect on physical activity levels in terms of the total time spent and frequency of walking.

Each of the four studies that aimed to influence exercise-related knowledge reported positive effects, demonstrating that social marketing can have a positive effect on this outcome. There were 11 studies that aimed to impact upon psychosocial variables, such as self-efficacy or perceived social support to exercise regularly. Of these studies, six reported a positive effect on at least one variable, whereas five had no effect. Of the six that showed an effect, one example was the San Diego Family Health Project, a school-based intervention developed for American-Indian children in the United States. Evaluation data showed that self-efficacy to exercise was significantly higher among the treatment group than the control group (Caballero et al., 2003).

Of the physical activity social marketing initiatives, 14 reported physiological outcome results using a range of measures, including BMI, cardiovascular disease (CVD) rates, cholesterol level, and blood pressure. Only four studies reported a positive effect, four reported mixed results, and six reported no effect, suggesting that there is weaker evidence that social marketing initiatives tackling physical activity can improve physiological outcomes. One of the few interventions that did have an impact on physiological outcome measures was the Pawtucket Heart Health Program, directed towards lower-income adults in a Rhode Island city in the United States. The study reported a bigger reduction in CVD rates among the initiative group than the control group, and although BMI increased significantly among the control group, no increase was seen among individuals in the initiative condition (Gans et al., 1999).

Workplace interventions

There is increasing appreciation of the impact that work can have on the general health and well-being of employees—and conversely, that poor health can have on workplace productivity, job satisfaction, and absence (Pelletier, 1997; Proper et al., 2002; Mimura and Griffiths, 2003; Aust and Ducki, 2004). Against this backdrop, a review was conducted to explore the potential of social marketing approaches to promoting workplace health and well-being. There was particular interest in exploring the value of participatory approaches—ones in which employees themselves are involved in programme planning and implementation.

Evidence from 15 systematic reviews showed that workplace initiatives in general can positively influence health behaviours and related outcomes such as smoking cessation, physical activity, and diet. Intensive initiatives were found to be more effective than those that were less intensive and, in general, participation was found to be a challenge, with many initiatives having low participation rates or attracting more motivated and healthier employees.

Reanalysis of the systematic reviews found 14 individual workplace health interventions that met all or five of the social marketing criteria and could, therefore, be described as using social marketing principles in their design and implementation. Only two of these 14 initiatives actually used the label 'social marketing' to describe their approach. Most of the social marketing initiatives targeted CVD risk factors: diet, smoking, or physical activity, either singly or in combination. Only one initiative addressed job-related well-being (job satisfaction and self-esteem). Many interventions emphasized intervening at both an individual level (e.g. support and counselling) and the workplace environment level (e.g. policies on smoking and healthier canteen menus).

There was evidence that social marketing initiatives could be effective, although the effects were sometimes short lived or not found to address all desired outcomes or target groups. Intensive and multifaceted interventions tended to produce better results. The ways in which the interventions were 'consumer oriented' and participatory included use of formative research with employees to explore their needs and interests, pretesting intervention elements, and employee involvement in the planning and implementation of programmes, through mechanisms such as task forces and employee advisory boards. It was not always clear how genuine were some forms of employee participation. Many programmes were initiated from outside the workplace (e.g. by researchers or health organizations), and it is unclear how the management were persuaded to initiate or support the programmes.

Illustrative case studies (gathered from grey literature and company websites) were also included in the review. The initiatives featured in these had a range of objectives, including those related to both health (e.g. smoking, diet, physical activity) and well-being (e.g. stress, satisfaction, employee engagement). Like the interventions reported in the academic literature, they typically combined both individually targeted approaches, such as health checks and fitness coaching, and approaches targeting the workplace environment, such as creating cycle routes and targeting managers' own behaviour. A particularly important environmentally focused approach in several initiatives was the adjustment of working patterns to allow more flexible working and leave, leading to increased satisfaction. The initiatives contained several examples of creative use of the 'marketing mix', such as providing bicycles and fruit-based snacks. The case study initiatives claimed a range of benefits, including reduced sickness levels, improved employee engagement, and increased fitness. However, it was not always clear how the outcomes were measured, nor was it clear to what extent the employees had been genuinely involved and consulted.

Overall, the effectiveness reviews for nutrition, substance misuse, physical activity, and workplace social marketing initiatives identified social marketing as a promising behavioural-intervention approach, and highlighted the potential for social marketing to be used as an approach in future behavioural-change efforts.

There were a number of common features of the successful interventions identified in the reviews. In addition to meeting Andreasen's six benchmark criteria for social marketing, they shared the following elements:

- *Clear goals*—Being absolutely clear about what the intervention is trying to achieve is one of the most important considerations when using social marketing. The setting of clear goals, aims, and objectives increases the likely success of the intervention and makes assessment of that success easier.
- *Evaluation*—This is a vital part of any behavioural-change intervention. It is important from the outset to be clear about what is to be measured, what specific measures will be used, and how findings and knowledge will be disseminated and used. One common problem encountered when reviewing evidence of effectiveness is the lack of use of universal measures to allow cross-comparability.
- *Based on theory*—Several of the successful interventions identified made judicious use of theory, which brought a level of structure and understanding to the behavioural-change approach pursued (see Chapter 4 for a more detailed discussion of how you can use behavioural-change theory in your social marketing).
- *Well implemented*—The quality of implementation is another vital component of the intervention process. A good intervention should be able to deliver on the ground, in real-life settings with well-trained and motivated delivery agents who are clear about the programme goals.

A broader view of social marketing evidence

These four reviews of social marketing effectiveness make a substantial contribution to building the social marketing evidence base. In their reliance on existing systematic reviews and systematic review methods, however, it could be argued that they perpetuate some of the narrow methodological limitations that the start of this chapter explored. Against this, it should be pointed out that the reviews strove to be flexible and inclusive in how they defined social marketing initiatives. Rather than be restricted to one single initiative type, one single setting, or one single set of intervention methods, the reviews were designed to include any initiative that adopted the social marketing principles of consumer-centeredness, mutually beneficially exchange, addressing the competition to the behavioural change, and so on. In doing this, they provide a model for how a systematic approach for gathering and selecting evidence can be applied even to an intervention approach that potentially encompasses a diverse range of methods, tools, and applications. In the case of the workplace review, the inclusion of illustrative case study examples, reflecting contemporary workplace initiatives in the United Kingdom and further afield, helped show what a social marketing approach to workplace health promotion might look like in practice.

Future efforts to examine the effectiveness of social marketing can build on this work. It may be helpful to refine the criteria further—how exactly, for instance, do we assess an intervention as having provided a meaningful exchange? It would also yield valuable learning for social marketing to have a sense of the relative importance of the criteria: is there a stronger relationship with effectiveness for some of the benchmarks—say, consumer research—than others? Or is it the presence and synergy of all the criteria that are important?

Assessing the effectiveness of social marketing requires us also to look at the bigger picture. As the first part of this chapter argues, narrow behavioural outcomes are not everything (even assuming they can be meaningfully measured at all). Processes and practitioner perspectives must also inform our understanding of what it means to do social marketing effectively. A broader view of social marketing effectiveness should incorporate the following questions:

- *Acceptability to target groups*—Do target groups engage with, like, appreciate, and trust social marketing initiatives? These 'softer' outcomes are often neglected in the traditional approaches to assessing effectiveness, but they are absolutely crucial to bringing about behavioural change. If the target consumers refuse to engage with an initiative in the first place, mistrust it, or only engage grudgingly and with little pleasure, they are unlikely either to persist with any changes in behaviour or to recommend the intervention to their friends and family.
- *Acceptability and feasibility to implementers*—Another important element, which is often neglected in the traditional approaches to assessing effectiveness, is the perspective of the implementer. Is the intervention acceptable to them, is it practicable to run, can it be fitted into routine practice, do implementers perceive any immediate benefits to themselves, or do the hassles and difficulties outweigh any positives? This underlines the need for any measurement of outcomes to also evaluate processes. In the event that an intervention shows no change in outcomes, process evaluation can assess whether it did not do so because it was inherently faulty (failure of design or theory) or because it was poorly delivered (failure of implementation; Dane and Schneider, 1998; Stead et al., 2007b). Process evaluation also sheds light on the factors that impede or facilitate initiative implementation, yielding valuable learning for the future rollout of activities and for how evidence-based programmes can be put into real-life practice (e.g. Buston et al., 2002).
- *Appeal to stakeholders*—Because social marketing programmes are developed and delivered in the real world, stakeholder perspectives on their appropriateness are also important. There is often a careful balancing act to manage here: although it is desirable to build stakeholder approval for particular approaches, this does not mean that 'anything goes'. Stakeholders and funders may favour approaches that are unsound, that offer 'quick fixes', or which are effective only in narrow ways (e.g. a highly graphic advertising campaign may be 'effective' in terms of recall but may raise ethical and moral concerns; Hastings et al., 2004).
- *Tackling disadvantage*—In a public health social marketing context, the search for evidence of effectiveness cannot be blind to inequalities. It is not enough for an intervention to be effective with its general target population: it must be *more* effective with disadvantaged groups if it is to narrow inequalities (Jackson and Waters, 2005). An intervention that is 'effective' at the expense of widening the gap between the better and worse off in society cannot be said to be effective.
- For those funding programmes and developing strategies, effectiveness research will only ever be one of several factors that must be considered (Macintyre et al., 2001). Other factors include that it will fit with government, funding, or other priorities; that the programme or strategy will bring benefits not solely related to health outcomes; that it will be unlikely to do harm; and that it will be easy and/or relatively inexpensive to implement (Macintyre et al., 2001). In some fields, there are no unequivocal answers about 'what works' (ibid.) Furthermore, to be hesitant about effectiveness can be dangerous. Continually stating that

no conclusions can be drawn because the perfect study has not yet been conducted defers decision making (or leads to very wrong decisions). At some point, decisions have to be made on the basis of the evidence that already exists (McDonald, 2003; Livingstone, 2005). It is perhaps wise to view the situation as a potential collision with an evidence iceberg, in which we know and can see a little bit (the tip) about what is going on and can react accordingly but much of which remains hidden beneath the surface.

Conclusion

As this chapter has shown, evidence for the effectiveness of social marketing interventions does exist and is growing, despite many challenges. Clearly, there is a need to move beyond the narrow biomedical approach to evaluation, and to recognize that complex, real-world, and flexible approaches to change require equally complex, pragmatic, and flexible methods of assessing effectiveness. Sometimes, it is simply not possible to achieve the perfect study or an unequivocal evidence base. This does not mean that efforts to establish effectiveness should not continue to be refined. It does mean, however, that narrow interpretations of effectiveness should not always be the primary factor informing what and why social marketers do what they do.

In practice, decision making at the political, policy, and practice end is influenced by a much wider range of factors—including values and beliefs that may not be based on evidence at all, emotional engagement, pressure from external sources, experience, and even intuition. The challenge for social marketers is to bring these equally valid factors to bear in shaping a more inclusive and meaningful view of the social marketing evidence.

References

Alcalay, R. and Bell, R.A. (2000). *Promoting Nutrition and Physical Activity through Social Marketing: Current Practices and Recommendations.* Sacramento, CA: Davis Center for Advanced Studies in Nutrition and Social Marketing, University of California.

Allison, K.R. and Rootman, I. (1996). Scientific rigor and community participation in health promotion research: are they compatible? *Health Promotion International*, 11(4): 333–340.

Andreasen, A.R. (1995). *Marketing Social Change: Changing Behavior to Promote Health, Social Development, and the Environment.* San Francisco, CA: Jossey-Bass.

Andreasen, A.R. (2002). Marketing social marketing in the social change marketplace. *Journal of Public Policy and Marketing*, 21(1): 3–13.

Aust, B. and Ducki, A. (2004). Comprehensive health promotion interventions at the workplace: experiences with health circles in Germany. *Journal of Occupational Health Psychology*, 9(3): 258–270.

Baldwin, S., Wallace, A., Cruncher, K., Quilgars, D. and Mather, L. (2002). *How Effective Are Public and Private Safety Nets in Assisting Mortgages in Unforeseen Financial Difficulties to Avoid Arrears and Repossessions?* York: University of York.

Biglan, A., Ary, D., Smolkowski, K., Duncan, T. and Black, C. (2000). A randomised controlled trial of a community intervention to prevent adolescent tobacco use. *Tobacco Control*, 9(1): 24–32.

Boaz, A., Ashby, D. and Young, K. (2002). *Systematic Reviews: What Have They Got to Offer Evidence Based Policy and Practice? Working Paper 2.* London: Economic and Social Research Council UK Centre for Evidence Based Policy and Practice.

Buston, K., Wight, D., Hart, G. and Scott, S. (2002). Implementation of a teacher-delivered sex education programme: obstacles and facilitating factors. *Health Education Research*, 17(1): 59–72.

Caballero, B., Clay, T., Davis, S.M. et al. and Pathways Study Research Group (2003). Pathways: a school-based, randomized controlled trial for the prevention of obesity in American Indian schoolchildren. *American Journal of Clinical Nutrition*, 78(5):1030–1038.

Cabinet Office (1999). *Modernising Government.* London: Cabinet Office. Available at: http://archive.cabinetoffice.gov.uk/moderngov/download/modgov.pdf [accessed 29 April 2008].

Campbell, M.K., Motsinger, B.M., Ingram, A. et al. (2000). The North Carolina Black Churches United for Better Health Project: intervention and process evaluation. *Health Education and Behavior*, 27(2): 241–253.

Clark, N.M. and McLeroy, K.R. (1998). Reviewing the evidence for health promotion in the United States. In J.K. Davies and G. MacDonald (eds.) *Quality, Evidence and Effectiveness in Health Promotion*, pp. 21–46. London: Routledge.

Dane, A.V. and Schneider, B.H. (1998). Program integrity in primary and early secondary intervention: are implementation effects out of control? *Clinical Psychology Review*, 18(1): 23–45.

Davies, J.K. and MacDonald, G. (eds.) (1998). *Quality, Evidence and Effectiveness in Health Promotion.* London: Routledge.

DoH (2004). *Choosing Health: Making Healthy Choices Easier.* London: Department of Health.

Fawcett, S.B., Lewis, R.K., Paine-Andrews, A. et al. (1997). Evaluating community coalitions for prevention of substance abuse: the case of Project Freedom. *Health Education and Behavior*, 24(6): 812–828.

French, J. and Blair-Stevens, C. (2005). *Social Marketing Pocket Guide.* London: National Social Marketing Centre.

Gans, K.M., Assmann, S.F., Sallar, A. and Lasater, T.M. (1999). Knowledge of cardiovascular disease prevention: an analysis from two New England communities. *Preventive Medicine*, 29(4): 229–237.

Gordon, R., McDermott, L., Stead, M. and Angus, K. (2006a). The effectiveness of social marketing interventions for health improvement: what's the evidence? *Public Health*, 120(12): 1133–1139.

Gordon, R., McDermott, L., Stead, M., Angus, K. and Hastings, G. (2006b). *A Review of the Effectiveness of Social Marketing Physical Activity Interventions.* Stirling, Scotland: Institute for Social Marketing. Available at: http://www.nsms.org.uk/images/CoreFiles/NSMC-R1_Physical_Activity.pdf [accessed 29 April 2008].

Hastings, G., Stead, M. and Webb, J. (2004). Fear appeals in social marketing: strategic and ethical reasons for concern. *Psychology and Marketing*, 21(11): 961–986.

Heiser, P.F. and Begay, M.E. (1997). The campaign to raise the tobacco tax in Massachusetts. *American Journal of Public Health*, 87(6): 968–973.

Higgins, S., Hall, E., Baumfield, V. and Moseley, D. (2005). A meta-analysis of the impact of the implementation of thinking skills approaches on pupils. In *Research Evidence in Education Library.* London: EPPI-Centre, Social Science Research Unit, Institute of Education, University of London.

Jackson, N. and Waters, E. (2005). Criteria for the systematic review of health promotion and public health interventions. *Health Promotion International*, 20(4):367–374.

Kennedy, M.G. and Abbatangelo, J. (eds.) (2004). *Guidance for Evaluating Mass Communication Health Initiatives: Summary of an Expert Panel Discussion.* Sponsored by the Centers for Disease Control and Prevention Office of Communication, Atlanta, GA, May 3–4, 2004. Available at: http://www.healthcommunication.net/Evaluating_Mass_Comm.pdf [accessed 29 April 2008].

Learmonth, A. and Mackie, P. (2000). Evaluating effectiveness in health promotion: a case of re-inventing the millstone? *Health Education Journal*, 59(3): 267–280.

Livingstone, S. (2005). Assessing the research base for the policy debate over the effects of food advertising to children. *International Journal of Advertising*, 24(3): 273–296.

Lowe, C.F., Horne, P.J., Tapper, K., Bowdery, M. and Egerton, C. (2004). Effects of a peer modelling and rewards-based intervention to increase fruit and vegetable consumption in children. *European Journal of Clinical Nutrition*, 58(3): 510–522.

Luepker, R.V. Perry, C.L., McKinlay, S.M. et al. (1996). Outcomes of a field trial to improve children's dietary patterns and physical activity: The Child and Adolescent Trial for Cardiovascular Health (CATCH). *Journal of the American Medical Association*, 275(10): 768–776.

Macintyre, S., Chalmers, I., Horton, R. and Smith, R. (2001). Using evidence to inform health policy: case study. *British Medical Journal*, 322(7280): 222–225.

McDermott, L., Stead, S., Gordon, R., Angus, K. and Hastings, G. (2006). *A Review of the Effectiveness of Social Marketing Nutrition Interventions*. Stirling, Scotland: Institute for Social Marketing. Available at: http://www.nsms.org.uk/images/CoreFiles/NSMC-R2_nutritioninterventions.pdf [accessed 29 April 2008].

McDermott, L., Stead, M. and Hastings, G. (2005a). What is and what is not social marketing: the challenge of reviewing the evidence. *Journal of Marketing Management*, 5(6): 545–553.

McDermott, L., Stead, M., Hastings, G. et al. (2005b). *Systematic Review of the Effectiveness of Social Marketing Nutrition and Food Safety Interventions*. Stirling, Scotland: Institute for Social Marketing.

McDonald, G. (2003). *Using Systematic Reviews to Improve Social Care*. London: Social Care Institute for Excellence.

McKinlay, J.B. (1993). The promotion of health through planned socio-political change: challenges for research and policy. *Social Science and Medicine*, 36(2): 109–117.

McQueen, D.V. (2001). Strengthening the evidence base for health promotion. *Health Promotion International*, 16(3): 261–268.

Mimura, C. and Griffiths, P. (2003). The effectiveness of current approaches to workplace stress management in the nursing profession: an evidence based literature review. *Occupational and Environmental Medicine*, 60(1): 10–15.

Mulrow, C.D. (1994). Systematic reviews: rationale for systematic reviews. *British Medical Journal*, 309(6954): 597–599.

NCC and DoH (2005). *National Social Marketing Strategy for Health: Realising the Potential of Effective Social Marketing*. London: National Social Marketing Centre.

Neiger, B.L., Thackeray, R., Merrill, R.M., Miner, K.M., Larsen, L. and Chalkley, C.M. (2001). The impact of social marketing on fruit and vegetable consumption and physical activity among public health employees at the Utah Department of Health. *Social Marketing Quarterly*, 7(1): 9–28.

NICE (2007). *Interventional Procedures Programme Methods Guide*. London: National Institute for Health and Clinical Excellence.

Ogilvie, D., Egan, M., Hamilton, V. and Petticrew, M. (2005). Systematic reviews of health effects of social interventions: 2. Best available evidence: how low should you go? *Journal of Epidemiology and Community Health*, 59(10): 886–892.

Pelletier, K.R. (1997). Clinical and cost outcomes of multifactorial, cardiovascular risk management interventions in worksites: a comprehensive review and analysis. *Journal of Occupational and Environmental Medicine*, 39(12): 1154–1169.

Pentz, M.A., Dwyer, J.H., MacKinnon, D.P. et al. (1989). A multicommunity trial for primary prevention of adolescent drug abuse: effects on drug use prevalence. *Journal of the American Medical Association*, 261(22): 3259–3266.

Perry, C.L., Williams, C.L., Veblen-Mortenson, S. et al. (1996). Project Northland: outcomes of a communitywide alcohol use prevention program during early adolescence. *American Journal of Public Health*, 86(7): 956–965.

Petrosino, A., Turpin-Petrosino, C. and Buehler, J. (2002). 'Scared straight' and other juvenile awareness programmes for preventing juvenile delinquency. *Cochrane Database of Systematic Reviews* [online], 4, Art. No.: CD002796.

Price, N. (2001). The performance of social marketing in reaching the poor and vulnerable in AIDS control programmes. *Health Policy and Planning*, 16(3): 231–239.

Proper, K.I., Staal, B.J., Hildebrandt, V.H., van der Beek, A.J. and van Mechelen, W. (2002). Effectiveness of physical activity programs at worksites with respect to work-related outcomes. *Scandinavian Journal of Work, Environment & Health*, 28(2): 75–84.

Reger, B., Cooper, L., Booth-Butterfield, S. et al. (2002). Wheeling Walks: a community campaign using paid media to encourage walking among sedentary older adults. *Preventive Medicine*, 35(3): 285–292.

Rychetnik, L., Frommer, M., Hawe, P. and Shiell, A. (2002). Criteria for evaluating evidence on public health interventions. *Journal of Epidemiology and Community Health*, 56(2): 119–127.

Sackett, D.L., Rosenberg, W.M.C., Gray, M.J.A., Haynes, B.R. and Richardson, S.W. (1996). Evidence-based medicine: what it is and what it isn't. *British Medical Journal* 312(7023): 71–72.

Samuels, B. and Glantz, S.A. (1997). The politics of local tobacco control. *Journal of the American Medical Association*, 266(15): 2110–2117.

Solesbury, W. (2001). *Evidence Based Policy: Whence It Came and Where It's Going*. London: Economic and Social Research Council UK Centre for Evidence Based Policy and Practice.

Stead, M. and Angus, K. (2007). *Review of the Applicability and Effectiveness of Social Marketing as an Approach to Workplace Health and Well-being*. Stirling, Scotland: Institute for Social Marketing.

Stead, M. and Hastings, G.B. (1997). Advertising in the social marketing mix: getting the balance right. In M.E. Goldberg, M. Fishbein, and S.E. Middlestadt (eds.) *Social Marketing: Theoretical and Practical Perspectives*. Mahwah, NJ: Lawrence Erlbaum Associates.

Stead, M., Hastings, G. and Eadie, D. (2002). The challenge of evaluating complex interventions: a framework for evaluating media advocacy. *Health Education Research*, 17(3): 351–364.

Stead, M., McDermott, L., Gordon, R., Angus, K. and Hastings, G. (2006). *A Review of the Effectiveness of Social Marketing Alcohol, Tobacco and Substance Misuse Interventions*. Stirling, Scotland: Institute for Social Marketing. Available at: http://www.nsms.org.uk/images/CoreFiles/NSMC-R3_alcohol_tobacco_substance.pdf [accessed 29 April 2008].

Stead, M., Gordon R., Angus, K. and McDermott, L. (2007a). A systematic review of social marketing effectiveness. *Health Education*, 107(2): 126–140.

Stead, M., Stradling, R., MacNeil, M., MacKintosh, A.M. and Minty, S. (2007b). Implementation evaluation of the Blueprint multi-component drug education prevention programme: fidelity of school component delivery. *Drug and Alcohol Review*, 26(6): 659–664.

Tones, K. (2000). Evaluating health promotion: a tale of three errors. *Patient Education and Counselling*, 39(2–3): 227–236.

Turner, W., MacDonald, G.M. and Dennis, J.A. (2005). Cognitive-behavioural training interventions for assisting foster carers in the management of difficult behaviour. *Cochrane Database of Systematic Reviews* [online], 2, Art. No.: CD003760.pub2.

Victora, C.G., Habicht, J-P. and Bryce, J. (2004). Evidence-based public health: moving beyond randomized trials. *American Journal of Public Health*, 94(3): 400–405.

Chapter 7

Generating 'insight' and building segmentations – moving beyond simple targeting

Dominic McVey and Lynne Walsh

Errors like straws upon the surface flow: Who would search for pearls must dive below.
John Dryden

Learning points

This chapter

- Introduces the concepts of 'insight' and 'segmentation';
- Gives an overview of how to generate insight;
- Provides an understanding of the importance of segmentation to social marketing initiatives; and
- Uses case studies to demonstrate what can be achieved by social marketing when insight and segmentation theory are put into practice. More details on segmentation methods can be found in Chapter 11.

Introduction

One of the most important elements of the social marketing process is developing the in-depth understanding of the customer or citizen which forms the foundation for the choice of the target group and the construction of the intervention.

The development of insight is becoming more widespread across the UK government. Nearly every government department has it own 'insight unit' developed as a consequence of David Varney's Review of Service Transformation (2006).

The review concluded that *we need to exploit customer insight as a strategic asset.*

One measure of whether the UK public sector makes use of insight is how much is invested in looking for it. The UK commercial and public sectors have always had a good reputation for investing in consumer and social research and developing innovative research methods. Much of the government-funded consumer research and campaign evaluation is commissioned by Central Office of Information (COI) on behalf of most government departments. In 2004/05 spending was £13.2 million which increased to £22.6 million in 2007/08 (COI, 2008). The public sector spending on consumer research and evaluation may appear considerable and may be increasing, but this is a fraction of what industry spends. It is estimated that the UK commercial market-research industry is worth £1.8 billion a year (Advertising Association, 2009) and a significant proportion of this will be spent on improving the sales of health-damaging products such a junk food, tobacco, and alcohol.

Developing customer insight still has a long way to go in the public sector. A recent report on the use of consumer data by primary-care trusts working with deprived communities in the UK revealed that, despite a desire to develop a greater understanding of people living in deprived communities and some excellent example of interventions aimed at marginalized groups, there was a clear need for guidance training and resources on how this could be done (Mathrani, 2008).

Defining 'insight'

If you were to stand out in a busy street and conduct a survey on the meaning of the word 'insight', you would probably elicit a variety of responses. Some respondents would, no doubt, opt for 'perception' or 'understanding', others for 'the discovery of deeper or hidden meanings'. If you happened to be standing outside a conference of etymologists at the time, you might even get the dictionary definition:

> The capacity of understanding hidden truths etc., esp. of character or situations.
>
> The Concise Oxford Dictionary, Eighth Edition 1991 OUP

> The clear (and often sudden) understanding of a complex situation.
>
> www.wordreference.com/definition/insight

So far, so good. Well, perhaps the word 'sudden' may be misleading in the context of social marketing. Creating insight based on a sudden thought sounds rather whimsical – perhaps more of an 'inkling' than an insight. Which brings us to several key questions:

- Does an 'insight' have to be fresh?
- Should it be something we have never considered before, or could it be a confirmation of what we have known for some time?
- Is it an epiphany?
- Does it come from deduction, observation, or from intuition?

The NSM Centre conducted a brief survey, and here are the responses from some of the respondents questioned:

> An understanding or knowledge of the workings of a subject or situation.
>
> A more informed and intuitive understanding of given subject. A useful light shone on a hitherto relatively murky subject. A doorway.
>
> A breakthrough, into a situation or issue, which is new and takes people by surprise or attracts their curiosity.
>
> Knowledge: something that other people might not know. An insight into someone's life gives me an experience of them that means I can understand a bit more about why they are how they are.
>
> Getting closer to your target audience by understanding their needs or aspirations.

And here is the advice from the Hong Kong-based company Building Brands (2009):

Next time you think you've got an insight, check it against this definition:

> An insight is a fresh and unexpected perspective. It gets the following reaction from those involved: *"Wow, yes, you're right.' I'd never thought of it like that before, but you're absolutely right. You really understand what's going on here."*

Although we may be able to accommodate most of these definitions within social marketing, this last one might present social marketing professionals with some problems. It may be exciting to get a 'wow factor' or 'light-bulb moment' from an individual, but if they are unable to support their revelation with some sound research, we would strongly suggest that you put the brakes on.

As Professor Merlin Stone, Bryan Foss, and Alison Bond highlight in *Consumer Insight: How to Use Data and Market Research to Get Closer to Your Customer*, insight does not just happen.

> Customer insight has two forms. Firstly, there are Insights [plural] – flashes of inspiration, or penetrating discoveries that can lead to specific opportunities. Market research or customer databases can deliver these, and often do. However, much bigger than this, and central to what companies need today, is Insight [singular], defined as 'the ability to perceive clearly or deeply', a deep, embedded knowledge about our consumers and our markets that helps structure our thinking and decision making.
>
> (Stone et al., 2004, p.1)

A useful working definition of customer insight in the context of social marketing is provided by the Government Communications Network's *Engage* Programme which classes insight as *a deep 'truth' about the customer based on their behaviour, experiences, beliefs, needs or desires, that is relevant to the task or issue and 'rings bells' with targeted people* (GCN, 2006).

Insight is also defined by the way it is collected and used, and by two attributes in particular:

1. it draws on multiple sources of information, using these to build up complete pictures of customer needs and behaviours; and
2. it is essentially a business process, aimed at creating something which has value to the organization.

The 'Insight' section of the government's *Engage* Programme's website (www.comms.gov.uk) includes information on the methodology and tools needed to generate insight. It also provides case studies of interventions that have effectively inspired behaviour change using psychological truths revealed by consumer-insight activity.

However, we should be wary of inferring that the use of insight is systematic across government. A recent review of service transformation by David Varney concluded that, whilst a number of government departments and agencies had established insight functions, *only a few [treat] insight as a strategic asset and [manage] it in a systematic way* (Varney, 2006, p. 88). One of the many recommendations in the report was that 'every department be required to appoint a Contact Director to carry overall responsibility within that organization for creating and exploiting insight as a strategic asset' (*ibid.*, p. 3).

Generating insight

So, how do we generate consumer insight? Here we provide an initial response to that question, but greater detail on the stages that contribute to insight generation are presented in Chapter 11. There is usually no single source of insight generation but a combination of sources cross-referenced and triangulated to support recommendations. Example sources include:

- Frontline staff and other stakeholders;
- Surveys (a guide to the more than 80 surveys of the UK population can be found at www.nsmcentre.org.uk/images/CoreFiles/NSMC-R11_compendium.pdf);
- Data mining of customer databases; e.g. Tesco Clubcard data;
- Customer-journey mapping;
- Customer-immersion techniques (living with the target group for a few days);
- Usability testing and website analysis;

- Qualitative research with the target group– focus groups, in-depth interviews, paired depths, deliberative workshops, etc.;
- Ethnography (the scientific description of peoples and cultures);
- Public consultations;
- Formal and informal contact with representative bodies;
- Agents or intermediaries;
- Written correspondence;
- Media coverage;
- Sales data;
- Media analysis of press and broadcast coverage to understand the social, political, and cultural context;
- Process evaluations, and;
- Reviews of the effectiveness of interventions.

Descriptions of some of these methods can be found in Chapters 11, 13, and 14. Another useful source is the Customer insight in public services – 'A Primer', (Cabinet Office, 2006, p.9) produced by the Customer Insight Forum.

Before we take a look at some examples of customer-insight strategies, we should remind ourselves of a basic difference between the commercial and social marketing use of such strategies.

Commercial and social marketing use of insight

Business guru Peter Drucker gets to the point quickly: *The aim of marketing is to know and understand the customer so well that the product or service fits him and sells itself* (Nantel et al., 1996). This is true – at least, for the private sector. But as Rob Donovan and Nadine Henley point out:

> A basic distinction between social and commercial marketing is that social marketing campaigns are often not based on needs experienced by consumers, but on needs identified by experts. This is true. Communities might prefer their resources to be spent on hospitals rather than on disease prevention, and on tough prisons rather than rehabilitation. On the other hand, whereas epidemiological evidence indicates smoking and physical inactivity are greater causes of morbidity and mortality, a government might allocate far more resources to anti-drug campaigns because a majority of voters considers drug-taking a more important issue.
>
> (Rob Donovan and Nadine Henley, 2003, p. 23–24)

Bradley (2007) has highlighted that a recent development in the world of business is the emergence of Consumer Insight Departments. He believes that this development stemmed from the realization of the need for a shift from drawing on the results of individual research projects to working from a wider understanding of the dynamics operating in the full market place. He also points to the impact of developments in information technology which have led to the increasing accessibility to the vast amounts of information found in databases. For the corporate world, there are savings. By making use of all existing information, through insight management, there is less need to consult customers, thereby minimizing unnecessary contact and costs. For example, the data collected as part of the Tesco Clubcard provides a vast source of information on shopping patterns and preferences and clearly has value for suppliers and retailers.

Although these may be important considerations for the commercial sector, social marketing demands are somewhat different, and in many ways greater.

Social marketing, inequality, and understanding the disadvantaged

Social marketing tackles big social concerns such as health and crime and requires an understanding of disadvantaged and marginalized groups in society, not only the mainstream audiences targeted by the commercial sector. To create interventions that work with these groups requires greater understanding of their social circumstances and their ability to change. Interventions also need to build empathy and develop trust to sustain a continuing customer relationship with people who are not normally valued by commercial marketers as potential clients.

Interventions targeted without adequate understanding of the groups they are meant to serve can result in a widening of the health inequalities between the rich and the poor in society.

For example, despite the evidence of effectiveness of polices and interventions aimed at reducing smoking prevalence, there is little available evidence that these polices reduce inequalities. A review of systematic reviews undertaken by the Health Development Agency (HDA, 2004) showed little evidence of effectiveness of interventions to reduce inequalities.

Whilst health promotion and social marketing in all its forms may contribute to the decline in overall prevalence of risky behaviour, there is evidence that some interventions may indeed be contributing to widening the gap in health inequalities. Smokers who live in more deprived neighbourhoods with high levels of smoking prevalence are less able to respond and change their behaviour in response to health-promotional interventions (Acheson, 1998). This does not mean to say that vulnerable groups do not exhibit resilience and change their behaviour, many of them do, but proportionately there is less change amongst these groups compared to the better-off smokers and this can result in a widening of the gap in health inequalities.

The paradigm supported by The Acheson Report (Acheson, 1998) stated that health inequalities were embodied in the structure of society and the wider social determinants of health rather than the unhealthy behaviours of individuals. Furthermore the report made key recommendations to promote healthier lifestyles, particularly with issues exhibiting a strong social gradient in prevalence. Targeted social marketing was viewed as one of the many approaches capable of addressing this.

However, the lack of insight and understanding of the lives of vulnerable and disadvantaged groups and the wider social determinants operating on the individual has lead to inappropriately targeted interventions. Interventions based solely on individual choice are unlikely to overcome the structural factors promoting inequalities in health. General-population approaches, whilst working with the better-off groups, will generally have less affect on those that need them the most.

Properly applied social marketing and health-promotional techniques based on a deep understanding of peoples lives, circumstances, and aspirations can help ensure that interventions are appropriately targeted. This coupled with a mix of approaches – behavioural, fiscal, legislative, and environmental – can mitigate the possibility of widening the gap in health inequalities and may even narrow it.

The position of social marketing in the publics' mind

Mass media and social marketing interventions operate within a very crowded marketplace with commercial marketing competing with public sector campaigns and public sector campaigns competing with each other for the audience's attention. Assuming the intervention is a well-constructed, emotionally involving, creative narrative (as all good advertising should be) a public health intervention tends to get higher recall and awareness than advertising for commercial products – assuming the investment in both are equal. Health and social issues will always be more emotionally relevant to people than their choice of soap powder. Of course, there has to be a minimum threshold of investment in media buying so people have the opportunity to be exposed to the intervention, otherwise all that creative development and research will count for nothing. Another reason why mass public education can outperform similarly funded commercial advertising is the provenance of the advertising, i.e. they are branded from government departments, the NHS, non-governmental groups (NGOs), and the not-for-profit sector. Even with a public increasingly sceptical about government and civil servants, these sources still tend to be trusted more to give accurate information and advice, especially when the increasing levels of commercial misinformation about health and well-being continue to confuse people.

The values attached to the issues covered by social marketing provide an advantage over the commercial marketers; however, this is far outweighed by the complexity of the social issues to be addressed and the barriers to behaviour change within materially deprived communities.

Quantitative and qualitative insight

As mentioned earlier, there is usually no single source of insight generation but a combination of quantitative and qualitative cross-referenced data. What is clear is that we cannot understand the complexity of people's lives by just asking them questions. If we are to gain understanding of where the customer is starting from – their knowledge, attitudes, and beliefs, along with the social context in which they live and work – we will be required to see life from their perspective. There are many useful statistical techniques available to explore large quantitative datasets, e.g. cluster analysis and multi-level modelling, all of which will reveal insights into people lives; however, if we are to uncover insights into how consumers' thoughts, feelings, objectives, and coping strategies influence their behaviour, we also need more open, qualitative techniques employing in-depth interviews, observation, and ethnography.

The issue which interests a social marketer may not seem relevant to the target group and consequently will not be an obvious driver of the behavioural change under consideration. It may be more appropriate to address the person's more immediate situational needs or the more upstream psychosocial determinants of the behaviour as a way of addressing the behaviour of interest. Box 7.1 includes examples of insights drawn from looking beyond the immediate health behaviour and into peoples' lived experience.

Box 7.1 Using Insight

Smoking amongst single mothers

The prevalence of smoking amongst single mothers living in more deprived communities has always been higher than the average for that community. Survey research reveals they are aware of the risks, want to give up, and many have tried to give up but failed. Using ethnographic research to study the lives of single mothers reveals that smoking has a much more important meaning for this group. Social isolation, financial worries, and the challenges of raising children alone means that smoking is one of the few pleasures left to them and provides a few minutes' break from life's stresses. Smoking is more that just a habit or addiction, it is a stress-coping mechanism and it's a reward; smoking is more a 'friend' than an 'enemy'. If interventions are to be effective, they need to take account of this social and psychological context.

A description of ethnographic research in this area can be found in the chapter by Hilary Graham. 'Surviving by Smoking' in *Women and Health: Feminist Perspectives* by Sue Wilkinson, Celia Kitzinger Taylor, and Francis 1994.

Sex workers and condom use

In the 1990s in the UK, studies of sex workers revealed that condom use with their clients was much more common than condom use with their partners. The partners were usually their pimps and these men had several partners. The women were aware of the risks of unprotected sex: many protected themselves with clients. But many did not use condoms with their partners who also clearly posed a risk to them. The pimps sometimes refused to use condoms, but there were also other factors at play. Research conducted by anthropologists revealed that sex workers needed to make a distinction between clients and partners, i.e. between work and private life. We all consciously or unconsciously make distinctions between our work and private lives but with sex workers these boundaries clearly need to be demarked more explicitly. Within the context of sexual behaviour this was achieved by not using condoms when they had sex with their partners to maintain a clear boundary between work and private life. This qualitative research contextualized behaviour within the lives of sex workers and provided valuable insights for addressing this group.

For further reading on this issue see: *Sophie Day, On the Game: Women and Sex Work: Pluto Press 2007.*

Smoking cessation programme for pregnant women in Sunderland

This project aimed to increase the uptake of smoking cessation services and quit rate among pregnant women in Sunderland, mainly from deprived areas and social class C2DE. Its development was underpinned by qualitative research which explored what it was like to be a pregnant smoker in Sunderland and provided insights into the particular issues facing pregnant women who smoke. The focus-group research with pregnant women found that many feel that their baby is seen as the priority (not them) when they are pregnant, that they are information poor, that the body language of the health professional can be inhibiting, and that they do not want to be nagged (as it makes them feel worse than they already feel about smoking). These barriers to recruitment of women were compounded by poor existing information, and the lack of enthusiasm amongst health professionals. The intervention was developed based on these insights. It included proactive recruiting and support for smoking women via a dedicated worker, home visits, design and pre-testing of new marketing/information material, role-play training of health professionals to engage more effectively with smoking women, and consumer-friendly cessation support – including dedicated health professionals. The impact of the project was impressive. During the intervention, there was a 10-fold increase in the number of women setting a quit date and quitting whilst pregnant – this was higher than both the preceding year in Sunderland and in neighbouring primary-care trusts which did not use a social marketing approach.

Smoking Cessation in Pregnancy – Innovative Success in Sunderland, December 2002.
A Qualitative Study report., Dr Ray Lowry, University of Newcastle; Christine Jordan and Gillian Wayman, Sunderland Teaching Primary Care Trust

Before we consider segmentation (see below), we should remind ourselves that consumers do not care much about the decisions we take or the segments we place them in. Their demands – in the commercial sector – would probably be 'meet my needs, provide the product [or service] I want, persuade me to stay with you, or I'll go to a rival'.

In social marketing, it is insight which helps us to understand consumers' internal drivers and barriers to change. Segmentation helps us to reach them with the most persuasive tactics via the best possible route.

Since we cannot offer customers a one-on-one service, we need to segment audiences into homogeneous groups and tailor the proposition (see Chapter 11) to their needs, to the extent possible.

One of the challenges in social marketing is that consumers are constantly developing and adapting to life around them. Segmentation needs to do the same – it needs to be comprehensive and dynamic to take account of these changes and to spot shifts and trends in the lifestyles of customers.

Segmentation

Segmentation can be a powerful tool in understanding consumer groups and focussing resources where they are most needed. It is, therefore, a valuable addition to the insight toolbox. This section introduces the concept of segmentation, but you will find more detailed information about how to segment your target audiences in Chapter 11.

Segmentation is a process of looking at the audience or 'market' and seeking to identify distinct, manageable sub-groups (segments) that may have similar needs, attitudes, or behaviours. We all regularly segment people into groups. We talk about adults who are working and adults who are unemployed, single mothers who smoke and those who do not; and we subdivide these further by e.g. social class, ethnicity, level of income, use of public services, and neighbourhood type.

Traditionally, segmentation has focussed on the use of demographic (age, sex, class, etc.) geodemographic (type of neighbourhood), and epidemiological data (mortality and morbidity) data. However, factoring in attitudinal and psychographic data to provide a rounder picture of the segments is a good starting point for developing tailored interventions. 'Psychographic' variables describe the individual in terms of their overall approach to life, including personality traits, values, beliefs, and preferences.

There are a wide range of segmentation techniques: sociodemographic, geodemographic, behavioural, epidemiological, psychographic and attitudinal, service utilization, and social network analysis, to name a few. However, as Table 7.1 shows, they all draw on a pool of common factors.

When segmenting populations, the aim should be to define a small number of groups so that:

- all members of a particular group are as similar to each other as possible; and
- they are as different from the other groups as possible.

It is important for social marketers to know what differentiates one group from another; but, what is more important are the similarities between people in a particular group. These allow us to create clusters of people and target our interventions at priority groups.

Some of the key attributes of a good segmentation are listed below:

- Segmentations should build on current knowledge
- Should get us a step closer to knowing our audience
- Provide a language for understanding people
- Utility/Applicability – the segments should exist in the real world rather than be just statistical constructs; the segment descriptions should make sense to the people who have to apply

Table 7.1 Factors common to segmentation approaches

Behaviour/Current status	Demographics	Geographic	Activities and lifestyle	Attitudinal/ Psychographic
Dependency/addiction issues	Age/Life stage	Urban/rural	How do they spend their money?	Needs, desires, aspirations
How engrained is the behaviour – how long has it been sustained	Gender	Geodemographic	Where do they socialize and what do they do	Beliefs and values
Frequency of behaviour e.g. Regular, occasional, hardly ever, experimenting stage	Family size	Proximity to services	What do they read, watch and listen to, and what engages them most	Personality type
Occasion – e.g. social smoker, smoke after meal, never smoke at work	Income	Area deprivation		Self-esteem, self-efficacy, locus of control
Stage of change: e.g. contemplating change or have tried to change and relapsed	Social Class/ Occupation	Social Capital		Key influences in their life – parent, peers, partner, religion, and the media, role models
Health status	Education			Attitudes towards the issues in question, the service, the product, the organization, the government, health professionals' e.g. contemplating a behaviour change, or tried and relapsed
Are they in serious debt?	Religion			attitudes towards services (NHS, local councils, etc.), customer satisfaction
Have they just experienced a major life event	Ethnicity			
Use of services – how often? What for?				
Habits				

NHS: National Health Services

them; and the segmentation should add value and greater sophistication when developing and targeting interventions

- Replicability – practitioners should be able to identify or recreate the segments in their own research.
- Stability – the segmentation definitions should be fairly stable but the size of the segments may change over time as people move in and out.
- The segmentation should create a focus for our time and money
- Segmentations should not be too complicated – some of the most powerful segmentations are the simplest
- The segmentation should not be the final word but should allow room for new insight.

Most segmentations within public health use 'quantitative' (measurable) data (e.g. surveys, epidemiological data, or hospital-episode data). However, there are some good examples of 'qualitative' segmentations (based on people's views, needs, and behaviours) which have drawn on in-depth interviews and focus groups to produce typologies of particular groups (e.g. see the alcohol case study later in this chapter). Although they cannot provide accurate estimates of the size of each segment, they do provide a rich description of the various groups and types emerging from the qualitative analysis and are very useful for developing propositions and defining the 'exchange' (see Chapter 11). The qualitative segments can be sized subsequently using quantitative survey research.

The type of segmentation you use will depend on what you are trying to achieve. Irrespective of the approach used, the resulting segmentation should be clear and actionable and should help the team visualize the people one is trying to reach. A good strategic segmentation of all your customers, mapping behaviour, service use, and attitudes can provide you with a much clearer understanding of your priority groups and be a valuable asset to your organization in planning programmes.

Segmentation starts with the consumers and how they should be served, instead of focussing on the product on offer. Messages, products, or services should be designed or redesigned around the priority segments. If executed well, this will produce more satisfied consumers and a more efficient delivery of your intervention.

Segmentations do not last for ever. They need updating as media, services, and attitudes towards them change. However, a well-constructed segmentation – which visualizes customers with clarity and insight – will result in buy-in from within your organization and its delivery partners and can drive activity for years.

Box 7.2 Geodemographics

Geodemographics has been defined as the 'analysis of people by where they live' (Harris et al., 2005) .i.e. using geography to help us draw general conclusions about the characteristics and behaviours of the people who live in defined, small areas – usually postcode areas. The underlying premise is that similar people live in similar places, do similar things, and have similar lifestyles.

The complex interplay between deprivation, the housing market, environmental issues, and access to services ensures that 'place' remains an important factor in public health and health inequalities (Blackman, 2006.) Using geodemographics to segment populations is gaining currency in the public sector as a means of examining spatial patterns of crime, health, and other social issues, and designing services to address them. There are many geodemographic database available e.g. ACORN (A Classification of Residential Neighbourhoods), MOSAIC, OAC, etc., which classify areas into different types with varying levels of detail and granularity. For example, ACORN identifies 56 neighbourhood types including, e.g. *Flourishing Families*, *Aspiring Singles*, *Settled Suburbia* and *Inner City Adversity*. A technical briefing, produced by the public health observatories for England and the NSM Centre, examines the various applications of geodemographic systems in the health sphere (APHO, 2009).

Geodemographics have been successfully used to segment populations and identify at-risk groups. A study by Powell et al. (2007) sought to establish whether geodemographic segmentation could effectively pinpoint heavy episodic drinkers, in order to target them with a social marketing programme. MOSAIC codes were added to Hospital Episode Statistics (HES) data on admissions for alcoholic liver disease. The admissions proved to be concentrated in a few geodemographic groups, typified by low levels of income, social class, education, and social cohesion. Interventions could be targeted at these groups right down to the postcode level.

Geodemographics is only one approach to segmenting populations and should be considered in the context of the wide range of other segmentation methods available – some of which will be better suited to your organizational needs.

Case studies

These case studies illustrate various approaches to developing insight and building segmentations, some are examples of single-issue interventions with a local focus, and others include national segmentations which look at several health issues with common attitudinal and behavioural factors.

Each case study features its own insight or segmentation challenges. You might ask yourself whether the segmentation factors or the target audience selected are the ones you would have chosen.

Case study: Trident

Source: Author's interview with Andy Nairn, planning director, MCBD, London, March 2008.

Trident is an anti-gun crime-partnership set up in 1998 by the Metropolitan Police and members of London's black communities to help bring an end to a series of shootings and murders among young, black Londoners.

Context

- In 75% of London's gun crime, the victim and suspect both come from the capital's black communities.
- Suspects and victims have become younger, and are increasingly likely to be British born.
- Girls and young women are also beginning to become involved by carrying guns, drugs, and cash for their partners.
- Police research has also shown that guns are increasingly being used to sort out what might be considered relatively 'trivial' or 'disrespect' issues.

Generating insight

The campaign targets teenagers and young people (street-wise black males; age range: 14–24) in gun-crime priority areas because of the need to influence attitudes and behaviours *before* youths get involved in gangs and criminal activity. A secondary audience included girlfriends and family, whilst a third group comprised younger teens, and finally stakeholders, including the police themselves.

One of the key elements of insight generation was the acknowledgement that witnesses are reluctant to provide evidence because of the fear of reprisals and distrust of the police. But, importantly, the problem being targeted is closely intertwined with a whole host of other social problems:

- Many commentators have focussed on the family, pointing out that young black offenders often have a non-traditional family life.
- Meanwhile, other observers concentrate on education, noting the perceived underperformance of black boys in school.
- In addition, most experts acknowledge the role of deprivation, emphasizing that young black Londoners are more likely to live in poverty than other groups.
- Finally, almost everyone recognizes gun crime's strong links with broader criminal activities such as drug dealing and gang conflict.

Nairn also hints at an issue which Trident has had to tackle early on. *I think there might be a kind of white, liberal stance which is reluctant to point the finger and say this is a black issue. The black community, though, has always been very, very clear that this is a significant problem for them.* It was, therefore, vital to engage with the community – both via established groups and informally.

This initiative faced significant competition from a multi-million-pound media industry which constantly depicts guns as glamorous and powerful. If this was not challenge enough, there was also a relatively low budget of around £247 000 a year, and the core audience was extremely difficult to recruit to formal research.

Some creative approaches ensued, including commissioning a photojournalist to go out and about to capture images of life on the streets of the key boroughs. In a new move, dubbed 'webnography', some young people gave up their passwords for social networking sites such as MySpace. The team was able to wander in the young people's space, which revealed the music they were listening to, videos they liked, and thus helped uncover the kind of language they would respond to.

Greater understanding of the audiences also came from talking to club-owners, DJs, and ethnic media journalists, as well as police officers, victims' families, community-leaders and members of the Trident Independent Advisory Group. The agency also interviewed academics to gain an understanding of the psychology of fear.

The intervention

The intervention's key messages were designed to 'de-glamorize' gun crime and challenge young people's perceptions of violent crime as cool and deserving of respect. The Trident campaign runs in the five London boroughs with the highest level of gun crime, and uses 'niche' and mainstream media, including billboards, school packs, and specialist radio stations with a predominately black audience.

Rappers' collective *Roll Deep* produced a track, 'Badman', as a message to those who might have been seduced by the glamour of guns. The music video ran online and was played on music channels as programme content, initially in the autumn-2006 phase of the campaign. Directed by Jake Nava (famous for Beyonce's 'Crazy in Love' video), it highlighted the grim reality of gun crime, its effects on people's lives, and the endless cycle of violence it promotes.

Intervention delivery was tailored to the audiences' perceptions: the music track was rolled out first, via clubs and e-mail, with no branding whatsoever. People loved the track: they were raving about it. It ran for six weeks, and then the video came out – with only a subtle acknowledgement that the Metropolitan Police were involved. The target audience loved the track and the video. The track was being played on pirate radio, a medium which would otherwise be highly unlikely to run anything associated with the police, and certainly one in which the Metropolitan Police would never advertise.

To target secondary audiences, particularly friends and family of victims of gun crime who wanted the shooting to stop, the intervention took up the plea and issued *Stop the guns* as a rallying cry. Building on this, they then focussed on the implications of doing nothing: the notion that individuals could end up with *blood on their hands.*

In February 2007, three teenagers were killed because of gun crime, and the Met police decided to rerun the Don't Get Blood on your Hands campaign, which was originally run in 2005 as part of Trident and was only shown on limited cinemas. It carried the message: *If you know someone has got a gun but don't report it, you could have blood on your hands.* As Fig. 7.1 shows, one of the ads featured 7-year-old Toni Ann Byfield, shot in September 2003, in North West London. The second running of the campaign brought greater exposure, as it was shown on music TV channels MTV Base, MTV Dance, Channel U/Fizz, and Passion TV and online on Channel U, Choice FM, RWD, and Jumpoff.tv.

More recently, Trident's campaigns feature radio and TV advertisements that were produced using views from real prisoners. Under the headline, *Don't blow your life away*, runs the text: 'Bang goes your liberty, your mates, your girlfriends, your clothes, your sex life, your

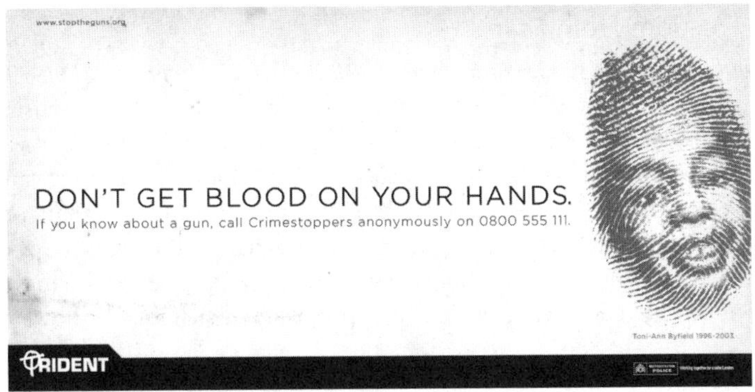

Fig. 7.1 Advertisement from the Don't Get Blood on Your Hands campaign.

Reproduced with permission ©Metropolitan Police.

phone, your mum's cooking, your fun'. TV and online advertisements also show the reality of a prison cell – a tiny space with no privacy, uncomfortable bed, and meals very far removed from mum's home cooking.

This phase of the Trident campaign drew on insights into teenagers' 'selfishness' that had been revealed in the early stages of the initiative. So campaign materials referred to the humdrum things teenagers would miss if they were imprisoned, such as going to McDonalds. In addition, there was the emphasis on the fact that gang members would drop them the minute they were no longer useful to the gang.

In another creative stretching of a restrictive budget, police officers toured the target boroughs in November 2007 with a 'real cell' (in reality, Perspex) showing the grim reality of a prison sentence. This also enabled officers to talk with young people, who were drawn by sheer curiosity to the event.

Thousands of magazines were placed in barbershops frequented by the target audience – each publication pierced through with a hole. On the final page, an insert revealed to the bemused reader: gun crime tears through whole communities. It encouraged readers to come forward with information: a simple (anonymous if they wished) call to the Crimestoppers could make a difference.

Results

Gun crime is falling in London. Trident officers, however, are also arresting many more offenders, as well as seizing more guns, ammunition, drugs, and cash.

In the year from its launch in November 2006, the 'Badman' video has been viewed online by more than 694 000 people.

'Actionable calls' – those which contain high-quality intelligence, capable of forming the basis for an arrest – to Crimestoppers have risen by 86% since the Trident campaign was launched in October 2004, based on London Crimestoppers figures.

We feel that Trident is a powerful example of campaigns which target disparate audiences linked by behaviour which may be amongst the toughest to change. It is a keen reminder that, in social marketing, the initial response is that consumers do not want what we are selling. This is where we depart from the existing theories within commercial marketing. With the challenges we face in persuading people to change behaviours which may be ingrained, inevitable, or seemingly inescapable, the least we can do is to try to understand their lives and communicate messages in a language and tone that is relevant and appealing.

Case study: Freedom From Fear

Source: Donovan and Henley (2003) and Donovan RJ, Paterson D, & Fracas M (1999).

Western Australia's Freedom From Fear campaign created mass media advertising to promote a men's domestic violence helpline and to encourage violent and potentially violent men to call. The Freedom from Fear is relatively unusual amongst domestic violence campaigns in its empathy for the key audience. Finding ways through a blame culture, so that communication was really persuasive and encouraging, has resulted in real change. It may seem easier to communicate with women suffering domestic violence – since they want change, and may be persuaded to play a part in taking action. Whether this is appropriate or sustainable, however, is another matter.

Donovan and Henley point out:

> While usually attracting little sympathy, violent men also suffer psychologically via guilt and remorse, feelings of helplessness, anxiety and depression, often resulting in suicide or murder-suicides.
>
> (Donovan and Henley, 2003)

Many campaigns on domestic violence have encouraged women to report assaults, to leave the home, take children to refuges, take out restraining orders, and so on, leading to prison sentences for some men.

However, if we include the women and children as consumers, we should acknowledge their needs and emotional investment. Not all women want to leave the home, nor see the perpetrator in prison. They want the violence (and threat of it) to end. They do not want to live in fear, waiting for a release date from prison, or for an ex-partner to find their new location.

Generating insight into the target audiences

Part of the 'insight challenge' here is to balance the needs of two target audiences – perpetrators and victims/survivors.

As Davina James-Hanman, Director of the Greater London Domestic Violence Project (GLDVP), stated in an interview with the authors of this chapter:

> One of the main reasons that domestic violence is dealt with so ineffectively is because we focus on the survivors' response to the problem rather than the perpetrator and his behaviour. Ironically, this has meant that most domestic violence campaigns have focussed on telling abused women what to do, which mirrors the behaviour of the abuser. Traditionally, campaigns have urged abused women to turn their whole lives upside down, to lose their homes, leave their partners and let an array of strangers into their lives, with little consideration of the consequences of such actions for abused women and children's lives.
>
> (Davina James-Hanman, interview)

However, if we listen to survivors, what *they* overwhelmingly tell us they want is for the violence to stop and for their partners to get help with changing their behaviour. Campaigns such as Freedom From Fear not only focus on the person whose behaviour is actually the problem, encouraging them to voluntarily seek help, but also manage to encompass the desires of their other audience in a respectful and non-abusive way.

Research started with 15 focus groups conducted with men with ages ranging between18 and 40. The subjects were told only that they would be discussing important social issues; domestic violence was not mentioned at the recruitment stage. Three group discussions were also held with violent men, all of whom were in treatment programmes. From these latter sessions, key points began to emerge, all of which are familiar to those who work in this area.

The first occasion of physical violence is a watershed, regarded by some as a 'point of no return', or an act which eases the way to subsequent violence. Many of the men in the campaign research expressed shame and guilt, but did not know where to get help without legal implications. Many perpetrators showed a 'siege mentality' and felt persecuted. In fact, when campaigners tried out a 'social disapproval' message idea, they found that perpetrators reacted angrily. They already felt that it was unfair for them to be apportioned all the blame for being violent.

A pivotal moment in planning seems to be the acknowledgement that men did not care enough about the effects of violence on their partner to change their behaviour towards them. The effects on their children, however, were a different matter. Even more than that, such a theme was significant for men who did not have children.

A secondary target audience was all other men aged between 18 and 40. A third was those who might encourage the primary target audience to seek help (victims, family, friends and doctors, police officers, and counsellors). The intervention also targeted members of the community, to keep domestic violence a community concern and to support men not engaged in domestic violence.

Segmentation

In terms of segmentation, the definition of the primary target audiences was male perpetrators and potential perpetrators who were ready to do something about their violence or potential violence. Hardcore perpetrators, in a strong state of denial, were not therefore part of the prime audience. Potential perpetrators were defined as those who subjected partners to nonviolent forms of abuse, such as emotional abuse, social isolation, or financial deprivation.

The intervention

In response to the insight that had been generated, the intervention team acknowledged that encouraging perpetrators – and those who feel they may be violent – to take the first step in calling a helpline, and then the next in attending counselling programmes, may be more effective than approaches used in previous interventions. It recognized that many of the men were, naturally, worried that calling a helpline may result in the police arriving at their door. Anonymity was offered, and there was no pressure for callers to give their details.

Specific tactics included TV advertising, particularly in sports programmes, and posters sent to workplaces – where key professionals (usually health and safety officers or human resources managers) were briefed about the campaign. Trades unions participated by distributing information packs.

Since many men lived outside cities and larger towns, the campaign developed further phases to tackle the problem of accessing counselling services. Services were also scheduled so that working men could attend outside their hours of employment. The helpline was staffed throughout the night.

Aware that advertising may make contact with another audience, albeit an unintended one, the team ensured that advertisements showing effects on small children would run at times when children could not see them. More than this, they tried out the materials with selected children at women's refuges, eager to make certain that they would not trigger stress symptoms among the youngsters, nor stimulate unintended actions, such as the children calling the helpline or believing that they should ask their fathers to do so.

Results

By late 1999, more than 3600 calls had been made, 63% of which were from the target group. Of these calls, 205 ended in referrals to counselling (50% of self-identifying perpetrators).

Beyond this success itself, the fact that more men have entered counselling programmes meant that there is an increased focus on measuring the outcomes of the programmes – an area in which there has previously been a paucity of such evaluation.

For more information, visit http://www.freedomfromfear.wa.gov.au.

The final two case studies look at building segmentations – both segmentations are health related.

Case study: Targeting harmful drinkers

Source: Department of Health (2008)

To inform its marketing strategy on alcohol harm-reduction, the Department of Health (DH) commissioned research to:

- provide a detailed qualitative segmentation of hazardous and harmful drinkers, accounting for discrepancies between claimed, perceived, and actual behaviour;
- provide a detailed understanding of the attitudes and motivations driving hazardous and harmful drinking and the key barriers to reducing alcohol consumption;
- identify and explore a strategy for influencing alcohol reduction; and
- generate insight for key interventions or communication.

Hazardous and harmful drinkers were defined as: women who drank 21–35 units per week and men who drank 21–49 units per week.

Methods

This was a qualitative study which employed a range of techniques to assess attitudes, beliefs, and behaviour including:

- drinking diaries and focus groups;
- 12 in-depth interviews; and
- four participant observation sessions (e.g. going shopping for drink with respondents, drinking with people at home, and drinking with them on a night out).

Segmentation

This research generated many interesting insights into the role of alcohol and the social context of drinking amongst target groups. Rather than focussing on the individual insights unearthed, we will set out the segmentation that emerged from the research. The segmentation was based on several principles:

- unravelling the core underlying needs driving behaviour underpins the most powerful way of segmenting and audience;
- this needs-based segmentation is based on a model of human motivation, identifying segments by the primary need behind harmful drinking;
- the needs and motivations behind harmful drinking are not always fixed: they can change over time or in different situations;
- the 'intensity' of the need (frequency and depth of experience) and the extent to which alcohol is believed to satisfy it account for drinking to harmful levels; and
- demographic differences should be accounted for where they exist.

These principles led to the creation of nine segments, as illustrated in Table 7.2.

Each of these segments was fully described by the researchers. Two examples are set out in Box 7.3.

Table 7.2 The nine segments of hazardous and harmful drinkers

Name	Characteristics	Key motivations
Depressed drinker	Life in a state of crisis, e.g. recently bereaved, divorced, or in financial crisis	Alcohol is a comforter and a form of self-medication used to help them cope
De-stress drinker	Pressurized job or stressful home life leads to feelings of being out of control and burdened with responsibility	Alcohol is used to relax, unwind, and calm down and to gain a sense of control when switching between work and personal life. Partners often support or reinforce behaviour by preparing drinks for them
Re-bonding drinker	Relevant to those with a very busy social calendar	Alcohol is the 'shared connector' that unifies and gets them on the same level. They often forget the time and the amount they are consuming
Conformist drinker	Traditional guys who believe that going to the pub every night is 'what men do'	Justify it as 'me time'. The pub is their second home and they feel a strong sense of belonging and acceptance within this environment
Community drinker	Drink in fairly large social friendship groups	The sense of community forged through the pub-group. Drinking provides a sense of safety and security and gives their lives meaning. It also acts as a social network
Boredom drinker	Typically single mums or recent divorcees with restricted social life	Drinking is company, making up for an absence of people. Drinking marks the end of the day, perhaps following the completion of chores
Macho drinker	Often feeling undervalued, disempowered, and frustrated in important areas of their life	Have actively cultivated a strong 'alpha male' image that revolves around their drinking 'prowess'. Drinking is driven by a constant need to assert their masculinity and status to themselves and others
Hedonistic drinker	Single, divorced, and/or with grown-up children	Drinking excessively is a way of visibly expressing their independence, freedom, and 'youthfulness' to themselves. Alcohol is used to release inhibitions
Border dependents	Men who effectively live in the pub which, for them, is very much a 'home from home'	A combination of motives, including boredom, the need to conform, and a general sense of malaise in their lives

These segments informed the development of a needs-based segmentation model, which included two axes – the first included the socially based attributes around the desire to 'belong' and connect with others or the need to stand out and display personal power.

The second axes included individually based attributes revolving around the need to 'control' and regulate their day or the need to release and escape.

Plotting each of the nine segments on to the 'needs' axes produced the segmentation scheme set out in Fig. 7.2.

The Department of Health's qualitative research demonstrated that harmful and hazardous drinkers need to be described by more that just their age, sex, and social class. Using various qualitative techniques, exploring attitudes and social contexts, has resulted in a diverse set of segments. People will move between some of the segments during the course of their lives with

Box 7.3 Examples of segment definitions

Conformist drinkers

- Aged 45–59, social grade C2DE, males.
- Very traditional values and attitudes, with the pub being a core part of their weekly, habitual behaviour.
- Drinking in the same place, at the same time, with the same drink most days of the week.
- Choose male-dominated drinking environment (the local or working men's clubs).
- Go straight from work or after finished 'tea' with their families, often on their own, with no arrangement to meet friends.
- Spend time chatting with other regulars, other 'blokes like them', or watch the big screen, play pool, for example.
- Stick to their 'usual' (pints), drinking at a steady, slow pace over the course of a few hours.
- Unit consumption is 30–50 units in the week but can increase to higher levels if have social events at the weekend.

Boredom drinkers

- Typically single mums or recent divorcees, they have a restricted social life (e.g. they have young children and little money).
- Drinking is company, making up for an absence of people (e.g. at dinner or when sitting on the sofa watching TV).
- Drinking is something to do when they are alone in the evening time, and it marks the end of the day (e.g. it follows the completion of chores and can act as a 'reward' or constitute 'me time'.
- Lacking stimulation, they drink to relieve restlessness and develop a 'liking for the taste' that develops over their regular fixed consumption.
- Drinking is a reassuringly familiar activity that gives them something to do with their hands and to savour in the mouth.
- Although boredom drinker's rarely drink to hazardous levels, there is a danger they can gradually creep up to harmful levels during times of stress or as children get older.

transitions triggered by material circumstances, attitudinal change, life events, and changes in life-stage. For alcohol interventions, as with many social interventions, one size does not fit all. For social marketing interventions, the segmentation will inform the construction of more tailored, and hence more actionable, propositions for each group. The Department of Health is currently working with this segmentation scheme to size the segments in terms of population numbers and to set priorities for interventions.

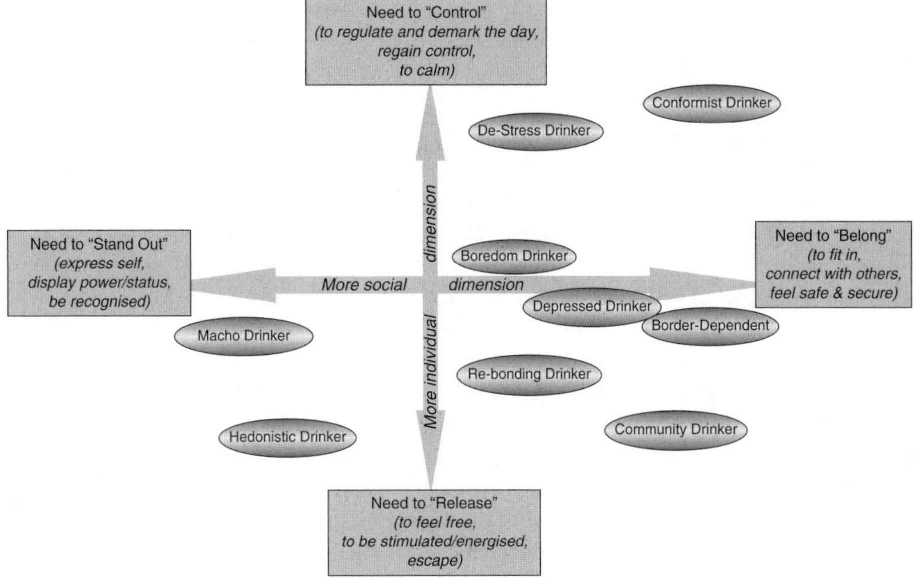

Fig. 7.2 Plotting the segmentation scheme.

Reproduced with permission ©Department of Health.

Case study: The Healthy Life Stage segmentation

Source: Department of Health (2008)

The Department of Health for England has developed a life-stage segmentation which builds on existing research and knowledge within the DH and academia to create a segmentation of the nation's health-related behaviour. The work focusses on the drivers of behaviour across the six Public Service Agreement (PSA) areas: smoking, obesity, alcohol, substance misuse, sexual health, and mental health (DH, 2008).

Methodology

If we were starting from scratch to produce a health-related segmentation of the general population, we would look at an existing general population survey which includes:

- health measurement across the PSA areas (e.g. using knowledge, attitudes, beliefs, and behavioural studies);
- an assessment of risk, self-esteem, and locus of control;
- indicators of motivation to change;
- environmental measurements – deprivation indicators and social norms;
- people's use of services and their views about services;
- Lifestyle indicators: social life, family life, aspirations, what people read, what they watch;
- their views about professionals and government; and
- demography: sex, age, class, ethnicity, etc.

Using this data, we would conduct a factor analysis and a cluster analysis[1] to produce segmentation. Unfortunately, no such dataset exists. Governmental surveys and campaigns tend to concentrate on single issues. Occasionally, some surveys on smoking ask about alcohol use or a survey on sexual health asks about alcohol use prior to sexual activity. The Health Survey for England covers many of the behavioural indicators of interest but includes very few attitudinal questions. Very few health surveys include attitude questions and fewer still ask about self-esteem, locus of control, or perceived social norms. Campaign-tracking studies usually have more detailed attitudinal statements, but again they are usually focussed on single issues. There are valid reasons for this deficit. Apart from the difficulty of getting buy-in from several governmental departments with different responsibilities and funding streams, there are considerable methodological challenges in condensing all the issues into an interview of between 45 and 60 minutes.

In the absence of this cross-issue survey with motivational and environmental indicators, the Healthy Life Stage hypothesis was created based on extensive desk research and stakeholder interviews.

At present, there is no consistent approach to segmentation across different health areas. One main outcome of the current project is to develop a segmentation framework or model that can be applied across issues and can develop insight in a consistent manner across life-stage groups. Once tested and validated, the model will be used as a building block for a customer-focussed approach to the development of behavioural change interventions.

To develop the hypothesis researchers identified more than 80 reports as relevant to the study. Behavioural 'drivers' and 'barriers' were then mapped to identify any commonalities across existing target audiences and health issues with regards to:

- behaviour/lifestyle;
- attitude towards health, decision-making priorities, aspirations (and other shared attitudes which may affect health behaviour); and
- knowledge, attitudes, and beliefs forming the basis of current behaviours.

Additionally, this mapping process revealed the behavioural or demographic groups for whom information was weak or missing.

To validate the first stage of analysis, researchers interviewed DH stakeholders who have an expert understanding of the target audiences currently addressed in campaigns to:

- confirm whether the drivers identified matched the stakeholders' own understanding;
- identify which of the drivers had the greatest priority and significance; and
- identify any further research or evidence that needed to be considered.

Subsequent workshops with key members of DH, health professionals, and academics were used to review the research analysis and identify attitudinal drivers common across different audience groups and issues.

Segmentation

Following this process of sharing of these common factors, three overarching 'dimensions' were highlighted as having the greatest significance when identifying population segments that are most likely to adopt 'at-risk' behaviours in relation to health. These are:

- the circumstances/environments in which people live;

[1] Factor analysis and cluster analysis are statistical techniques commonly used to analyse survey data into a number of segments.

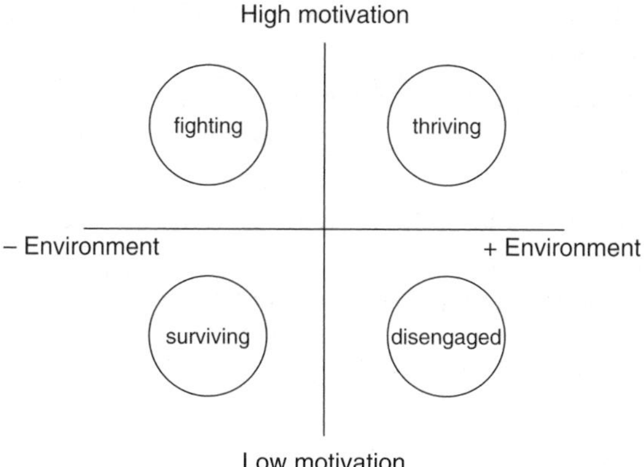

Fig. 7.3 The four quad segmentation.

Source: Department of Health (2008).
Reproduced with permission © 2008 Department of Health.

- their attitudes and beliefs towards health and health issues and the sense of control they have over their health; and
- age/life-stage.

Combining the first two axes, the environmental controlling factors (labelled the environment axes) and the individual controlling factors (labelled the motivation axes), produces a basic four quadrant segmentation (see Fig. 7.3).

These segments have been given names to indicate the principal dynamics of their circumstances: note that this segmentation is a hypothesis based on existing research. Although the description of the segments make intuitive sense, the exact descriptions and the size of each of the segments will not be known until the hypothesis is validated by survey research.

1. **Survivors** – people living in negative health environments who have a low level of motivation to look after their health. Within this group there will be many people with unhealthy behaviours, and many of these will have poor health. Their position on the motivation scale indicates that they feel they have less control over their health and have less confidence in their ability to do anything about improving it or preventing ill health. Their position on the environment scale indicates that they will be living in more deprived circumstances, which will make it more difficult for them to change their lifestyle. Moreover, in some of the most deprived communities in England the social norms for some behaviours make it difficult for those wishing to change. Levels of smoking prevalence can be over 60% in some areas, making the process of giving up much more difficult. If one of the main purposes of segmentation is to target resources where they are needed, this segment would clearly be a priority for properly tailored interventions and services.
2. **Fighters** – people living in negative health environments but who are standing above their norms, and who have a higher level of motivation to look after their health. This segment exists in the same conditions as the surviving group; indeed, some of them may be in the same family. There may be a number of reasons why they have managed to maintain a healthier lifestyle and exhibit a degree of 'resilience' to the deprivation surrounding them. Whatever the reasons which emerge from research, this group has great potential to influence their 'survivor group' peers.

3. **Disengaged** – people living in positive environments who for a variety of reasons have a low level of motivation to look after their health.
4. **Thrivers** – people living in positive environments who have a high level of motivation to look after their health. People in this group appear to be on the right track, and are probably the least in need of attention.

Although this is a basic four-segment solution, it has generated a number of issues for discussion around targeting and exploring resilience within particular segments. It also highlights major challenges relating to social inequalities in health and questions the degree to which encouraging individual behavioural change in deprived communities can really have an effect – unless efforts are made to address, simultaneously, the environment and social inequalities within which people exist.

However, this is not the final segmentation. Life-stage is an important driver for many behaviours. For example, moving from school to college, school to work, having children, getting divorced, looking after relatives, and the whole landscape of retirement can create positive and negative health opportunities for people, and this has to be factored into the segmentation.

Pulling the three dimensions (environment, motivation, and life-stage) together creates a richer segmentation. It should be acknowledged that working with three dimensions rather than two is relatively unusual in segmentation, but it is clear from research data that the ambition of the task (looking across the entire population on a range of health issues) requires this extra level of sophistication if the work-streams are to be relevant and sufficiently compelling.

The life stages in Fig. 7.4 should cover everyone in the population from the cradle to the grave. They have been given intuitive names and will be validated with survey research. Within each

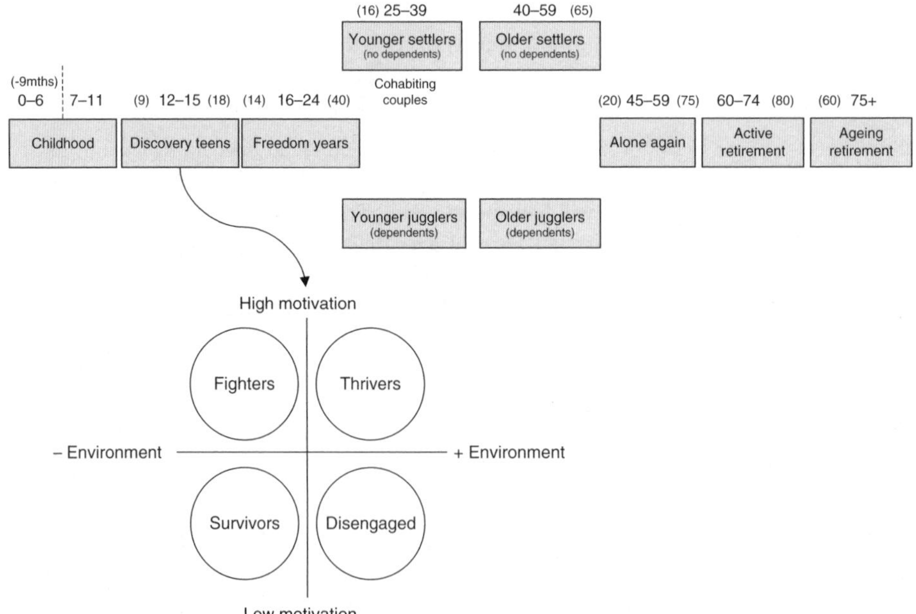

Fig. 7.4 The segmentation hypothesis generated from existing knowledge and expert opinion.

Source: Department of Health (2008).

life-stage, the basic four segment solution can be generated and used to understand the priorities within that group.

The schematic in Fig. 7.4 is the segmentation hypothesis generated from existing knowledge and expert opinion; it is *not* the finished product. At the time of writing, the hypothesis is currently undergoing validation with large-scale survey work to fully build the three axes with numerous scales and measures to describe and size the resulting segments.

What is captured in this simple and intuitive segmentation schema is the interaction between 'structure' and 'agency'. The debate surrounding the influence of 'structure' *and* 'agency' on human thought and behaviour is one of the central issues in sociology. In this context, 'agency' refers to the capacity of individuals to act independently and to make their own free choices; 'structure' refers to those factors such as social class, religion, gender, ethnicity, and customs which seem to limit or enhance the opportunities that individuals have.

To a fair degree, the two axes of the segmentation (Motivation/Environment) reflect the personal agency/structure variables and, therefore, capture a key feature neglected in many segmentations: the influence of social deprivation and social inequalities on personal motivations to change and vice versa.

One of the primary objectives of this segmentation is to locate the greatest need in the population, to identify what can reasonably be achieved by typical intervention approaches and to articulate what interlocking environmental and motivational factors have to be taken into account when designing new approaches.

Some of the existing individual approaches to prevention may not work with *some* subsets of the socially and materially deprived groups. More upstream approaches looking at, e.g. reorientation of service provisions may be the most productive route. One of the key features of the segmentation will be to articulate these nuances at the general population level. The population level analyses will not provide the detailed regional analysis but rather the overarching analysis of the relationship between life-stage, environment, and personal motivation and the detailed description of the segments that emerge from this framework. Furthermore the research programme will explore the possibilities of people moving between segments. This macro analysis will be useful locally by providing a backdrop to local research and implementation strategies. The tested methodologies employed nationally could be replicated locally using standardized instruments.

Amongst the many uses of this 'strategic' segmentation will be the exploration of the possibly of cross-issue interventions. So, for example, rather than just target people's smoking behaviour or drinking behaviour separately via different interventions or services, it may valuable to explore the common drivers for both behaviours within each segment and address them concurrently.

Conclusion

Developing an in-depth understanding of your audience using research and segmentation underpins effective social marketing. Many programmes jump too quickly into the design and implementation stage without taking enough time to study the target group at the programme-scoping stage (see Chapter 11 on 'Scoping'). Social marketing, social advertising, and health promotion are littered with examples of interventions which display little understanding of the beliefs and aspirations of their target audiences and why they behave as they do, often within socially and materially deprived communities. Talking to people and 'walking in their space' for a while develops an appreciation of the challenges they face every day. Having this insight and knowledge will help with understanding the audience 'exchange' and building strong message propositions which will be relevant and salient to the target group. If applied appropriately, this will result in interventions with the best chance of success. At the very least, it will help avoid the costly errors associated with poorly conceived programmes which did not take the time to listen and understand their audience.

References

Acheson D. (1998). *Independent Inquiry into Inequalities in Health – Report*. London: Department of Health.

Advertising Association (2009). *The Marketing Pocketbook*. p.177. London: Advertising Association.

Trident Advertising campaign (2007). Available at: www.stoptheguns.org (accessed 28 March 2008).

Association of Public Health Observatories (APHO) and the National Social Marketing Centre (2009) *Geodemographic Segmentation: APHO:Technical Briefing 5*, April 2009.

Author's interview with Andy Nairn, Planning Director, Miles Calcraft Briginshaw Duffy (MCBD), London, March 2008.

Author's interview with Davina James-Hanman, Director of the Greater London Domestic Violence Project, London, March 2008.

BBC News – Health (2008). *Drinkers fall into 'nine groups'*. Available at: http://news.bbc.co.uk/1/hi/health/7619508.stm. (Accessed: March 2009).

Blackman, T. (2006). *Placing Health*. Bristol: The Policy Press.

Bradley, N. (2007). *Marketing Research. Tools and Techniques*. Oxford: Oxford University Press.

Building Brands: Marketing Definitions. Available at: http://www.buildingbrands.com/definitions/04_marketing_insight_definition.php (accessed February 2009).

Central Office of Information (COI) (2008). *The Central Office of Information Annual Report 2007–08*. London: COI. Available at: http://www.coi.gov.uk/documents/coi-annualreport2007-8.pdf. (Accessed January 2009).

Customer Insight in Public Service 'A Primer' (2006) Cabinet Office. Available at: http://www.cse.cabinetoffice.gov.uk/UserFiles/File/Customer_Insight_Primer.pdf (accessed February 2009).

Department of Health (2008) *Ambitions for health: a strategic framework for maximising the potential of social marketing and health-related behaviour. The Healthy Foundation Segemenation models*. Availble at: http://www.dh.gov.uk/en/Publicationsandstatistics/Publications/PublicationsPolicyAndGuidance/DH_090348 (Accessed February 2009).

Donovan, R., Henley, N. (2003). *Social Marketing: Principles and Practice*. Melbourne: IP Communications.

Donovan, R.J., Paterson, D., and Fracas, M. (1999). Targeting male perpetrators of intimate partner violence: Western Australia's Freedom from Fear campaign. *Social Marketing Quarterly*, 5(3): 127–143.

Government Communications Network (GCN) Engage Programme. Available at: https://www.comms.gov.uk/ (Accessed February 2009).

Harris, R., Sleight, P., and Webber, R. (2005). *Geodemographics, GIS and Neighbourhood Targeting*. London: Wiley.

Health Development Agency (2008). *The Effectiveness of Public Health Campaigns:* Consumers and Markets. Briefing No. 7, June 2004. London: Health Development Agency.

Mathrani, S. (2008). *Sharpening the Spearhead: Customer focused public health information to tackle health inequalities. A report to The National Social Marketing Centre*. London: The National Social Marketing Centre. Available at: http://www.nsmcentre.org.uk/images/CoreFiles/sharpening_the_spearhead.pdf (Accessed January 2009).

Nantel, J., Weeks, W.A. (1996). Marketing ethics: is there more to it than the utilitarian approach? *European Journal of Marketing* 30 (5): 9–19.

National Social Marketing Centre (2006). Compendium of Social and Market Research Sources. By Kristina Staley and Dominic McVey. Available at: http://www.nsmcentre.org.uk/images/CoreFiles/NSMC-R11_compendium.pdf (Accessed February 2009).

Powell, J., Tapp, A., and Sparks, E. (2007). Social Marketing in Action – Geodemographics, alcoholic liver disease and heavy episodic drinking in Great Britain. *International Journal of Nonprofit and Voluntary Sector Marketing*, 12:177–187.

Stone, M., Foss, B., and Bond, A. (2004). *Consumer Insight: How to Use Data and Market Research to Get Closer to Your Customer*. London: Kogan Page Ltd.

The Concise Oxford Dictionary, Eighth Edition (1991) Oxford: Oxford University Press.

Varney, D. (2006). *Service Transformation: A Better Service for Citizens and Business, a Better Deal for Taxpayers*. London: HM Treasury, The Stationery Office.

Word Reference dictionary definition of 'Insight'. Available at: www.wordreference.com/definition/insight (Accessed March 2009).

Chapter 8

Commissioning social marketing

Jeff French

Knowing is not enough, you must apply; willing is not enough, you must do.
Bruce Lee

Learning points

This chapter

- Provides guidance on how and when to commission social marketing scoping, development, implementation, evaluation, and follow-up initiatives;
- Provides an understanding of the fundamental concepts of commissioning social marketing projects and programmes;
- Highlights the essential elements of developing tender documents and managing the process of selecting potential suppliers;
- Gives guidance on how to manage suppliers and assess progress and value for money.

Chapter overview

This chapter sets out some practical considerations and tips for organizations considering investing in external suppliers to provide either elements of a social marketing initiative or a whole initiative, from inception through to evaluation and dissemination of results.

Introduction

What is 'commissioning'?

Piggot (2000, p. 156) defines commissioning as *the strategic activity of assessing needs, resources and current services, and developing a strategy to make best use of available resources.* In the public sector, commissioning is the means by which we secure the best value and quality in public services. 'Best value' means the best possible outcomes and the best possible value for investment.

To achieve this, public sector organizations have two key roles:

- To be the advocate for people; and
- To be the custodian of taxpayers' or donors' money.

The commissioning of social marketing initiatives and other activity that puts people at the centre of service delivery is part of this wider set of responsibilities. Effective commissioning of such initiatives should lead to

- Improved impact and outcome of social marketing programmes;
- Improved quality, responsiveness, and efficiency of service delivery; and
- Improved understanding of service users or target audiences through building relationships and deep understanding of the service users' or target audience's needs.

For example, the NHS commissioning framework (NHS, 2007) sets out the need for commissioners to place more emphasis on developing services based on a greater understanding of people's needs and providing public health services that are informed by market research.

Commissioning is essentially transformational, and not just transactional. It incorporates 'contracting' and 'procurement', but only as mechanisms for achieving higher commissioning objectives. Commissioners also need to display visionary leadership and to operate with tact, assertiveness, and skill.

> They draw legitimacy from being seen to be engaged with communities, with service providers and with partner agencies drawing complementary views into a credible and coherent plan to which all sign up—putting the 'mission' into commissioning.
>
> Increasingly commissioners will be locally perceived as investors; that is, they commission to achieve the greatest health gains, return on investment and reduction in inequalities at best value. The process is often referred to as 'commissioning for improved outcomes'.
>
> (NHS, 2007, p. 5)

Commissioning can take place between public sector organizations, where one branch of the service acts as an executive commissioning agency and another acts as a delivery arm. However, in social marketing, commissioning often involves outsourcing or buying in specialist services from external private sector or third sector suppliers. 'Outsourcing' can be defined as the provision, generally by a third party, of defined services and activities, typically involving a transfer of assets, intellectual property, and/or staff. Organizations across the private, public, and third sectors are increasing the number of functions they outsource and are becoming the holders of a variety of outsourcing contracts. As outsourcing increases, and with it the interdependence between commissioners and suppliers, the nature of contractual arrangements is changing from being prescriptive and punitive (driven by bottom-line performance) to a situation that is more relational, and based on greater transparency, trust, and working towards a common goal over time.

Decisions about what to commission should be informed by answers to questions such as

- Can suppliers provide the service at lower cost?
- Are specialist suppliers needed for a defined time period?
- Do suppliers have skills that are not available internally?
- Are there opportunities to reduce risk by using suppliers? and
- Is there is a need to reduce core organizational running costs or simplify internal systems?

Think strategy and operational tactics

One of the key issues for commissioners is deciding whether they are going to apply a social marketing approach to their overall strategic development and/or to specific behavioural challenges and interventions. The following set of questions is designed to help you think through which approach you wish to take.

You will be adopting a 'strategic social marketing' approach if you answer yes to most of these questions

- Do you want to help inform your organization's wider policy context and/or related strategic plans?
- Are you wanting to look at behavioural challenges as a whole, rather than just focusing on a single behavioural area?
- Do you want to identify and consider potential connections and synergies between different topics or issues and their related behaviours?
- Do you want to develop a fuller understanding and insight into the audiences or 'customers' you are addressing that goes beyond a particular topic or issue and related behaviour?
- Do you believe that there is an opportunity and value in looking at behaviour 'in the round' before selecting a specific topic or issue?

If you answer yes to the majority of the following questions, you will be adopting more of an 'operational social marketing' approach

- Have you (at this time) ruled out taking a 'strategic social marketing' approach to look beyond a specific topic or issue area?
- Have decisions already been taken to tackle a specific topic or issue that you want to address?
- Are you clear about what type of operational social marketing research, development, or intervention you want to commission/develop?

Characteristics of excellence

There are a number of characteristics that are shared by efficient commissioners of social marketing initiatives, regardless of whether they are taking a strategic or operational approach. These are shown in Box 8.1.

Box 8.1 Characteristics of commissioning excellence

Excellent commissioners

- Collaborate with organizations that share the same strategic and operational goals, and share intelligence and collaboratively plan with partners and stakeholders;
- Are guided by what works and foster communities that contribute to the design, delivery, and evaluation of social marketing interventions;
- Specify behavioural outcomes and ethical processes to be followed;
- Systematically use information from target audiences alongside other forms of data and evidence to inform and shape social marketing interventions;
- Rigorously monitor and hold suppliers of social marketing interventions to account for delivering programmes to agreed levels of quality, value, and impact; and
- Have a mindset that moves from 'not invented here, so won't work here' to one of maximizing the use of best practice 'wherever invented'.

This list of characteristics was informed by but goes beyond characteristics for effective health sector commissioning developed by Dr Foster Intelligence (2007).

Writing a tender document

Having decided whether you are taking a more strategic or operational focus, the next step is to develop a tender document (a 'brief') that sets out what you wish to commission. The way that tenders need to be put together varies significantly between organizations, and the form and focus of the document will vary depending on what type of service you are commissioning and what stage of the initiative you are at. However, the first thing to do is speak with whoever is in charge of approving and monitoring such documents, if you work in an organization with such a function, to ensure that you are following the correct procedure and including all the elements your organization requires.

The time spent developing your brief is time well spent. It will save time and money later and help to build a better relationship and gain respect from your professional advisers. Sometimes, however, less can be more: do not clutter the brief with unnecessary background information or statistics that are irrelevant.

Some examples of what tender documents might focus on are contained in Fig. 8.1.

Tender documents range in length and complexity, but there are common features that should appear. The following checklist has been developed from the guidance given in the CD-ROM 'CDCynegy Social Marketing Edition Three ' (CDC, 2006). Before applying it, however, you should also make a judgement about the scale and focus of the work that you are intending to commission, as this will also help inform how comprehensive your tender needs to be.

Scoping tenders

- Desk based evidence reviews
- Desk based data reviews
- Desk based policy reviews
- Stakeholders surveys and interviews
- Target audiencce knowledge, attitude and behaviour surveys
- Target audience service experience surveys or obeservations
- Development of initial segmentations
- Development of propositions
- Competition analysis
- Review of existing social marketing case studies on similar topics and/or target audiences
- SMART objectives

Development tenders

- Development of intervention methods and materials
- Pilot of services changes, products and campaigns
- Development of segmentations and user understending
- Development of insight and testing propositions
- Testing creative executions
- Coalition building
- Community engagement
- Development of evaluation plans and systems
- Risk analysis

Delivery tenders

- Service delivery contact
- Community engagement programme delivery
- Stakeholder engagement programme delivery
- Media campaign delivery
- Partnership building and coalition formation and management
- Policy lobbying
- Organisational change
- Programme management

Evaluation tenders

- Evaluation of intervention processes
- Evaluation of short term intervention impact
- Evaluation of knowledge and attitude change
- Evaluation of behavioural change
- Evaluation of physiological change
- Evaluation of partnership and coalition
- Evaluation of specific programme and/or campaign elements
- Cost benefit analysis
- ROI analysis

Follow up tenders

- Project publicity
- Project write-ups
- Conference presentations
- Publications
- Evaluation launches
- Political dissemination strategies

Fig. 8.1 Commissioning tenders in social marketing.

General information

- *Overview of tender and issue being addressed*—This is an explanation of why you are producing a tender and the issue(s) being addressed. As well as providing a description of the issues, you should set out relevant research data, evidence, and research.
- *A clear statement of aims and objectives*—What are your initiative's aims and objectives? Include a description of your organization's current and past work and research in the area.
- *Budget/funding level*—You may choose to give an indicative budget or not, depending on your organization's approach. There are advantages in indicating the scale of your available budget, as this helps applicants tailor their proposals. But some organizations prefer not to disclose the available budget in the belief that this will help promote cost competition and keep cost lower.
- *Project timescale*—The contract period, start date, and end date.
- *Anticipated outputs* (such as reports, presentations, and reviews) and dates for their delivery. This should also include the timetable for application and decisions.

Scope of work

- *Detailed description of the work to be completed.*
    - Specific activities to be undertaken.
    - Products to be delivered or developed
    - Research or pretesting activities to be carried out.
    - Evaluation to be designed or carried out.
    - Number of items, workshops, staff, or other quantities you expect to be delivered.
- *Reports and/or updates you require* during the course of the work and the means for delivering these.
- *Follow-up and dissemination activity required.*
- *Ethical considerations.*

Requirements

- *Eligibility criteria*—Who may apply (you may have a requirement that the service is provided by a local supplier or one that has specific skills such as language skills, PR, media buying and planning, direct marketing, merchandising, new media, creative development, research or survey design, and delivery)? You may require submissions only by agencies with certain experience (e.g. marketing, public relations, marketing research, specific ethnic group marketing, youth marketing and public education, grassroots organizing, crisis management, and special events).
- *Invoicing*—Includes requirements for invoicing arrangements, timing, and process.
- *Acceptability of joint applications or consortium bids*—You may accept a lead agency affiliated with other agencies with relevant experience (e.g. lead agencies without ethnic marketing experience may still be considered as long as they make it clear in their proposal which subcontractors they would partner to create the plans for ethnic minorities).
- *Potential/perceived conflict of interest*—You should require a statement of disclosure of affiliation or contractual relationships, direct and indirect, with any agency that you feel

is incompatible with your organization's values and/or the aims of the initiative you are funding. You should also ask for details of any other current or previous relationships with such organizations.

- *Applicant questionnaire*—This should include
  - Questions regarding agency mission and philosophy;
  - CVs of the staff who will be working on the project and agency;
  - Years in business;
  - Relevant social marketing experience;
  - Health-related accounts, including past pro bono work;
  - Track record (ask for accounts);
  - Examples and contacts for references;
  - Examples of accounts that demonstrate the agency's experience and skill in the area of the tender results; and
  - Information about how the agency uses research in developing, executing, and evaluating campaigns.
- *Performance requirements*—Set out the expected performance required and over what time frame it is to be delivered. Also set out any penalty clauses, incentives, and contract break points that you wish to include.
- *Format for the proposal*—Set out headings that you want the proposal to address. These may include ideas for how the work will be developed and delivered, including
  - Supplier name and address;
  - Tax and company reference numbers;
  - Lead contact information;
  - The rationale;
  - Proposed approach;
  - Mix of interventions and tasks;
  - Timetable;
  - Stakeholder and partnering arrangements;
  - Research and evaluation elements;
  - Outline of budget allocations;
  - Approach to ongoing tracking and reporting; and
  - Examples (include the standard format for cover sheet, budget, and action plan, e.g. as appendices).

A standardized approach to submissions will also help prevent glossy or lavish applications that may distract from a systematic assessment of the applications based on their content.

Process for preparing and submitting proposals

- *Application deadlines*—including for letters of intent (confirming intent to submit full proposal) and complete proposal package.
- *Key contact information at your organization*—including information on how to submit questions and how they will be responded to. It is good practice to make a public record of all questions submitted by potential suppliers and the answers given, so that these can be seen by

all potential suppliers. It is also a good idea to include a question-and-answer sheet with the tender documentation, as this will help reduce the number of subsequent enquiries.

- *Instructions for how to submit application*—This should include a date and time, the number of copies required and whether fax or email versions are acceptable. You should also include instructions for oral presentations, including the time, date, location and form of presentation or pitch interview.
- *Instructions for how to withdraw application.*
- *Reasons for disqualification*—These may include
  - Incomplete or late submission;
  - Failure to meet requirements;
  - Submitting application with false, inaccurate, or misleading statements; and
  - Unwillingness or inability to fully comply with proposed contract provisions.

Review, evaluation, and selection

You will need to set out the criteria for evaluation and, ideally, the respective weighting given to each criteria. You can use the guidance in this chapter concerning the assessment of suppliers and their proposals as a basis for agreeing what factors you are looking for.

Other inclusions and issues

As stated in the preceding, you will need to be clear of your organization's rules about how contracts should be signed and who can sign them. Other issues that should be built into tender documents include

- Reasons for termination of contract;
- The right to remove or replace subcontractors;
- The responsibility or liability for costs incurred by bidders prior to contract award;
- Confidentiality policy; and
- Your organization's terms and conditions (e.g. intellectual property rights, payments, indemnity, liability, insurance, termination, and records maintenance).

Creating a positive pitch environment

When conducting a pitch with a possible suppler, it is important to remember that a pitch is not a solo performance but a dialogue; it might also be the start of a long-term relationship. As a potential client, you need to create a positive experience in which the potential suppler and your organization can gain the best possible sense of what is on offer in terms of skills, experience, and ideas. When you are planning pitch meetings, consider the following questions:

- Do you need a facilitator for the meeting?
- Did you answer all of the agencies' questions prior to the pitch?
- Have you provided all the research reports and other background material that the supplier might need?
- Are you going to hold a single meeting or a set of meetings before you make decisions?
- Have suppliers had a reasonable amount of time to prepare?
- How will you react to challenges to the brief from the supplier?

- How will you evaluate the pitch process?
- Do you have a set of explicit written criteria that all those people on the selection panel will use to evaluate each pitch?
- What system have you put in place to debrief all those who pitched?
- Are you putting in place a system for suppliers to give you feedback on the process?

It is simply good practice to treat with respect all those suppliers that have put effort and expense into pitching for work and ensure that good relations are maintained for the future. Even if a given supplier did not win the contract, you may want to work with them in the future.

Assessing social marketing suppliers and proposals

Organizational capacity

If you are supporting specialist commissioners to commission social marketing initiatives, or are commissioning on their behalf, you may be using approaches and tools that differ from those the commissioner usually uses. They need your input and support to critically assess the suppliers that are pitching for work and the proposals they bring forward. You need to be aware, and to make colleagues aware, that there are many suppliers who do not have a deep understanding or track record in delivering successful social marketing programmes but who are skilled in pitching for work. Therefore, it is important that companies bidding for work are interviewed consistently and rigorously to ensure that what they plan to deliver is actually what you require and that you yourself are satisfied that they can deliver it. It is also important that you have systems and resources in place to ensure the ongoing management and monitoring of supplier organizations throughout the contract period, and not just at the start.

Assessing potential suppliers

There are several important issues to consider when assessing the competence and track record of potential social marketing suppliers (Government Communications Network, 2007):

- Establish that the potential supplier understands your aims and objectives—do they understand the strategy behind them and how the work you are commissioning will add value?
- Look for a track record of effectiveness as well as attractiveness. Were previous initiatives 'fit for purpose' rather than just looking good? Look for evidence of clear behavioural change.
- Consider supplier size, resources, and position in the market, including the strength of the proposed project team and organizational management team.
- Can they demonstrate a professional understanding of social marketing principles and concepts? How does what they are proposing match up with the national social benchmark criteria (see Chapter 3)?
- Can they demonstrate an ability to use research techniques to segment, target, and design interventions that meet the needs of distinct target groups?
- Check for strong evidence of an ability to customize solutions. Is there evidence of the supplier's submission that they can understand your challenge, or are they just applying an approach they have used before?
- Have they provided evidence of genuine audience and stakeholder engagement, partnerships, and collaborative delivery?

- You will usually want to appoint an organization that has a track record of collaborative delivery and ability to manage local stakeholders and partners. Ask for references and evidence of such work.
- Does the supplier demonstrate a good understanding of your sector and the issues you are concerned with?
- Is the supplier committed to delivering against your targets and are they clear about the consequences of failing to deliver?

Assessing social marketing proposals

You can use the checklist set out in Table 8.1 to assess the strength of social marketing proposals.

Table 8.1 Checklist for assessing social marketing proposals

Programmes displaying these characteristics are likely to be effective.	Yes	No	Unsure
A systematic scoping and development phase has been built into proposal.			
Proposal contains the need to gather and synthesize insight into the proposed target audience.			
The supplier aims to develop a clear 'exchange proposition' through which advantages of the proposed behavioural change will be spelt out in a way that the target group believes is attractive and achievable.			
Measurable behavioural goals have been or will be set, and there is a clear process for this.			
Interventions proposed are informed by relevant theoretical models.			
Interventions proposed are informed by a review of evidence about effectiveness.			
Data reviews have been used to inform the development of the proposed strategy.			
Systematic short-, medium-, and long-term planning is clearly set out.			
If appropriate, the plan includes action to establish multisector delivery coalitions to assist in development, delivery, and evaluation.			
The proposed budget allocation is realistic enough to develop, deliver, and evaluate the aims and objectives of the initiative.			
Competitor analysis has been or will be undertaken, and measures to address competitive factors feature in the proposal.			
The proposal sets out a multicomponent strategy that can be delivered in an integrated way.			
There are clear plans to involve the target group in intervention development, implementation, and evaluation.			
Mechanisms will be put in place to coordinate international, national, regional, and local action if appropriate.			
The proposed initiative is complementary to the current policy and delivery environment.			
The plan sets out how any relevant ethical issues will be addressed			
A comprehensive evaluation strategy is proposed covering process, impact, and outcome evaluation.			

Other recommendations for commissioning suppliers

Avoiding conflict of interest

It may be worth checking out other clients of your proposed supplier to ensure that there is no conflict of interest with your eventual intervention. This is particularly pertinent if agencies work for both commercial and public sector organizations.

Beware of 'add-ons'

In pitching for your commission, an organization may include a few promotional freebies, contests for kids, free-phone or help lines, for example. Although these ideas may appear to offer value for money, they may not actually help you archive the results you want; so question how such 'add-ons' will contribute to the overall initiative.

Ongoing management of the organization you commission

Once you have commissioned a supplier and have agreed to clear objectives, it will be necessary to ensure that the supplier is monitored and managed in terms of their performance and that a strong two-way flow of information is maintained over the contract period.

Normally, some form of management group or programme board, consisting of key commissioners and representatives from the supplier agency, will agree to meet to keep the initiative under review, monitor progress, and agree to changes as the programme proceeds. Such a group should work to an agreed set or terms of reference that indicate to whom the group reports to in the commissioning organization. The group should also be the forum for resolving issues and challenges that arise as the programme proceeds. The group or committee should meet at appropriate intervals and receive milestone reports from the agency.

It is important not to let the supplier lead the intervention down a route that is not based on hard evidence or goes against what you want. At all stages of an initiative, commissioners should be able to evaluate progress against the original brief to ensure that the initiative remains focused on the original aims and objectives.

Making the most of current evidence

It is widely recognized that investments in social marketing are hampered by a lack of clear and consistent measures of their impact, which leads to inadequate funding (Bennett, 2003; Jackson, 2005; Hay, 2006). However, there is also a growing evidence base that proves that social marketing not only works but also is cost-effective (Hornick, 2002; McDermott et al., 2006; Gordon et al., 2006; Stead et al., 2006; Lister, 2007), see also Chapter 6.

A key task for any social marketer is to assess the current evidence base. Rather than undertake a systematic review of the evidence, it is usually more practical to search the evidence reviews and 'reviews of reviews' that have been carried out by others and to draw on case study databases. There are a number of such services and sites on the Internet. For a list of relevant links, visit the National Social Marketing Centre's (NSMC) website at www.nsmcentre.org.uk.

Using information gathered from these and other sources will help you answer questions about the probable effectiveness of your eventual intervention. However, commissioners must be aware that only by undertaking a thorough development phase and field testing process with the intended target groups a more accurate assessment of impact can be arrived at. For more information regarding drawing on current evidence, field testing, and evaluation, see Chapters 6, 12, and 14, respectively.

Ensuring return on investment (ROI)

One of the central issues facing any marketing agency or marketing manager is demonstrating that investment in marketing makes a direct impact on the bottom line of the organization they work for. The same is true for those marketers working on social issues in the public, private, or third sectors.

The plain fact is that we are all competing for investment in our initiatives. It is right that senior management in any organization should ask the three key tough commissioning questions:

1. Will it work?
2. What return do I get for my investment?
3. Is it value for money?

Those seeking to attract investment into marketing initiatives to address social issues are going to have to get smarter about setting out clear answers to these questions and being held to account for delivery against any investment made.

In the private sector, the ROI is the annual financial benefit of an investment minus the cost of the investment. In the public sector, the ROI is the cost reduction or cost avoidance obtained after an improvement in processes or systems, minus the cost of the improvement. In recent times, the ROI has been enhanced by the notion of the 'triple bottom line'. This equates to an expanded baseline for measuring organizational performance, adding social and environmental dimensions to the traditional financial 'bottom-line' results. Marketers will need to set out the likely impact on the environment and the wider social impact of their intervention to build a picture of the total impact of the intervention.

Focusing purely on the financial aspects of ROI, Box 8.2 sets out the kind of ROI analysis that social marketers should include in their proposals for funding. These kinds of assessments are also helpful as tools for tracking programme performance. Such assessments not only set out a clear economic case but also provide commissioners with hard numeric measures for assessing ROI.

Box 8.2 Example estimates of ROI on a proposal to extend social smoking cessation clinic opening times

Numbers of current attendances annually	1 000
Percentage increase projected by increasing opening time	10%
Number of new clients	100
Percentage of new clients expected to quit	25%
Number of additional quitters	25
Average cost saving per quitter	£3 000
Annual gross cost of savings (25 × £3 000)	£75 000
Annual costs of providing extended opening	£20 000
Net cost savings	£55 000
ROI (£20 000–75 000)	3.5:1 OR 350%

Is it value for money?

Value-for-money audits are non-financial audits, usually built into summative evaluation strategies, to measure the effectiveness, economy, and efficiency of investing in marketing. They do not question the policy itself; they examine the focus on the efficiency and implementation as measured against the initiative's goals and overall scale of the project. Value-for-money audits should also be accompanied by a cost–benefit analysis, which is a technique to compare the various costs associated with an investment with the benefits that it proposes to produce.

Both tangible and intangible returns should be addressed and accounted for. Marketers should use cost–benefit analyses to assess the return they get in terms of behavioural change for each of the investments made in a programme. For example, what generated the most contacts from the public about advice to recycle? The website? The telephone advice line? The drop-in centre? And what was the cost of each of these contacts (the number of contacts against the cost of providing the service)? Clearly, how the benefit is defined will be specific to the intervention.

Avoid panic buying

In circumstances where additional funds become available at short notice, and they must be spent rapidly, try to avoid spending for its own sake. Rather, try to reinforce or increase effort in those areas that are demonstrating payback in terms of behavioural shifts.

Two final points about funding and cost assessment

When investing in social marketing, there is a threshold point that must be reached in terms of population awareness and action before the ROI can be measured. In an environment in which there is increasing competition for attention and engagement, social marketing programmes are often not funded to a sufficient level so that they can 'cut through' to their intended groups. Low levels of investment are often compounded by stop–start approaches to investment. Consequently, and importantly, the amount to be invested to achieve measurable impact on behaviour in target groups is a key factor to be determined in the development stage of any social marketing programme (for more detailed guidance on the development stage, see Chapter 12).

A second key recommendation for commissioners is the timeframe over which investment needs to be maintained to achieve the targets of the programme. If investors are not able to commit sufficient funds over the required period, they must be made aware that the impact of their more limited investment may be reduced further by a lack of perseverance. Impact over time is a key issue to be addressed when putting together a full business case for investing in social marketing.

A three-step process for commissioning and budget allocation

The NSMC (2006) recommends that budgets are allocated in three steps, rather than allocating a fixed amount at the start of an initiative, to ensure that a rigorous marketing development process is adhered to.

Step 1

First, allocate a budget to scope an issue (see Chapter 11), understand the issue to be tackled, understand the audiences and assets that exist or that could be brought into play, and define the obstacles to success. As Chapter 11 sets out, the key output from this scoping phase is a 'scoping report', which outlines the initial insights that will be taken forward into the development stage and explains how these insights were generated.

Step 2

On completion of the scoping stage, and based on the scoping report, commissioners should allocate a budget for a development phase (see Chapter 12). During the development phase, suppliers should work up the proposals, undertake field testing, and refine (or, if necessary, redesign) the proposed interventions so that they meet the initiative's requirements and are acceptable to the target group(s).

Step 3

From the development phase, a full business plan can be developed. This should form the basis of funding allocations to scale up and fully implement the recommended interventions (see Chapter 13) and evaluate their impact (see Chapter 14).

If commissioners apply this three-step approach to funding and it is complemented by marketers in the public sector, setting out evidence for their recommendations, estimates of projected savings, and a value-for-money analysis, the chances of well-executed social marketing interventions will increase. We will also start to build a robust, costed evidence base for social marketing that will inform future planning and delivery, which will itself lead to greater investment in social marketing. Building this virtuous circle of practice should be a primary concern for all marketers.

Conclusion

Commissioning social marketing is a key activity for an ever-increasing number of public service workers. Commissioning is a straightforward process, but it does demand a systematic approach and the proactive management of prospective and successful suppliers. Commissioning social marketing can be a highly cost-effective way of drawing on the necessary specialist skills that may not be present within public or third sector organizations. Commissioning is, however, not without risk. Commissioners need to dedicate sufficient time and resources to constructing a thorough and fair process and actively managing the chosen suppliers, while evaluating their delivery against the brief that they successfully competed for.

Review exercise

Use the following briefing template to set out a programme of work that you wish to put out to tender. If possible, use it for a real project, but if this is not appropriate, select a project that you would like to commission. Set a budget for the work and then attempt to fill in as much of the form as you can. If you get stuck at any point, refer back to the advice in this chapter and others in the book that deal with specific issues.

- Title of project/programme
- Background, context, and rationale for the project/programme
- Purpose (focus of the project, scoping, development, implementation, evaluation, follow–up, or a full end-to-end programme)
  - Aim(s)
  - Objective(s)
  - Target audience(s)
- Requirements (brief description of project/programme)
- Timeframe (programme start and end date)

- Organizational, technical, and/or scientific requirements or standards such as compliance with national guidelines
- Intended audiences
  - Primary
  - Secondary
  - Tertiary
  - Intermediate
- Explicit skills and experience that the agency must have
- Key partnerships and stakeholders that will need to be engaged
- Ethical issues and requirements (involvement of ethics committee in research activity)
- Incentive, bonus, and/or penalty schemes
- Declaration of any conflict of interests
- Branding requirements
- Sign-off procedures
- Reporting arrangements and milestones
- Evaluation required
- Financial arrangements, payment, and invoicing
- Specific contractual and legal clauses including intellectual property rights
- References and examples of similar or relevant work

References

Bennett, J. (2003). *Investment in Population Health in Five OECD Countries.* Paris: Organisation for Economic Cooperation and Development.

CDC (2006). *CDCynegy Social Marketing Edition Three.* Atlanta, GA: Centers for Disease Control and Prevention.

Department for Education and Skills and DoH (2006). *Industry Techniques and Inspiration for Commissioners.* Available at: www.everychildmatters.gov.uk/planningandcommissioning [accessed March 2009].

Dr Foster Intelligence (2007). *Intelligent Commissioning. Intelligence*, Issue 2, September, London.

Gordon, R., McDermott, L., Stead, M., Angus, K. and Hastings, G. (2006). *A Review of the Effectiveness of Social Marketing Physical Activity Interventions.* Stirling, Scotland: Institute for Social Marketing.

Government Communications Network (2007). *Engage.* London: Cabinet Office. Available at: www.comms.gov.uk/engage [accessed March 2009].

Hay, D.I. (2006). *Economic Arguments for Action on the Social Determinants of Health.* Ottawa: Public Health Agency of Canada.

Hornick, R.C. (ed.) (2002). *Public Health Communication: Evidence for Behavior Change.* New Jersey: LEA.

Jackson, T. (2005). *Motivating Sustainable Consumption: A Review of Evidence on Consumer Behaviour and Behavioural Change.* Surrey: Network Centre for Environmental Strategy, University of Surrey.

Lister, G. (2007). *Prevention Is Better Than Cure: Cost-effectiveness of Interventions Aimed at Promoting Health and Reducing Preventable Illness.* London: National Social Marketing Centre.

Mayo, E. (2005). *A Playlist for Public Service.* London: National Consumer Council.

NHS (2007). *World Class Commissioning: Competencies.* London: NHS Commissioning Team Directorate.

NSMC (2006). *It's Our Health!* London: National Social Marketing Centre.

McDermott, L., Stead, S., Gordon, R., Angus, K. and Hastings, G. (2006). *A Review of the Effectiveness of Social Marketing Nutrition Interventions.* Stirling, Scotland: Institute for Social Marketing.

Pigott, C.S. (2000). *Business Planning for Healthcare Management.* Buckingham: Open University Press.

Stead, M., McDermott, L., Gordon, R., Angus, K. and Hastings, G. (2006). *A Review of the Effectiveness of Social Marketing Alcohol, Tobacco and Substance Misuse Interventions.* Stirling, Scotland: Institute for Social Marketing.

Chapter 9

Ethical issues in social marketing

Aiden Truss and Paul White

Only through embedding respect in our system at the level of the individual encounter as well as in the institutional fabric, will our health service regain its proud position as the best in the world.
Sir Liam Donaldson

Learning points

This chapter

- Explains how influencing people's behaviour presents a range of ethical issues and principles;
- Shows how a better understanding of ethics can strengthen the impact and effectiveness of work;
- Helps prevent misunderstandings about the ethical basis of social marketing and addresses potential criticisms; and
- Provides a framework for a practical code of ethics for social marketing.

Chapter overview

This chapter discusses the ethical decisions that need to be considered when applying social marketing. It raises important questions such as 'is it ever ethical for the state to intervene in the private lives of citizens?' that we, as social marketers, need to identify and address when scoping an intervention (see Chapter 11). Although there is a wealth of literature concerning ethics in public health and marketing, the unique position of social marketing as a discipline implies that we also need a broader understanding of the issues. There are many areas of society in which a plurality of social, cultural, and even religious practices may be at variance with an identified behavioural issue. Simply stated, there are few straightforward ethical decisions when dealing with so many cultural and demographic variables in many interventions.

It is not enough to rely on the Kantian imperative of rational altruism to frame our idea of ethical good. And, as Bill Smith points out (Andreasen, 2001), even the 'do unto others ...' admonition may present us with dilemmas in certain circumstances where it may weigh the rights of individuals against the needs of society.

In this chapter, we hope to provide an understanding of what ethics are and at what stage of the social marketing process they should be applied. In addition to discussing the key debates in public-policy intervention, we illustrate many of them with an example of a successful, yet from an ethical viewpoint highly controversial, initiative.

Finally, we will put our learning into an 'ethical checklist' to help highlight the key considerations that you might need to explore when scoping an intervention.

Introduction

Ethical debates around social marketing

As social marketers, it could be argued that our entire *raison d'être* is to contribute towards social good. Just exactly what defines 'good', and more importantly who decides what 'good' is, is a matter for debate and discussion. We need to be sure where this imperative is derived from and what its direction and authority actually are. Are we being asked to intervene on behalf of the government out of concern for the welfare of its citizens? Or are we, in fact, trying to remove barriers to promote positive behaviour that people would really like to pursue for themselves? Either example might be seen as ethical or even noble on the face of it, but at the same time the former might be open to accusations of paternalism and the latter to accusations of outright state interference.

In *Social Marketing: Influencing Behaviours for Good* (2008, p. 46) Philip Kotler and Nancy Lee provide a snapshot of some of the current debates on this subject. With reference to the discussions held on the Social Marketing Listserv (http://www.social-marketing.org/aboutus.html), they reveal that a wide spectrum of ethical perspectives inform the way in which we work. These range from the notion of social marketers as 'hired guns', who should use personal value judgements to shape the direction of an initiative, to suggesting that public consensus or even the United Nations Declaration of Human Rights might be used as a baseline measurement.

This is not the place to explore the concept of ethics in any abstract sense. We all have some notion of a code of moral standards and how they should be applied to our working practices – particularly in the public sphere. One dictionary definition describes ethics as *a system of moral principles governing the appropriate conduct for a person or group* (Encarta, 2008). It could be argued that this is all we need as a theoretical basis for our exploration of the subject. The problem lies in the fact that there can sometimes be a tension between diverse ethical standpoints and moral principles for change. This can be seen clearly in the debates on the use of condoms to prevent the spread of HIV/AIDS and the 'moral' rejection of this by the Catholic Church, particularly in Africa. From a public health viewpoint this is possibly a cut-and-dried issue, but where does that leave the right of individuals and organizations to hold an opposing ethical viewpoint?

This is a perennial problem. In the 1970s, in a study into the ethics of social marketing, Laczniak, Luscha, and Murphy identified three main areas of concern:

- Social marketing is a two-edged sword that is perceived to have major beneficial elements, but it also contains the potential to cause significant ethical controversies.
- The accountability of social marketers will be a major societal concern, but the initiation, at this time, of professional licensing or governmental review of such activity is undesirable or premature.
- When judging social marketing from an ethical standpoint, it appears to be difficult to separate the ethics of applying marketing techniques to social ideas and programmes from the ethics of the ideas themselves (Laczniak et al., 1979).

These areas articulate an ongoing problem with the perception that some individuals have of social marketing: if it can be used effectively for good, might not some agencies, authorities, or corporations seek to use it for less worthy purposes? The notion of social marketing as a tool of equal use for good and bad in society still pervades today. As one of the responses to the aforementioned survey worriedly posited, *Social marketing could ultimately operate as a form of thought control by the economically powerful* (*ibid*).

Social good?

It is perhaps inadequate to say that in defining social marketing we are underlining the fundamental and intrinsic characteristic that we are attempting to do 'social good' and that social marketing for social ill is not social marketing. The question is asked and perhaps provides a reason for the problematic association with potential harm: whether the same marketers who apply their craft to slick electioneering campaigns, spin, and pleasing focus groups are really the best people to be involved in selling change to society? Of course, this is not always the case, but it is an issue of negative association which needs to be dismissed with a clear articulation of ethical probity.

Donovan and Henley highlight this problem in their exploration of consequentialist and non-consequentialist ethics. Consequentialist thought encompasses the utilitarian concept that ethical choices should be weighed in favour of producing the greatest good for the greatest number of people. Non-consequentialists do not attempt to quantify results, but hold that some actions are intrinsically good. They see a distinction in the motivation between different types of social marketers:

> Social marketers with a strong commercial background appear, for the most part, to subscribe to the consequentialist school, whereas those with a public health background may be more likely to subscribe to the non-consequentialist school.
>
> (Donovan and Henley, 2003, p. 165)

Donovan and Henley go on to illustrate the issue of negative association by looking at a Nike advertising campaign which advocated a positive message that girls who took part in sports experienced fewer negative and more positive events in their lives. The ads were screened for students and involved positive slogans and positive image enforcement around the benefits of physical activity. The only visible sponsorship branding was the Nike 'swoosh' symbol. All very laudable, but many of the students took the ethically non-consequentialist view of the campaign as having little value, tainted as it was by association with what they perceived as a company with a poor ethical track-record and which allegedly employed cheap labour in developing countries (*ibid*).

This is a great example of the way in which people with the best of motives attempt to be ethically good but arrive at completely different views of the same issue. Social marketers can, for the most part, only really afford to be consequentialists.

When initiating a behavioural intervention, it is very seldom the case that an ethical statement is included in its principles to inform development of the intervention. We might again argue that an ethical stance is implicit in social marketing, but perhaps this is not sufficient when attempting to convince the sceptical of what we are trying to achieve. It is also an inherent problem that when working with so many cultural and societal variables there are seldom any clear-cut issues that lend themselves to clear-cut ethical solutions. As all interventions carry the burden of ethical considerations, it might be prudent to outline an ethical policy or stance from the very beginning of the initiative (National Social Marketing (NSM) Centre, 2007). This would need to take into account the various positions informed by the different stages of the initiative. This is the area of 'applied ethics', where there is a connection of the 'discipline of moral philosophy to areas of human concern and endeavour, including professional and occupational action' (Cribb and Duncan, 2002, p. 272).

Professional standards for commercial marketing include ethics, but how often do we see this manifest itself in the marketing activity of businesses (consider, e.g. 'pester power' and the sale of products through children). However, with the growing voice of the consumer through the Internet and online social networking tools, ethical issues are becoming a greater debating theme for brands and reputation management. The ground rules are rapidly changing for business.

For social marketing, and for those responsible for delivering social policy through its application, ethical issues must have pride of place in the early phases of thinking to a much greater extent than they do in business.

Intervention and control?

Social marketing has been attacked in some sections of the media as some kind of sinister attempt at social control, even to the extent of being part of some covert government agenda. In the UK, apparently, the government is now *in the business of behaviour modification* (Furedi, 2008). We might argue that this is a lazy and even alarmist interpretation of the aims of social marketing, but it is nonetheless one that needs to be addressed from an ethical standpoint.

We posed the question at the beginning of this chapter whether it is ever ethical for the state to intervene and interfere in the lives of its citizens. In reality, this is all just a matter of context and perception. The fact is that, through its democratic mandate, the state already attempts to modify behaviour of its citizens in all sorts of areas. At the most basic level, needs dictate that we have legislation to ensure the smooth running of society, and most of us readily accept a degree of management in our daily lives. So why do some baulk at the idea of social marketing as a means of producing positive behaviours? Michael Rothschild suggests that if we, as participants in society, already accept a level of behavioural management, then the question we should be asking is not whether social marketing in itself is ethical but rather *What is the ethicality of marketing when compared to education and law as alternative tools of behaviour management?* (Rothschild, 2001, p. 17). He further suggests that we need to ask ethical questions as to when to apply each of these three forms of management (marketing, education, and law). This moves the ethical consideration to other areas of exploration, such as determining which form of intervention is appropriate for a problematic behaviour, what the motives are behind the intervention and what people will gain from it in the long term.

Voluntary versus involuntary approaches

Perhaps we can reduce the problem slightly by looking at the comparison between these three forms of approach to behavioural change. From an ethical standpoint, how does using marketing to promote positive behavioural change compare to regulation (law), and awareness raising (education)?

Social marketing techniques seek to avoid recourse to legislation where possible, but they do not rule out the possibility of this ultimate sanction where necessary. A key ethical question, however, is when does a situation justify a non-voluntary approach. Traditionally, we have often rushed to 'non-voluntary' solutions when we have not really examined and ruled out effective voluntary encouragements and support. Arguably, it is social marketing's customer understanding and insight that can provide the ethical basis and legitimacy for non-voluntary behaviour change, and this can be especially effective when a public consultation is linked with the development of regulation. A good example of this is the Conversations on Health Consultation in Canada (see http://www.bcconversationonhealth.ca), which gives citizens the opportunity to play an active role in the shaping of their health system.

Being able to examine and rule out the potential of voluntary approaches is key to considering the ethical implications of when to use non-voluntary approaches. Sometimes, a two-tiered approach is necessary: first to enable voluntary change and then to sweep up those who cannot or will not change.

Overriding many of these concerns is the idea of autonomous and free citizens, who, many would argue, should be allowed the freedom to make their own mistakes. A forceful argument for this comes from McDonough and Feinberg in which they articulate the right of the individual to respect:

> you may rank my survival over my autonomy, hoping, perhaps, that once the crisis is over you can persuade me that you have done the right thing. This may be an especially plausible choice if you have a special responsibility for my health [...] But even if you make this choice, it should be clear that you have done so against the weight of an important consideration: respect for me, treating me with dignity, surely entails respect for the reflective choices I make, even when they are mistaken.
>
> (McDonough and Feinberg, 2005, p. 62)

This is perhaps all well and good for an individual, but what happens when your autonomous and libertarian rights of self-determination have a detrimental effect on your fellow citizens? Individuals who indulge in harmful activities like smoking or alcohol abuse divert resources away from essential services. If we cannot, at least at the outset, force people into positive behaviours, then we need to be more effective in understanding them and helping people to change for themselves. Factored into this is the long-held perception, particularly in the area of public health, that individuals actually have direct control of their health-related behaviours (Mann, 1997). Societal determinants and barriers to behavioural change have been largely ignored in favour of awareness-raising campaigns. This would indicate that the individual's rationalization of their own circumstances and decision-making process is not sufficiently informed.

One response to these issues is the idea of a government 'stewardship' model for public health. This recognizes that it is sometimes necessary to intervene in a proportionate fashion when other methods to elicit change have failed. It seeks to be *more sensitive to the need to respect individuality, by seeking the least intrusive way of achieving policy goals* (Nuffield Council on Bioethics, 1997, p. 25). This is ethically perhaps where social marketing finds its role: in that space where paternalism is too strenuous and libertarianism is found wanting in its wider regards for society.

Who should we be trying to reach?

As Chapter 11 sets out, the initial stages of an initiative will involve scoping and background research into the challenge in question. This may involve quantitative and/or qualitative research into targeted demographic samples and groups of people. Immediately, there are considerations to be made about which groups to target with an intervention.

It is a recurring problem: do we go for the long haul and sustainable solution where the results may take months or even years to come to fruition, or do we go for the quick fix and the 'low-hanging fruit'? For example, a programme of behavioural change may be charged with achieving a 10% rise in the number of people engaging in regular physical exercise within a certain area. In certain more affluent areas, this may not be such a difficult goal to achieve. But where does this leave people in the neighbouring postcode with lower living standards, less access to services, and higher levels of obesity? What happens when a national fitness campaign sets out to achieve a 20% increase overall but does nothing to gain insight into the barriers preventing large swathes of the population from getting fit? Of course, the corollary of this problem is that (and we are making general assumptions here) reasonably fit, affluent, and literate people should not be excluded from the opportunity of health improvement. Any group that is excluded from an intervention is going to raise ethical concerns. This may, of course, all be decided by funding and resources.

With limited budgets, it is often the case that we can only tackle the hard-to-reach in a very limited way, or else we have to maximize the outcomes from those who are easier to reach. This is perhaps where it could be argued that social marketing's impetus to explore funding partnerships with wider improvement agendas for hard-to-reach communities comes into its own.

Partnerships

In the UK, the government sees working in partnership as key to *positively influencing people's lifestyle decisions [and] influencing the nation's health* (Department of Health (DH), 2007). In an environment where financial and resource constraints mean that we can rarely, if ever, compete on a level playing field with big business, partnerships are the obvious way to engage them and to tap into their marketing expertise.

This is an area which needs careful consideration. In conducting stakeholder analysis at the scoping stage of an initiative, we may identify a number of potential partnerships with the business sector. What are the risks we face? How ethical are the businesses we are considering?

A good starting point is to explore if there is a robust and active corporate and social responsibility policy. Do they have an active community engagement programme? Do they conduct marketing activity (e.g. marketing to children) which could tarnish public perception of a potential partnership? A recent report commissioned by the NSM Centre suggests several areas which need consideration in order to create a successful partnership (Eagle, 2009):

- Agreement on specific goals
- Relevant complementary expertise
- Long-term benefits for all stakeholders
- Equitable contribution of expertise and resource
- Transparent arrangements
- Agreed ethical codes

Working with business can add significant benefits to an intervention. A good example of an effective partnership is the Big Noise Snack Right Campaign which aims to improve the healthy-snacking behaviours of children under the age of 4 living in deprived areas of north-west England. The ChaMPs Public Health Network formed a partnership with the food retailer Aldi. The retailer had a policy of local supply of fresh produce, had signed up to the Healthy Start scheme, and had planned a campaign to promote fruit and vegetables, on which ChaMPS could 'piggyback'. The director of public health for Knowsley PCT commented *without these partners we just couldn't run this type of campaign* (DH, 2007, p13).

Unintended consequences

We also need to think about the unintended consequences of an intervention. A successful intervention might, e.g. use social marketing techniques to achieve a result in one area that then has a knock-on effect in another. A classic example of this is a smoking-cessation programme which successfully lowers the number of smokers within a particular area only to result in the replacement of one health issue for another. The effects of nicotine as an appetite suppressant are well known. If a significant proportion of these former smokers now become obese, whose fault is it? One might argue that, to the greatest extent possible, good research should leave very few unexplored variables that might lead to unintended consequences. Then there is the issue that the participants of a control group do not receive the benefit of an intervention, which is problematic from an ethical viewpoint. We might argue along utilitarian lines that the 'greater good' is being served, but we are still excluding a section of society from the benefits of the intervention. Of course, this is a problem in many areas and not just social marketing.

Working with the competition

In our efforts to achieve and encourage beneficial behaviour, there will be times when we come up against a different kind of 'competition'. By this, we mean groups that mean well, but whose actions and ethical direction may be at variance with what we are trying to achieve. An example of this might be found in the work of religious groups and their attitude towards contraception and sexual health (e.g. the Catholic Church and condom use). We might both be trying to prevent teenage pregnancies, but whereas part of a social marketing intervention might be to push for better sex education and wider access to sexual health and family-planning resources, the well-meaning competition might be advocating messages that preclude such options. Do we then employ our time in trying to combat their methods or do we seek ways of actively working with them?

As with the other ethical dilemmas we have explored, there is no easy answer to this. We have already stated that the consequentialist approach of social marketing really means that we are accountable to the greater societal good rather than working to appease minority interests and harmful behaviour that may be informed by other moral or religious frameworks. We need to be sensitive, flexible, and constructive in our approach to these conflicts of interest, but this does provide an opportunity to be creative and to really put to good use the insight gained into the motivators, barriers, and circumstances of the audiences we need to reach.

Facing facts

It is a fact that tackling certain behaviours 'safely' may require the acceptance of illegal or socially unacceptable social behaviours (e.g. drug and alcohol misuse). Good examples of this are high-profile interventions like the UK government campaign *FRANK* (www.talktofrank.com) and *Road Crew* (which we will examine later), which acknowledge that people take illegal drugs and drink excessively. OD999 (www.od999.org), an effective intervention to prevent drug addicts from overdosing in the north-west of England, even has its helpline number printed on drug paraphernalia and promises not to disclose caller details to the police. These interventions take a pragmatic approach to some of our biggest problems, which in the eyes of some is tantamount to acceptance and almost acquiescence. This 'if you are going to do it, at least be informed about it' message has been highly effective but is unpalatable to certain sections of society.

Segmentation

Much like commercial marketers, social marketers will frequently look to segment audiences to target particular groups for an intervention (see Chapters 7 and 12). There are sophisticated tools available that allow us to build up detailed pictures of particular groups by different shared characteristics and help us to ensure that resources are most effectively placed. From an ethical standpoint, this throws up yet more problems for those looking to reach certain groups.

It is sometimes the case that the outcome of targeting certain groups might result in their stigmatization. They might have been identified as the cause or the victims of a certain behaviour, which may then result in them being ostracized or disadvantaged in comparison with other groups. This is already evident to some degree in the general population, where the political 'hot potatoes' of obesity and smoking have seen attempts to marginalize the groups involved. Sensitivity to the needs of these groups needs to be of paramount consideration when putting an intervention in place.

By its very nature, segmentation means that some groups are not going to receive the benefits of certain targeted programmes and interventions.

Ethics in practice

Example: Road Crew intervention, USA

In order to provide a practical exploration of the ethical issues around social marketing, we are going to examine a controversial intervention that has become a lightning rod for debates on this issue. Road Crew has been used on countless occasions and in many publications as a case study, but it is worth re-examining for the purposes of looking at the ethical questions and concerns that it still continues to raise.

The Road Crew intervention was launched in Wisconsin in the USA in 2001 by the National Highway Traffic Safety Administration. Cited as a community-based programme designed to reduce alcohol-related car crashes, the main aim was to achieve a 5% reduction in alcohol-related crashes within certain pilot areas. These areas were struggling with spiralling rates of accidents and fatalities, caused predominantly and disproportionately by young, male drink-drivers between 21 and 34 years of age. The objective was to be achieved via a 'ride service', which would give intoxicated drivers a ride home after a night of drinking. But a strategy had to be formulated to sell the idea to the target audience.

Comprehensive research was carried out. A literature review was conducted of 178 studies of drink-driving which were undertaken between 1996 and 1999. Focus groups were conducted with both expert observers of the target groups and with the target groups themselves to learn about pervading attitudes, values, and processes. Brand-name testing was undertaken to find something that would resonate with and engage the target audience, and partnerships were formed with local organizations and businesses. An ongoing programme of follow-up surveys were undertaken in order to evaluate the effectiveness of the programme (Road Crew, 2008).

What this resulted in was a service through which young male drinkers are picked up by chauffeur-driven limousines and transported between bars in the local area. They are then driven home again at the end of the evening.

According to an updated report at the end of 2007:

> As of September 30, 2007, Road Crew has given over 85,000 rides, and has prevented an estimated 140 alcohol-related crashes and six alcohol related fatalities. The costs incurred from an alcohol-related crash are approximately $231,000, but the cost to avoid a crash through the use of Road Crew is approximately $6200. This means that it is about 37 times more expensive to incur a crash than it is to avoid a crash. Total net savings through the use of Road Crew has been about $31 million.
>
> (Rothschild, 2006)

Road Crew fulfils nearly all of the social marketing benchmark criteria (see Chapter 3): it has met or exceeded all of its targets; it is saving lives; it is cost-effective; and it has produced a self-sustaining programme.

So where exactly is the ethical problem?

For many, the sticking point comes when looking at the bigger picture. Road Crew does nothing to address the behaviour which led to the problem in the first place. Young men are still drinking to an excess which leads to many other consequences. This culture of drinking is not addressed in any way, and neither are the peripheral issues such as alcoholism and the wide range of health issues, domestic violence, and possible economic problems due to sick days and lost productivity. In fact, we could ask whether the intervention is just encouraging a greater number of people to drink.

It must be stressed that Road Crew was not asked to tackle any problem over and above its mandate to cut alcohol-related driving accidents. But when involved in trying to do social good, can we ethically ignore the knock-on effect that our interventions might lead to? Indeed, are we actually doing any real good if we are encouraging and facilitating one set of bad behaviours in order to mitigate another?

There is also a wider issue that is worthy of scrutiny: one of the major partnerships in this scheme was Miller Brewing, the second largest brewer in the USA. Road Crew, as Gerard Hastings suggests, seemed to allow the people who would normally be seen as the competition to have a direct and unfettered channel to a set of their customers:

> From a competitive perspective it also enables the brewery to promote its products as actively as ever, with an undesirable implication that getting drunk is both acceptable and fun.
>
> (Hastings, 2007, p. 171)

Looking at this from an ethically neutral point of view, the intervention has achieved its purpose. But we have to ask again whether social marketing allows us ever to be neutral, if we are aligning ourselves with the notion of social good? What we may in fact be looking at here is the uncomfortable – and to some unpalatable – idea that lives may have been saved in one arena of public concern, only to have other potentially damaging or fatal problems moved into another behind closed doors. It is entirely possible that Road Crew has merely resulted in a displacement of undesirable behaviour for someone else to sort out.

Another area of concern is the disquieting feeling that interventions like this help give legitimacy to the corporate social responsibility agendas of companies that do not make easy bedfellows with public health and behavioural change interventions. This is not to place corporations into the normally dichotomous relationship with social good; there are plenty of examples of socially responsible corporations. But the very idea of linking a brewery into a programme that then allows the target audience to seemingly drink with impunity would raise questions in the broadest of minds.

The Road Crew intervention merits considerable reflection because of its controversial nature. There are few purer examples of social marketing that we can call upon that exhibit all the benchmarks of success while at the same time eliciting such cries of alarm and discomfort when presented to health professionals. Yet, to a degree, Road Crew does set out to do a great social good in preventing accidents, road deaths, and associated societal costs and impacts. It has sustained itself to date and has become established over a growing area. For all that, the best we can really say is: as an intervention it did exactly what it was asked to do, but it does not really stand up to close scrutiny from an ethical viewpoint. For some, one life saved might be enough to justify such an approach, but for many others a more balanced approach would have been desirable.

An ethical checklist

Social marketing is not a part of a social control agenda, and to be seen to be above such accusations we must ensure that there are ethical checks and balances at every stage of the process of behavioural intervention – from scoping through to evaluation. In order to provide a framework for a practical code of ethics for social marketing, we will finish with an attempt at formulating an ethical checklist. As a starting point, Laczniak and Murphy (1993) suggest that the following questions be asked in order to ethically assess an intervention:

- Is it legal?
- Is it contrary to society's generally accepted moral obligations?
- Is it contrary to moral obligations that are specific to that particular organization?

- Is the intent harmful?
- Is the result harmful?
- Is there an alternative action that produces equal or better benefits, and by implication, will cause fewer negative consequences?
- Will it infringe on the rights of the organization's stakeholders?
- Will it leave any person or group poorer? Will it especially reduce the well-being of an already underprivileged group?

These are a useful starting point for consideration, but to these we should add our own list which encompasses the areas of concern we have looked:

What are the right behaviours for people?	Who decides, on what evidence, what are the counter-arguments (e.g. freedom of choice)?
Who should we target?	For example, a small number of hard-to-reach, vulnerable society or large number of more accessible people?
Shouldn't the control group benefit?	What are the consequences regarding increasing inequality? What is fair?
Will the target group be stigmatized?	If so, what care should we take in messaging/targeting to minimize?
Should we deal with the voice of competition?	What are the dilemmas (ethical benefits and risks) of working with competition?
Should there be informed consent?	For regulatory actions and limiting behaviours by laws, how much should we enable consultation?
How does the intervention impact on inequalities?	Does the intervention have the potential to increase inequalities in health/access to services, for example? How can this be minimized?
Might there be any unintended outcomes or knock-on effects?	Will the intervention impact other areas that we need to be aware of; is it just displacing a problem?

Conclusion

We have looked at the various ethical issues surrounding behavioural interventions and have hopefully identified some of the potential questions, quandaries and stumbling blocks that might be encountered. Armed with a sense of exactly what we need to do, and the ethical impulses behind it, it is possible to have a clearer sense of purpose and the means to justify our efforts to stakeholders, to our partners and to those we are attempting to help. As our case study has shown, you can have a high level of success in reaching your behavioural goals, but this does not guarantee that everybody will be happy with the ethical makeup of your intervention. What can be done to limit and to mitigate any possible ethical conflicts and problems is to be rigorous in the planning stages and to take into account as many ethical variables as possible in as transparent a manner as possible. The suggested ethical checklist is merely one attempt to aid in this process.

Social marketing is about sustained, long-term behavioural change. As such, we might say that short-term solutions are not solutions at all but are merely the deferment of a problem, surely an unethical position in itself? To get a short-term result may fulfil the requirements of fiscal or even political expediency, but it might also be deemed to be an abdication of our responsibility to do lasting and effective social good.

Ethical considerations should be as intrinsic and fundamental to social marketing interventions as customer insight, exchange theory, and all the other facets which we use to define the discipline. Debates over libertarianism, paternalism, personal freedoms, and 'nanny-stateism' will continue. But in attempting to address some of society's most pressing problems, social marketing tries to tread the difficult middle ground between respecting the rights of individuals as actors in their own lives and the responsibility of government to act as steward of the well-being of the nation.

Review exercise

Review an intervention that you are working on, or have worked on in the past, and use the ethical checklist to consider the ethical implications of the project. How would/did you address any contentious issues that arose from your intervention?

References

Andreasen, A. (2001). *Ethics in Social Marketing*. Washington DC: Georgetown University Press.

Cribb, A. and Duncan, P. (2002). Introducing ethics to health promotion, in Bunton, R. and MacDonald, G. (eds.) *Health Promotion: Disciplines, Diversity, and Development*. London: Routledge.

Department of Health (2007) *Partnerships for better health*. London: Department of Health. Available at: http://www.dh.gov.uk/en/Publicationsandstatistics/Publications/PublicationsPolicyAndGuidance/DH_075758 (Acessed 23 January 2009).

Donovan, R. and Henley, N. (2003). *Social Marketing: Principles and Practice*. Melbourne: IP Communications.

Eagle, L. (2009). *Social Marketing Ethics*. London: National Social Marketing Centre.

Encarta Online Dictionary Available at: http://encarta.msn.com/dictionary_/ethics.html (Accessed 15 January 2008).

Furedi, F. (11.9.06). *Save us from the politics of behaviour*. Available at: http://www.spiked-online.com/index.php?/site/printable/1638 (Accessed 22 January 2008).

Hastings, G. (2007). *Social Marketing: Why Should the Devil Have All the Best Tunes?* Oxford: Butterworth-Heinemann.

Kotler, P. and Lee, N. (2008). *Social Marketing: Influencing Behaviors for Good*. Thousand Oaks, CA: Sage Publications.

Laczniak, G. et al. (1979). Social marketing: its ethical dimensions. *Journal of Marketing*, 43(2): Spring, 29–36.

Laczniak, G. and Murphy, P. (1993). *Ethical Marketing Decisions: the Higher Road*. Boston, MA: Allyn and Bacon.

Mann, J. (1997). Medicine and public health, ethics and human rights. *The Hastings Center Report* 27(3) Available at: http://www.questia.com/PM.qst?a=o&d=5002240458 (Accessed 24 January 2008).

McDonough, K. and Feinberg, W. (2005). *Citizenship and Education in Liberal-Democratic Societies: Teaching for Cosmopolitan Values and Collective Identities*. Oxford: Oxford University Press.

National Social Marketing Centre. (2007). *Big Pocket Guide to Social Marketing*, Second Edition. London: National Social Marketing Centre.

Nuffield Council on Bioethics. (2007). *Public Health: Ethical Issues*. Nuffield Council on Bioethics. Available at: http://www.nuffieldbioethics.org/go/ourwork/publichealth/publication_451.html (Accessed 23 January 2009).

Rothschild, M. (2001). *Ethics in Social Marketing*. Washington DC: Georgetown University Press.

Road Crew Research Report. Available at: http://www.roadcrewonline.org/research (Accessed 28 January 2008).

Rothschild, M., Mastin, B., and Miller, T. (2006). *The impact of road crew on crashes, fatalities, and costs*. Available at: http://www.roadcrewonline.org/files/researchpaper.pdf (Accessed 26 January 2009).

Chapter 10

The Total Process Planning (TPP) Framework

Denise Ong and Clive Blair-Stevens

Here is Edward Bear, coming downstairs, now, bump, bump, bump, on the back of his head behind Christopher Robin. It is as far as he knows the only way of coming downstairs, but somewhere he feels there is another way, if only he could stop for a moment and think of it.
A. A. Milne

Learning points

This chapter

- Introduces key principles of planning in the context of the Total Process Planning (TPP) framework;
- Considers how a five-stage framework can be a powerful approach to organize and manage the complexity involved in developing a programme, campaign, or intervention;
- Emphasizes that planning should always be about the people and stakeholders involved, helping them engage and contribute effectively, rather than being perceived as a separate technical exercise;
- Discusses how, while planning needs to be systematic and phased, it should also allow flexible, creative, and innovative approaches to be properly managed;
- Emphasizes the importance of undertaking proper Scoping, so that issues, resources, and interventional options are properly considered prior to development; and
- Considers the two critical success factors in planning:
  - Investing time and effort in a proper scoping stage
  - Ensuring the process of planning engages and mobilizes the relevant people/stakeholders

Chapter overview

This chapter introduces the Total Process Planning (TPP) framework (Blair-Stevens and French, 2005) – a simple but robust framework to support effective intervention planning, development and delivery of interventions. It draws on thinking and learning from two key areas:

a) established programme- and project-planning methods and approaches; and

b) behavioural intervention and social marketing-related intervention planning.

By the end of the chapter you should have a clear overview of the value of using a simple and straightforward framework for helping systematically manage the potential complexity involved with working through intervention planning, development, and delivery tasks. You should recognize that planning is about engaging and mobilizing people, taking them on a journey, and ensuring they can contribute effectively at each relevant stage.

Introduction

There are always different ways to plan and develop a programme, campaign, or intervention. This will be heavily influenced by a range of factors, such as:

- the type and complexity of the behavioural challenge being addressed;
- the level of resources and assets available (people and finance); and
- the social and political context at the time.

Inevitably this means that all planning processes need to be flexible and iterative since requirements and needs commonly develop and change over time.

Even a cursory look at the literature on planning surfaces a plethora of different planning approaches, models, tools, or frameworks to consider. Deciding which one to use in any given situation can be difficult. It is nevertheless possible to identify some key principles and common factors that assist and support effective planning. The Total Process Planning (TPP) summarized here is based on recognizing these common features and providing a framework within which some of the complexity and need to tailor tasks can be properly managed.

Distinguishing between planning 'Framework', 'Process', and 'Tools'

Before looking at the TPP framework itself it is useful to consider it within a wider context, and to distinguish between a planning 'Framework', a planning 'Process', and different planning 'Tools' (see Fig. 10.1).

The TPP is the first of these, a planning 'Framework'. It provides an overarching and sound structure for managing the planning process and for considering and staging the specific tasks that will be required. A planning 'Process' is how, within the framework, any key tasks necessary are scheduled and planned as a specific process. As such it always needs to be adjusted and tailored to the expectations, context, and resources available. Finally, planning 'Tools' are various practical resources to assist in the analysis and development of specific tasks and stages, and which commonly need to be adapted to the specific topic and context they are being used in. A list of useful planning tools can be downloaded from the National Social Marketing (NSM) Centre's website (http://nsmcentre.org.uk).

Distinguishing between a Conceptual Model (cycle) and a Planning Framework (linear)

It is possible to approach and present the five key stages of TPP both as 'a conceptual model' and also as 'a planning framework'. Shown as a conceptual model, TPP can be represented as a cycle, see Fig. 10.2. This can be appealing for those who like the idea that this shows the stages as more of a dynamic cycle. However, while it is acknowledged that some may find the initial representation of TPP as a more linear process problematic, we have done this specifically to indicate that this is not being shown conceptually but as a planning framework. Effective planning is ultimately about managing a progression through time, since we are all essentially living and operating within an essentially temporal world.

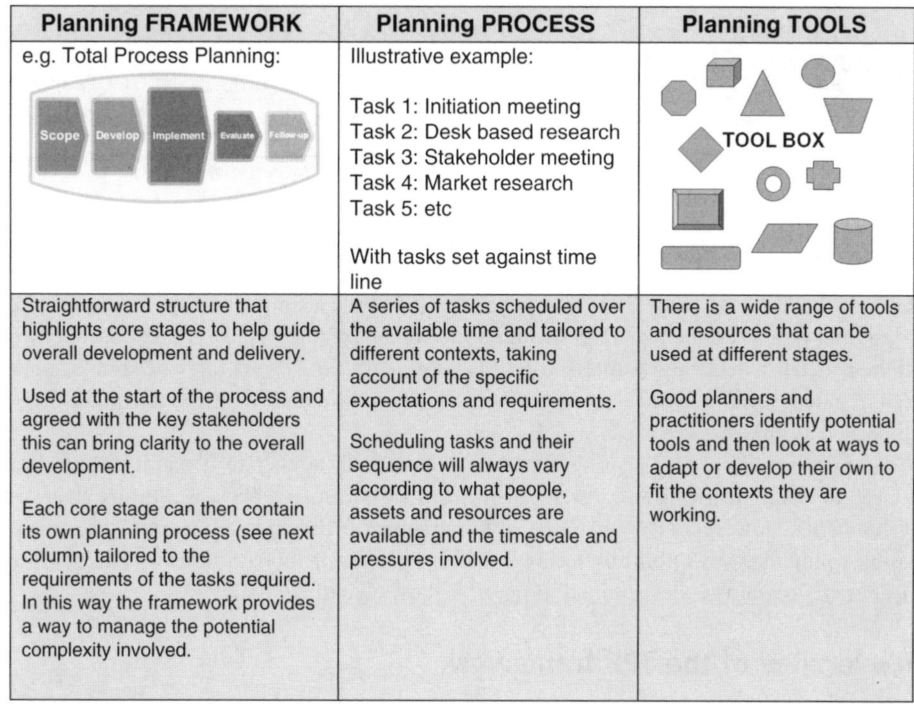

Planning FRAMEWORK	Planning PROCESS	Planning TOOLS
e.g. Total Process Planning: Scope, Develop, Implement, Evaluate, Follow-up	Illustrative example: Task 1: Initiation meeting Task 2: Desk based research Task 3: Stakeholder meeting Task 4: Market research Task 5: etc With tasks set against time line	TOOL BOX
Straightforward structure that highlights core stages to help guide overall development and delivery. Used at the start of the process and agreed with the key stakeholders this can bring clarity to the overall development. Each core stage can then contain its own planning process (see next column) tailored to the requirements of the tasks required. In this way the framework provides a way to manage the potential complexity involved.	A series of tasks scheduled over the available time and tailored to different contexts, taking account of the specific expectations and requirements. Scheduling tasks and their sequence will always vary according to what people, assets and resources are available and the timescale and pressures involved.	There is a wide range of tools and resources that can be used at different stages. Good planners and practitioners identify potential tools and then look at ways to adapt or develop their own to fit the contexts they are working.

Fig. 10.1 Planning frameworks, processes, and tools.

Source: Blair-Stevens, 2008.

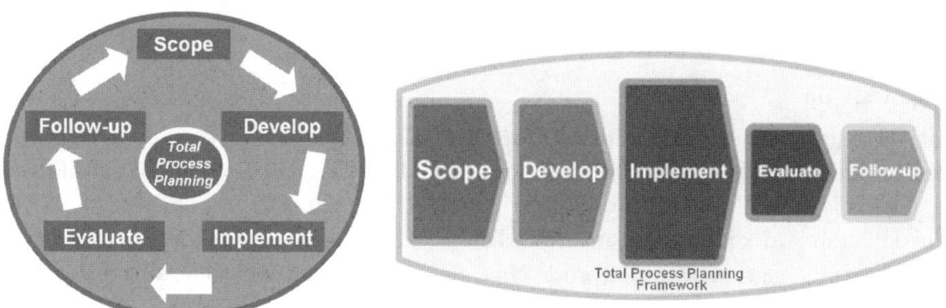

Fig. 10.2 TPP represented as a conceptual model and a planning framework.

Source: Blair-Stevens and French, 2005.

Approaching a linear representation as a strength not a weakness

When models are presented in a linear way, it is easy to criticize them as being unrealistic and impractical since we commonly operate in complex and variable environments, where simple sequential processes are rarely achievable. The TPP was developed recognizing this and while the core stages are shown in this linear way, the processes and tasks within individual stages are much more organic and flexible. This is because often the tasks required have to be undertaken in parallel with each interlinking at different stages and informing the other. An illustration of this would be considering tasks involved in behavioural analysis and in segmentation, and trying to answer the

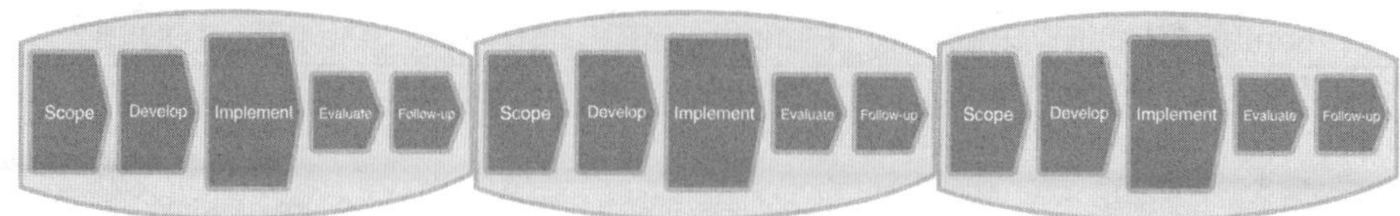

Fig. 10.3 Using the TPP framework to inform future scoping and development work.

question which should come first? In practice there is rarely a simple answer. The behavioural analysis may be a way to help segment an audience. Equally, segmenting an audience properly can help more detailed behavioural analysis of the key segments. Initial work often needs to be undertaken in parallel and then fed into each other in a more fluid and iterative way rather than be approached as rigid steps or stages.

One of the benefits of representing something conceptually as 'a cycle' is that it helps focus on the need to ensure learning and development from work can feed back into future stages and developments. However, even where the TPP framework is shown as a linear process, it is still possible to highlight this point by seeing linked campaigns or interventions forming part of a longer-term programme-development process, as illustrated in Fig. 10.3.

An overview of the TPP framework

The TPP framework has five primary stages.

1. Scoping
2. Developing
3. Implementing
4. Evaluating
5. Following-up

While these stages should be considered as sequential (as discussed above), the way tasks within each stage are undertaken requires a much more flexible and pragmatic approach, albeit handled in a systematic way.

The TPP framework is based on an acknowledgement that there are a number of different ways to undertake, manage, and develop work. No single checklist or tool will be able to cover every situation.

While many planning guides already exist, in practice, few people actually follow a guide as it is written. Inevitably the behavioural challenges being addressed can vary tremendously in complexity and scale and therefore it will always be important for people to tailor their approaches according to the particular circumstances and timeframes they are working within, in addition to drawing upon their own expertise.

The TPP framework takes this into account, and provides an adaptable approach within which more complex tasks and components can be effectively managed.

A short summary of how the TPP framework was developed

The development of the TTP framework (Blair-Stevens and French, 2005) came out of reviewing two distinct and important areas of learning:

1. programme- and project-planning methodologies and best practice principles; and
2. behavioural intervention- and social marketing-related planning and staging approaches.

These areas were explored as part of a government-commissioned independent review undertaken to examine effective behavioural intervention and social marketing approaches in England between 2005 and 2006 and subsequently published as *'It's Our Health!'* (NSM Centre, 2006). Through undertaking the review, it became apparent that there was a need to bring together and integrate learning from the two key areas of learning identified above.

The relationship between 'task' and 'process'

It is possible in looking at the different planning models and approaches presented across the diverse area of behavioural intervention and social marketing literature to see a strong focus on 'task' and how to 'stage' and 'plan' these over time. Such literature often places less focus on the handling of the overall and specific processes required – a consideration much more evident in the wider programme and planning literature. The TPP framework therefore seeks to bring these two areas together by providing a way of integrating the principles drawn from planning and managing work (in any context) together with those from behavioural intervention- and social marketing-related task planning.

Keeping the focus on engaging and mobilizing people, not just technical task completion

Ultimately the TPP framework recognizes that effective planning is essentially about engaging and mobilizing people rather than simply undertaking and managing a series of tasks. When done effectively, planning should help people engage and contribute successfully to the intervention. A common criticism when planning fails is that the people involved did not fully understand what they were part of, or why tasks were being undertaken, and therefore could not engage effectively or appropriately. In practice few people/stakeholders will be involved in a programme, project, or intervention from start to finish. Therefore, only relatively few people will actually have a full picture of all the tasks and components of the work as a whole.

On longer-term programmes where people can change and move on, there may sometimes be no-one with a complete picture and history of the full process. This highlights the importance of ensuring people can engage effectively at different stages, and understanding how what they are part of fits within a wider framework approach. People rarely need the detail, but they do need to understand the context and rationale involved to help them focus on the task or stage they are being asked to contribute to. This can significantly maximize the potential of their contributions to be valuable and appropriate to the overall development process. Ultimately this also helps support knowledge transfer and ensures that as people come and go within a wider programme the overall process is not lost.

The five primary stages of the TPP framework

The following provides an overview of the five primary stages of the TPP framework. Subsequent chapters expand on this and provide examples of the type of work within specific stages:

1. Scoping

- Examining the issue or challenge.
- Building an understanding of both the lives of the audience(s) involved, and specific relevant behaviours.
- Identifying and mobilizing available human and financial resources (or those that could be leveraged).

- Assessing and selecting options that are most likely to have a positive impact on the lives of those being addressed.
- **Primary output: a scoping report.**
- **Primary outcome: a decision on which intervention(s) to take into the Development stage.**

2. Developing

- Where the behavioural goals and audience insights gained during scoping are developed into a programme, campaign, or intervention.
- Includes specific pre-testing of ideas with the audience(s).
- Checking that the evidence, insights, and assumptions being made are relevant and actionable.
- **Key output: a development/marketing plan.**

3. Implementing

- The stage when things 'go live' (what this involves will necessarily vary according to what intervention approaches and methods were selected from the original Scoping & Development phases).
- Including an active process of live tracking, including:
  - opportunity spotting – looking for additional opportunities that might arise; and
  - risk watching and managing any potential threats that could undermine the intervention.
- **Key output: relevant interventions or 'products/services'.**

4. Evaluating

- Where the original aims and objectives of the work are revisited.
- Data and views collated on the impacts of the work.
- Evaluating process, impact, and cost-effectiveness.
- **Key output: the formal evaluation report.**

5. Following-up

- Where the results of any formal commissioned evaluation are specifically considered with:
  - those who have contributed – so they have a chance to comment on them;
  - wider stakeholders with an interest in the issue; and
  - key funders or decision-makers – to consider implications for the longer-term strategy and any potential follow-up work.
- Where proper consideration is given to thanking and demonstrating appreciation of the efforts and contributions of those involved e.g.: 'thanking strategies' (this is particularly important even where the impact of work may not have been immediately successful, since being able to continue to mobilize stakeholders will be crucial to future work).
- Where active consideration is given to communicating the learning from work to date, including writing up the work for articles and journals and getting on to potential databases.
- **Key output 1: articles and papers – promoting learning.**
- **Key output 2: recommendations and proposals for further work.**

Ensuring a systematic approach and avoiding the 'bear-traps'

The simplicity of the TPP framework should not be misinterpreted: in practice, keeping the framework simple and on track can be quite challenging. When reviewing how people take planning models and approaches and use and apply them in practice it is possible to identify some common bear-traps that should be avoided. These include:

1. undertaking no or only partial scoping, in a rush to progress to the development stage
2. putting creative communications before customer understanding and insight
3. seeing evaluation as just a stage and not a 'mind-set' through-out
4. not having a clear follow-up stage, leaving the evaluation report on the shelf, and failing to embed the learning into future work

Bear-trap 1: Undertaking no or only partial scoping, in a rush to progress to the development stage

Enthusiasm, experience, and pressure from funders can all put pressure on people to 'get going' before proper scoping has been done. Sometimes experienced and skilled people feel they already know the issues and therefore can bypass this stage and start developing the intervention. A simple example of this is the all too common rush to develop a communications awareness raising campaign 'to be seen to be doing something' before any one has really examined whether 'communicating a message' is likely to play a key role in influencing the behaviour.

Bear-trap 2: Putting creative communications before customer understanding and insight

While encouraging creativity and innovation should be an essential part of good programme, campaign, or intervention development, there can be a tendency for people to get caught up in clever and creative communications ideas and lose sight of the need to ensure all work is grounded in sound understanding and insight into what will move and motivate people. Proper investment of time and effort in scoping helps to avoid this and ensures where creative and innovative approaches are proposed they can be based on a strong audience/customer understanding and insight.

Bear-trap 3: Seeing evaluation as just a stage and not a 'mind-set' throughout

While evaluating is included in the TPP framework as a primary stage this does not mean it is only approached at that point. In fact one of the central reasons for undertaking proper scoping at the start is to ensure the rationale for proposing a particular method or interventional approach can be clearly and transparently identified at the very start. This allows appropriate baseline criteria and related data to be put in place that will then assist later evaluation and review. It can be tempting to see evaluation as a specialist skill that can be brought in, by perhaps commissioning an academic institution or other body to undertake, and not as a key underpinning 'mind-set' that needs to be part of the way the whole planning framework and processes are managed. Setting out the rationale for intervention option selection during scoping is a key support to effective evaluation, as is the crafting of clear aims and SMART objectives during the developmental stage.

Bear-trap 4: Not having a clear follow-up stage, leaving the evaluation report on the shelf, and failing to embed the learning into future work

In practice, it is common for the greatest efforts to focus on the developing and implementing stages, with evaluation 'tacked on' at the end and little proper handling of any follow-up stage to capture and embed the learning. This is a mistake, since all work needs to be seen in its wider context and timeframe. Most significant behaviours require sustained action in order not simply to promote adoption or change of behaviour but to maintain this over time. Having a dedicated follow-up stage is therefore a key factor. If handled well it provides an invaluable opportunity for stakeholders, and particularly key decision-makers/funders to examine the formal evaluation findings and to question and consider the findings. It is not uncommon for different stakeholders to have different views about the relevance or appropriateness of formal evaluation findings – capturing this at the end is invaluable in not leaving the formal evaluation report as the only record of the work. Without doing this, particularly where there may be disagreements, the pressure to leave the report on the shelf and move on and not embed the learning is strong. A proper follow-up stage therefore helps value people who were involved in the process and redirect attention onto how the learning from work undertaken can then be used to inform further work.

The value of investing in scoping

- Proper consideration is given to the people who need to be engaged and mobilized as part of the process (often needing to change within different stages).
- The presenting issue or challenge is properly assessed and the analysis of this is summarized to help people at all subsequent stages understand the rationale. underpinning the work being progressed, and to facilitate formal evaluation.
- The range of intervention options (and approaches) are properly considered, given the available resources – the balance or mix of interventions thought most likely to achieve and help sustain the desired behaviour.
- Ethical and practical implications of agreeing a particular intervention mix can be considered prior to moving into Development with these.
- The sharing and maximizing of learning. Handled well scoping can ensure the analysis underpinning the work can be made readily available to others maximizing its value. For example:
  - access to the analysis work of national programmes can be hugely helpful to smaller scale local programmes and help to ensure greater consistency, linking and integrating national and regional approaches; and
  - it helps reduce wasteful duplications of effort, a literature review undertaken by a national programme can save time and effort of local programmes having to reproduce the same task.

Conclusion

The literature on social marketing reveals a variety of different planning approaches. The TPP framework has been able to draw from these, and alongside the learning from established programme and project planning, provides a robust and flexible framework within which often complex sets of tasks can be effective managed and developed. While its initial presentation as five linear stages can appear simplistic, the integrity of the framework allows for a flexible and adaptable tailoring of plans and tasks to be able to respond to a diverse range of contexts and behaviours.

Effectively managing the complexity of tasks in a clear and transparent way can significant improve engagement of stakeholders and others throughout the process. Helping people appreciate what stage within the planning process they are in at any one time maximizes the ability to harness their efforts and contributions. Ultimately the TPP framework is a way of managing the complexity involved while keeping the overall drive of the work moving forward within a bounded framework.

Review exercise

Think about a project you have worked on in the past, or have come across in the literature. Sketch out the planning process used against the five stages of the Total Process Planning (TPP) framework. How similar (or dissimilar) was the process used? At which stage(s) was most time and effort spent? Consider how you might apply each of the five TPP stages in a project you are currently or will be working on.

References

National Social Marketing Centre (2006). *It's Our Health!* London: National Social Marketing Centre.

Chapter 11

Scoping

Lucy Reynolds and Rowena Merritt

Diligence is the mother of good luck.
Benjamin Franklin

Learning points

This chapter

- Provides a practical introduction to the scoping phases of social marketing;
- Outlines the processes, objectives, and outcomes involved in this phase; and
- Introduces key concepts, including customer insight, research, and audience segmentation.

Chapter overview

The first stage of the Total Process Planning (TPP) framework is 'scoping'. By the end of this chapter you will be familiar with the key components of the scoping stage and feel confident moving forwards into the second stage: 'development'.

Aims of scoping stage

- To consider and decide which intervention option(s) to progress
- To lay foundations for subsequent work

Objectives of the scoping stage

- To examine the issue or challenge
- To build understanding, of both the lives of the audience(s), and their behaviours
- To identify and mobilize available human and financial resources (or those that could be leveraged)

Primary output

- A scoping report

Introduction

'Scoping' is the first stage of the Total Process Planning (TPP) framework. It can be described as the most important single stage in any social marketing project and can make the difference between a powerful intervention that has strong, tangible impacts, and one that is ill-conceived and ineffective. The primary purpose of scoping is to examine and decide on which intervention(s) to take into the development stage, based on a sound understanding of the audience and their correct behaviours.

The scoping stage is all about building relationships with stakeholders, planning your project, collecting information, and making judgements which will drive the project forwards into the developmental stage. It is important to recognize that there is no single 'correct' way to go about scoping, as the scale, topic, resources and time available will vary in different contexts. However in the following chapter we set out key issues to consider, and propose a three phase approach.

The three phases of scoping

The scoping stage divides roughly into three phases. By progressing through these three phases, you will set secure foundations for your initiative. Not only will you gain an in-depth appreciation of the issue you are addressing, but you will also get insight into your 'customer' so that you understand:

- which segment of your target audience you will focus on;
- what moves and motivates them; and
- which barriers or incentives might prompt the positive behaviour you seek.

Further in this chapter, we provide a brief overview of the three phases. This is followed by a more in-depth discussion of the various steps required for successful scoping.

Phase 1

In the first phase of scoping you will form a steering group to oversee your social marketing project. Having done so, you will collect all the information that already exists about:

- the behaviour you are addressing;
- the locality you are working in; and
- the people you wish to influence.

It is advisable to synthesize all the data (as it is often voluminous) and write the findings up as a short report. This will help you identify any 'knowledge gaps' (areas where information is lacking) which remain after the collection of secondary data.

For example, the behaviour you wish to address may be the number of people currently using local stop-smoking services. By looking at local attendance figures, you may identify that middle-aged men are the group who use these services least. However, you may have no information available to tell you *why* these men are not using the service or how you might encourage them to do so.

In this phase of scoping you will also need to identify stakeholders you wish to engage in your initiative. You will aim to rank relevant stakeholders in terms of their influence over, and interest in, the project, and to engage them accordingly.

Phase 2

In Phase 2 you will build on the research findings from Phase 1 and, if necessary, fill any knowledge gaps with primary research (new research for a specific purpose). You will also do an asset mapping exercise to identify services, groups, or initiatives that are already operating in your area. By finding out about existing products and services (including when, where, and how they operate and who uses them), you will be able to identify potential sources of competition for your intervention and valuable opportunities for 'piggybacking' existing schemes.

Phase 3

Decision time! Where you consider and gain agreement for which intervention(s) to take into the next development stage. Here, you will roll together the findings from Phase 1 and Phase 2 to create a comprehensive overview of the situation. You will make informed decisions about the audience you will target and the intervention(s) that are likely to be most successful. You will also write a scoping report, outlining your research findings and key insights and suggesting which ideas will be taken forwards into the developmental stage.

Phase 1

Set up a steering group

The first task is to establish a steering group of people who will work with and support you for the duration of the social marketing process. The group will be made up of individuals who will take collective responsibility for the project: they will manage the process right the way through, drive things forwards, and ensure deadlines are met. It is advisable to keep the steering group reasonably small (between five and seven people). If you have colleagues or stakeholders who are very interested in the project but do not have time to commit to pushing the project forwards, it is preferable to involve them in the solution group rather than the steering group.

The steering group can be made up of individuals from inside or outside your own organization. They might be from the local authority, the county council, the primary care trust or the private sector – it will be up to you to consider who is most appropriate. It is important, however, to invite individuals who will bring a range of skills, experience, and relevant contacts to your project.

At the steering group's first meeting, you will develop a clear project plan, outlining your working budget and setting guide timescales. You will also define clear roles and responsibilities and allocate the work required to complete Phase 1 of scoping. Table 11.1 provides examples of how individual skills can translate into Phase 1 responsibilities.

If you do not have people in your steering group who can actually collect additional information, you may need to commission an external researcher to carry out certain elements, such as qualitative research, with the target audience. If this is the case, include this in your budget,

Table 11.1 Making the most of steering-group expertise

Individual's skills/knowledge	Phase 1 responsibility
Project management	Overseeing delivery
Knowledge of relevant stakeholders	Providing a full list of stakeholders to involve
Access to baseline behaviour figures	Providing baseline and other statistics
Knowledge of local service provision and uptake	Providing information on local assets and services
Contact with local community	Finding out as much as possible from the community itself
Knowledge of policy	Reporting on the policy context and flagging up previous or planned changes

and try to ensure that you have someone with experience in commissioning research sitting on the group. Be realistic about how much high-quality research costs. It may seem expensive, but conducting the research in-house can be unsuccessful as people may lack the relevant research skills and time to complete the final report. Poorly conducted research can be very misleading!

The steering group should meet at least once a month to report back on progress and keep the project moving forwards. At each meeting you should clarify who is doing what and when they are doing it by, and you should reiterate the final deadline for completion of scoping.

Review of the secondary research

You will rely on 'secondary data' to find out as much as possible about your target audience as quickly and easily as possible. That is to say, you will look for existing information that has been compiled for other reasons, but which is relevant to your own project. To find this secondary data, you may need to trawl through: data on the web, published literature in journals, newspapers, consumer surveys, national statistics, and data collected by government departments – in fact, anything you can think of that might be useful in providing an initial picture about the scope of the issue, the probable target audience, the competition, and previous attempts to tackle the issue. It is also valuable to interview key stakeholders who will be able to explain the issue from their viewpoint.

When looking at the secondary evidence, go further than just including data on spread and control of health issues (epidemiological data) and population (demographic data). Include data that can help build a picture of the target audience and their lifestyle. For example, information about people's shopping patterns collected by the commercial sector may be a valuable source of insight. Similarly, information with regards to social trends will enable you to work with, rather than against, social norms and trends. If you are working with limited resources to reduce teenage pregnancy rates, and you know that trends show the age of first consent is going down, you might choose to work *with* the behavioural trend by promoting safe sexual practices, rather than swimming against the tide and trying to promote abstinence or delay of sexual initiation.

Some of the most useful data may be qualitative in nature. However, finding qualitative research can be difficult (Dixon-Woods et al., 2001), as it is not usually indexed as well as quantitative research. Qualitative research is also often catalogued in the less well-known databases. However, the situation is improving and valuable insights can be gained from qualitative research. Some evidence may not be published, but it may be available on search engines which specialize in grey literature (printed reports, unpublished but circulated papers, unpublished proceedings of conferences, and printed programmes from conferences) such as System for Information Grey Literature in Europe Archives (SIGLE). A list of some commonly used search engines is given in Box 11.1.

Some of the information you find may be outdated, and some of it may not quite be relevant to the issue you are addressing. However, you will be amazed by the wealth of quantitative and qualitative information that is already out there.

Remember: there is no point re-inventing the wheel. If somebody's already done the research, use it!

Define the issue

Even if your steering group divides up the task, collecting secondary research data can seem an overwhelming task. It is therefore important to break the process down into manageable objectives. The first of these objectives is to 'define the issue' that you are hoping to address.

To do this, it helps to think of your behavioural issue as the gap between what *should* be happening in your community and what *is* happening. For example, the issue may be the gap

Box 11.1 Search engines for electronic bibliographic databases

CINAHL: provides access to virtually all English-language nursing journals and is also strong for qualitative studies.

MEDLINE: the world's largest medical database; has a focus on biomedicine and health.

EMBASE: provides access to the world's literature on pharmacology and biomedicine, and is also well respected for psychology and psychiatry literature.

PsycINFO: a useful database for psychology, psychiatry, and psychological research.

SIGLE: provides reports and other grey literature produced in Europe. Due to the nature of grey literature, searching this database is therefore likely to reduce the likelihood of publication bias.

Sociofile: since qualitative research is more widely dispersed than quantitative research and is catalogued on databases less familiar to medical researchers (Dixon-Woods *et al.* 2001), the database Sociofile was also searched.

National Research Register: a database of ongoing and recently completed research projects funded by, or of interest to, the NHS.

QUALIDATA: primary qualitative data is held on the ESRC Qualitative Data Archival Resource Centre (QUALIDATA), hosted by Essex University.

between the number of people you would *like* to be walking to work and the number of people who actually *do*. Or it may be the gap between the number of people you would *like* to have given up smoking by attending a NHS Stop Smoking Service and the number who actually *have*.

In order to define your issue, look for existing demographic, epidemiological, and socioeconomic data that has been collected. Once you have this information, briefly answer these four questions:

1. What should be occurring?
2. What is occurring?
3. Who is affected and to what degree?
4. What could happen if the issue isn't addressed? (CDCynergy, http://www.cdc.gov/healthmarketing/cdcynergy/)

Start by identifying all of the behaviours that are relevant to your area – including desired and problematic behaviours. An example appears in Table 11.2.

It can be difficult to decide exactly what desired behaviour you wish to focus on. For instance, with the kerbside, underaged binge drinking example, you would have to decide whether you wanted to reduce 'kerbside' drinking specifically or whether your aim was to reduce teenage drinking rates in general, with the resultant outcome being reduced levels of kerbside drinking. Each of these behavioural goals would be very different and would require different social marketing strategies.

Once you have defined the current and the desired behaviour for your project, go back to the four questions posed, and begin to consider the other aspects of issue definition. For example, if you are tackling a health issue, the first three questions can be answered by looking at health-status

Table 11.2 Current and desired behaviours

	Current	Desired
Behaviour(s)	**Current problematic behaviour(s):** kerbside binge drinking among underage people aged 14–17 in North Tyneside **(legal age for drinking in the UK is 18)**	**Desired behaviour:** reduce the amount of alcohol underage people aged 14–17 in North Tyneside drink in a single night
	Related problematic behaviour(s): unprotected sex, walking home alone	
	Beneficial behaviours of the current problematic behaviour: alcohol makes people feel more confident and attractive	**Existing beneficial behaviours to maintain:** feeling confident and attractive

indicators, nationally and locally, and identifying any differences between them. Health status indicators might include:

- rates of death, illness, injury, and disability;
- causes of death, illness, injury, and disability;
- number of health-related events (e.g. unintended pregnancies); or
- Access to/availability of community services.

To define what *should* be occurring, you can look for discrepancies between:

- local and national health-status indicators;
- local *subgroup* health-status indicators;
- targets that have been set at the national, regional, or local level; and
- health-status indicators from within your area (CDCynegy).

Once you have gathered this information, write a problem statement that defines:

- the existing behaviour you are hoping to challenge;
- how it compares to national trends and targets; and
- what the impact will be if behavioural change is not achieved.

Example: Smoking in Lewisham

The General Household Survey 2006 showed smoking prevalence of 22%. In contrast, the London Borough of Lewisham has a smoking prevalence estimated at 33%, and Evelyn ward has the highest smoking prevalence at 42%. Mortality rates in the Evelyn ward for cardiovascular disease and cancer are well above average. Quitting smoking using the NHS Stop Smoking Service has been shown to be 4 times more effective than willpower alone (Ferguson et al., 2005; West et al., 2000). However, the local data showed recruitment into stop-smoking services based in the area is not high. Given the negative impact of smoking on health, this is likely to lead to more chronic health problems within this population group and result in significant health inequalities both between and within Evelyn ward and Lewisham Borough.

Determine the cause of the issue

Now you have defined the behavioural issue you are going to address, do as much as you can to pinpoint the reasons why it occurs. At this stage, use your own knowledge and common sense, as well as existing information, to list the possible causes. You may wish to consider:

- psychological factors (e.g. embarrassment, fear, and inertia);
- genetic and biological factors;
- factors in the physical environment (e.g. lack of transportation and lack of cycle paths); and
- social factors (e.g. lack of social support and lack of prohibitive policy).

Once you start to list causes, you will probably be able to identify a whole host of them for any given behaviour. You will notice that some of these causes are direct (e.g. people do not eat enough fresh fruit because no local retailer sells fresh fruit), while others are more indirect (e.g. people do not eat enough fresh fruit because they do not know why it is important to do so or how to cook with it). Similarly, you will notice that some factors may increase an individual's risk of a certain outcome (e.g. episodes of stress will make people more likely to smoke), whereas others may protect against it (e.g. taking regular exercise may help to prevent weight gain).

Based on these distinctions, you will be able to categorize your list of potential causes according to whether they are direct or indirect, and whether they are risk factors or protective factors.

Once you have listed all possible causes and categorized them, you will be able to complete a problem analysis worksheet, as in the example in Fig. 11.1.

Health problem: childhood obesity

Indirect contributing factors

- Lack of relevant education (parents and children)
- Family-structure norms
- Killing with kindness
- Poverty
- Lack of safe exercise space
- Knowledge of physical activity benefits
- Knowledge of healthy diet benefits
- Availability of healthy food choices
- Affordability of healthy food choices
- Parent nutrition instruction
- Child nutrition instruction
- Low perceptual awareness of the problem
- Sedentary activity (computer games and TV)
- Car usage for short journeys
- Lack of perception of long-term health being dependent on risk behaviours (e.g. snacking and portion size

Direct contributing factors

- Family situation – chaotic, food as a treat
- Poverty
- Media coverage of obesity

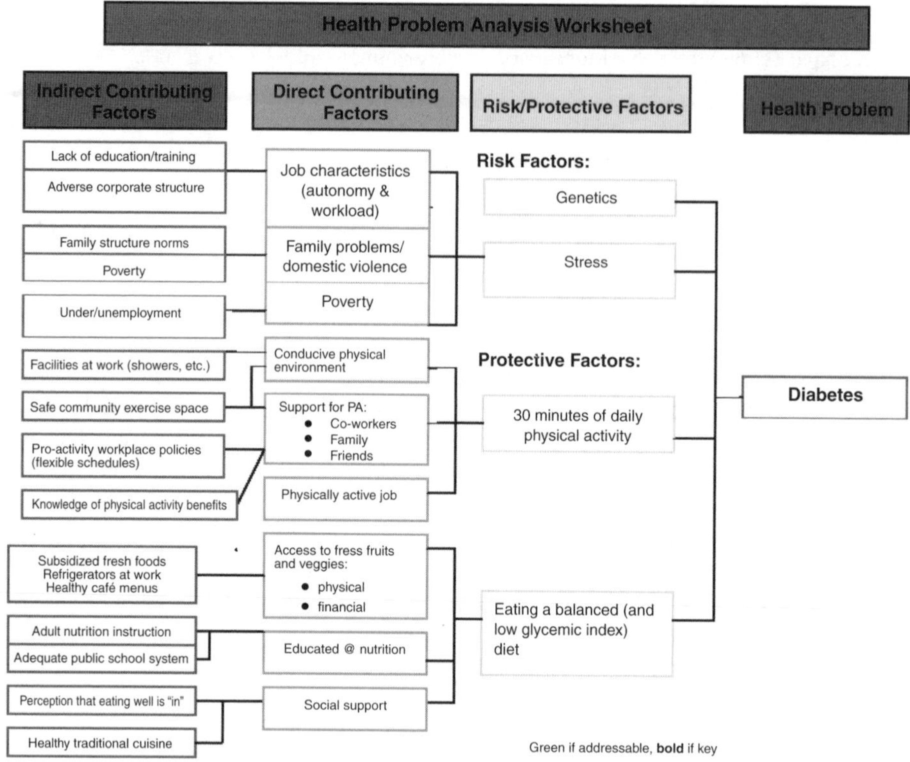

Fig. 11.1 Health problem-analysis worksheet.

Source: Adapted with permission from CDCynergy, http://www.cdc.gov/healthmarketing/cdcynergy.

- Conducive physical environment
- Support from government
- Support from schools
- Parental role modelling
- Access to fresh fruit and vegetables – physical, financial, and cooking skills
- Educated about nutrition and exercise
- Social support
- Parents' ability to gauge child's weight status

Risk factors

- Genetics
- Stress
- Rewarding children for good behaviour with unhealthy foods

Protective factors

- Eating a balanced diet and exercising regularly
- 60 min of out of school activity every day

- Reducing TV time to 2 hours a day
- Cutting out drinks with added sugar
- Three meals and two snacks a day
- Government's 5-A-Day campaign (Source: adapted from CDCynergy, http://www.cdc.gov/healthmarketing/cdcynergy)

Organizing causes in this way allows you to pinpoint the factors that are:

- most likely to affect the issue (e.g. is the lack of safe places to play likely to affect a child's ability to exercise more than their attitude towards exercise itself?); and
- most likely to be influenced by your initiative (e.g. a social marketing project cannot eliminate genetic risk factors or affect an individual's financial situation – but it might succeed in changing attitudes, physical environments, or support networks, which can then facilitate behavioural change).

By this stage, you should have a clear sense of what the behaviour is you are looking to change or sustain and of the primary reasons it occurs. Because you have been relying on knowledge and common sense and on existing information, there will probably be gaps in your understanding, and some of the assumptions you have made may be wrong. However, you will be able to refine your problem statement after you have gathered additional information in scoping Phase 2.

For now, you have a working understanding of the issue and its main causes, and the next step is to identify *who* is affected by, or involved in, the problematic behaviour.

Choose who to target

Using the secondary data you have collected, you will need to start identifying your potential target audience(s). Your choice can be refined following further research into the knowledge, behaviour, and needs of your target audience in Phase 2, but it is important at this stage to have a clear idea of the audience(s) you want to target. You will then break down this audience into 'segments' in Phase 3, so that you can shape your initiative according to the needs of each target segment.

Understanding people's behaviour

Individual behaviour contributes to wider health, environmental, and social issues. When considering the possible causes of the behaviour you are targeting, you probably listed at least one behavioural issue. For instance, 'people think it's cool to smoke', 'people don't think they'll be able to lose weight, so they don't bother trying', or 'none of my family thinks it's important to recycle, so I don't see why I should'. These attitudes sound simple enough, but they can be explained, understood, and predicted through the behavioural theories outlined in Chapter 4.

Social cognitive models (SCMs) attempt to improve understanding of consumer behaviour. SCMs are applied by anyone involved in a marketing initiative, whether it involves health or a commercial product. In the commercial world the marketer must consider how and why people buy and use products, how they react to prices, advertising, and other promotional tools, and what underlying mechanisms operate to help and hinder consumption (East, 1997). Thus the marketer must first understand consumer behaviour in the hope of ultimately influencing it. Models such as the Theory of Reasoned Action (Ajzen and Fishbein, 1980) may be applied to the consumption of anything, from computers to cornflakes.

In health care, the traditional view of the patient as a passive and obliging participant is increasingly being challenged, and the attitudes and beliefs of patients are now being recognized as central to treatment adherence (Kessing et al., 2005). As in the commercial sector, models such as the Theory of Reasoned Action are being applied in an attempt to explore the influence of different variables on an individual's health-related behaviour.

There are, of course, limits to any theoretical model, and no one model provides a full explanation. However, theoretical models try to unpack the relative importance of various factors, recognizing that what people say is not necessarily a guide to what they will do, and that there are numerous antecedent and situational variables.

When considering why your target segment behaves as it does, familiarize yourself with some of these theories and start looking for behavioural determinants such as those set out in Table 11.3.

An understanding and application of behavioural theory can have a significant impact on the success of a behavioural change initiative (Sheeran, 2006). By understanding the theoretical explanation for why people behave in certain ways, you will be able to:

- map out the possible causes of your given issue by referring to common patterns of behaviour and self-belief;
- refer to a theory checklist to make sure that important behavioural or psychological issues are not overlooked in focus groups and other market research;

Table 11.3 Factors determining people's behaviour

Internal	External
◆ Knowledge and beliefs	◆ Policies
◆ Attitudes	◆ Access
◆ Perceived risks	◆ Skills
◆ Perceived consequences	◆ Actual consequences
◆ Self-efficacy	◆ Cultural beliefs and values

Example: Understanding the target audience

Project Twin Streams is a 9-year, $39 million project to revitalize 56 km of stream banks in Waitakere (New Zealand). Although the focus is on streambank restoration, the vision of the project is much wider – it aims to build a sustainable catchment and it ties in to environmental, economic, social, cultural, and spiritual well-being.

The project applies a diffusion of innovation theoretical framework. Diffusion of Innovations Theory recognizes that people adopt new ideas or activities at different rates, and that once the 'innovators' and 'early adopters' have embraced something new, they will be followed in stages by the 'early majority', 'late majority', and 'laggards'. In Project Twin Stream, one of the main Diffusion of Innovation concepts applied is the use of opinion leaders – key local influencers who are selected to manage and implement the project at a local level.

Formative research informed the programme planners that communities wanted to engage at a local level to restore the stream banks. While residents were keen to learn about the causes of, and solutions to, stream degradation, they wanted learning to be fun. Most importantly, if they were going to give up their free time to plant trees, they wanted the process to be enjoyable.

In response to these findings, an intervention was developed (a large-scale, community-delivered weeding, planting, and maintenance project). The project is financed by regional government, managed by local government, and delivered via contracted community organizations that work with schools, businesses, local organizations, and the wider community to implement the requirements of the project and put the trees in the ground.

Since Project Twin Streams began in 2003, a total of 333 949 trees have been planted and over 13 000 volunteers have been actively involved in the project. The project has now expanded to engage with residents on issues of household sustainability. A $10.4 million walk/cycleway has also been developed under the auspices of Project Twin Streams.

For further information visit www.projecttwinstreams.org.nz

- understand your target segment(s) based on theoretical behavioural trends; and
- use theory to inform the interventional strategies you choose.

Find out what has already been done

No matter which behavioural issue you are addressing, you are probably not the first to tackle it. An important aspect of the first phase of scoping is to consider what other people have already done to address the behaviour, and to collect examples of what worked for them (see the examples in Table 11.4). With this in mind, always aim to publish findings from the initiatives you work on as well as drawing on findings from other people's work.

You may be able to find formal project evaluations online or in publications. Similarly, you may hear word-of-mouth accounts of successful initiatives. Whether official or anecdotal, all accounts of interventions are useful to spur on your project and provide valuable ideas for your own project. It is important to consider both successful and unsuccessful interventions, as lessons can be taken from both.

As well as reading reports about past interventions and researching what worked with similar audiences, it may be useful to ask the project managers who have attempted this work about:

- how they selected a target audience and target behaviour;
- what their budget was;
- the challenges they faced;
- data they have on their audiences;
- whether their programme was successful, and why; and
- what they would do differently in future.

By this point you are well positioned to start drawing conclusions from your Phase 1 scoping research. You will have a clear idea of the behaviour you are looking to address, its causes, your probable target audience, and the successes and failures of past interventions.

Table 11.4 Investigating the interventions that have been introduced to increase the uptake of school meals and fruit and vegetables in primary schools

Scope	Intervention	Lessons and questions to ask
Local	◆ Grasmere Primary School, Hackney: progressive changes to school menus ◆ Papdale Primary, Orkney: Early bird bar to get kids eating healthy breakfasts ◆ North East, Sunderland: after-school cookery club for parents and children ◆ St Joseph's, Yorkshire: whole-school approach to food supply and healthy eating	◆ Who was targeted? ◆ Why? ◆ Was it successful? ◆ Has it been thoroughly evaluated? ◆ Did uptake increase? ◆ What lessons could be transferred? ◆ What would they do differently?
National	◆ National Healthy Schools Programme ◆ Department of Health (DH) and Department for Children, Schools and Families (DCSF) Food in Schools Programme ◆ DCSF nutrient standards ◆ School Food Trust interventions and support ◆ Food Standards Agency cookery clubs ◆ 5-A-Day programme ◆ Free fruit in primary schools	◆ Who was targeted? ◆ Why? ◆ Was it successful? ◆ Has it been thoroughly evaluated? ◆ Did uptake increase? ◆ What lessons could be transferred? ◆ What would they do differently?
International	◆ Project LEAN, California: responding to the obesity crisis, using a social marketing approach to move local school board members to establish and enforce school nutrition policies in concert with the US Congress' Child Nutrition Act of 2004 ◆ North Carolina nutritional policy: using social marketing to move local school boards to establish and implement healthy nutritional policies	◆ Who was targeted? ◆ Why? ◆ Was it successful? ◆ Has it been thoroughly evaluated? ◆ Did uptake increase? ◆ What lessons could be transferred? ◆ What would they do differently?

Involve relevant stakeholders

Before moving to Phase 2 of scoping, you need to identify key stakeholders who should be engaged in the project. It is important to engage with stakeholders for a number of reasons.

1. They may work closely with the target audience, and therefore have valuable insight into current behaviours and interests. Examples of people in this group include community-workers and general practitioners (GPs).
2. Some of the stakeholders may have to deliver the intervention you develop. Therefore, making them feel part of the process and noting their views early on will help to reduce possible conflict at development and implementation stages.
3. External partners with a vested interest in addressing the issue, and who have the authority to represent their respective organizations, can add new points of view, resources, and experience.
4. Engaging external partners early in project planning helps create allies rather than competitors.

The first step in engaging stakeholders is to create a comprehensive list of all potential stakeholders (primary and secondary) and rank them according to their influence and interest in the project. Table 11.5 shows a list of potential primary and secondary stakeholders for an initiative to

Table 11.5 Potential stakeholders for an initiative to increase uptake of school meals

Primary stakeholders	**Secondary stakeholders**
Primary school children	Pre-school children Secondary school children Schools Council
Parents	Grandparents
Governors	
Union groups (teaching and catering staff)	
Local Authority Caterers Association	
Parent Teachers Association	
Head-teachers	Teachers Teaching assistants Bursars Administrative/office staff
Local Education Authority staff engaged in school food	Communications staff
Catering providers (private/local authority/in-house)	
Dieticians/nutritionists	Universities/Medical schools
Local food in schools groups (strategic or operational)	
Head cook/kitchen assistant	
Community groups	Sure Start centres
Healthy School coordinators	Wider Primary Care Trust (including health promotion and 5-A-Day)
	Health visitors and GPs
Various non-governmental organizations (NGOs)	Centres for Excellence
Local MPs	National MPs with a portfolio for food
Councillors	Portfolio leaders
Procurement officers	
Policy-makers	Department for Education and Skills/School Food Trust/Soil Association/Department of Health
Director of Children's Services	Government office Social Services
Media	
Private sector food producers/providers/suppliers/retailers	Wider private sector
Menu-analysis software providers	
Charities (Caroline Walker Trust/BHF/Sustain/National Heart Forum)	Big Lottery (Let's Get Cooking)
Action groups	
International school food reference (Finland/Sweden/Scotland)	
Celebrity chefs	

increase uptake of school meals. Primary stakeholders are those individuals who will have a *direct* influence over whether a child does or does not eat a school meal in primary school. Secondary stakeholders include those who will have some influence, and who will be relevant to the issue, but who will not hold as much power or exercise as much sway as the primary stakeholders.

Once you have compiled a comprehensive list of potential stakeholders, break it down into three stakeholder subgroups:

1. those affected by, or who significantly affect, the problem;
2. those with information, knowledge, and expertise about the problem; and
3. those who control or influence important factors related to the problem.

Table 11.6 shows how the potential stakeholders for a school meal uptake intervention might be subdivided.

Make sure you include a full range of different stakeholders – but make sure they are relevant and have a significant stake in your project. Do not just include everyone known to your organization.

Determining levels of engagement

Stakeholders are often busy people and may be involved in a number of projects. When first engaging with your stakeholders, ask what kind of involvement they want to have in your initiative. Then develop your stakeholder strategy based on this knowledge. You can use the Power and Interest Matrix tool to help with this process (Gardner et al., 1986). This offers a quick but highly effective way of prioritizing your stakeholders and will give you a clear view of how important it is to engage each stakeholder.

Plot your stakeholders in terms of how much power they have and how interested they are in your project (e.g. is it part of their day-to-day work and how far will their support impact upon the success of the project?). Figure 11.2 illustrates the stakeholders in the school meal intervention plotted by both their power and interest in the project.

Establishing your stakeholders' positions within the matrix will help you to define the level of relationship you want with them and, therefore, what type of engagement most suits your needs.

Clearly the higher up the power and interest scale the stakeholder is, the more time and energy you will want to invest in them. These are the people or organizations who could make or break your initiative and who you will probably want to secure as your partners.

Those stakeholders who have low interest and low power will need to be kept informed, but you do not need to devote the same levels of time and energy to them or communicate with them face-to-face.

Conduct strength, weaknesses, opportunities, and threats (SWOT) analyses

Armed with this information, you are now well positioned to conduct a SWOT analysis, which is a useful, structured way of looking at the internal factors (**s**trengths and **w**eaknesses) and external factors (**o**pportunities and **t**hreats) of a project to help you develop a clear plan of action. The objective of the analysis is to use the strengths of the organization to:

- take advantage of available opportunities;
- offset or improve the stated weaknesses; and
- minimize the risk of potential threats.

When considering strengths, weaknesses, opportunities, and threats, you will need to look at:

- potential sources of competition as well as existing opportunities and services that you may be able to exploit; and

Table 11.6 Categorization of primary and secondary stakeholders for a school meal-uptake intervention

Those affected by, or who significantly affect, the issue	
Primary	**Secondary**
◆ Primary school children ◆ Parents ◆ Head-teachers ◆ Head-cook	◆ Pre-school children ◆ Secondary school children ◆ Schools Council ◆ Grandparents ◆ Teachers ◆ Teaching assistants ◆ Kitchen assistants
Those with information, knowledge and expertise about the issue	
Primary	**Secondary**
◆ Head-teachers ◆ Local Education Authority staff engaged in school food ◆ Catering providers (private/local authority/in-house) ◆ Dieticians/nutritionists ◆ Local food in schools groups (strategic or operational) ◆ Healthy School coordinators ◆ Private sector food producers/providers/suppliers/retailers ◆ Menu analysis software providers ◆ Charities (Caroline Walker Trust/BHF/Sustain/National Heart Forum) ◆ International school food reference (Finland/Sweden/Scotland)	◆ Bursars ◆ Admin/office staff ◆ Communications staff ◆ Universities/medical schools ◆ Wider PCT (including health promotion and 5-A-Day)
Those who control or influence important factors related to the issue	
Primary	**Secondary**
◆ Head-teachers ◆ Governors ◆ Union groups (teaching and catering staff) ◆ Community groups ◆ GPs ◆ Various NGOs ◆ Local MPs ◆ Councillors ◆ Procurement officers ◆ Policy-makers ◆ Director of Children's Services ◆ Media ◆ Action groups ◆ Celebrity chefs	◆ Sure Start centres ◆ Health visitors ◆ Centres for Excellence ◆ National MPs with a portfolio for food ◆ Portfolio leaders ◆ Department for Children, Schools and Families (DCSF)/Ofsted/Food Standards Agency (FSA)/School Food Trust (SFT)/Soil Association/DH Chief Medical Officer (CMO)/Department for Environment, Food and Rural Affairs (Defra) ◆ Government office ◆ Wider private sector ◆ Big Lottery (Let's Get Cooking) ◆ Social Services

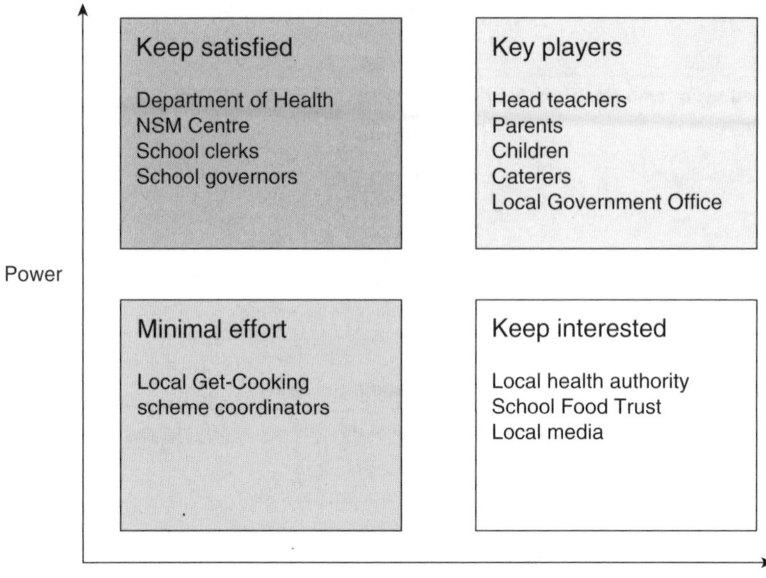

Fig. 11.2 Power and interest matrix for the school meal uptake project.

- internal or external factors which may hinder or promote your programme (e.g. funding, in-house capacity, and political resistance).

Table 11.7 shows a hypothetical SWOT analysis for an initiative to increase the number of mothers breastfeeding until their baby is 6-weeks old. As you will see, it highlights a number of areas towards which work could be directed to build on existing strengths and opportunities (e.g. mothers' existing sense of the health benefits of breastfeeding) or minimize weaknesses and threats (e.g. lack of support for promoting breastfeeding from the medical community). In this example you would probably not proceed with an advertising campaign to promote the benefits of breast milk, because of the aggressive infant formula advertising already in existence. You may, however, wish to run an intervention aimed at the medical community, encouraging and training GPs, nurses, and midwives to actively promote breastfeeding to new mothers.

Having evaluated the importance of the issues you identified, set out what you will do to address weaknesses, build on strengths, capitalize on opportunities, and deal with threats. You should include the steps to be taken, the people involved, the timeframes and the budget. Involve your steering group and key stakeholders in drawing up the action plan to get their commitment.

Summarizing Phase 1

You have now reached the end of Phase 1 of scoping, and should write a review of your work to date, summarizing your findings and suggesting any areas where further research is required. You will then be ready to progress to Phase 2.

To sum up, by the end of Phase 1 you should have:

- formed a steering group to guide the project;
- defined the behavioural issue you will target;
- defined different target audience and decided which you might focus on;

Table 11.7 SWOT analysis for an initiative to increase the number of women breastfeeding until their baby is 6-weeks old

Factors/ variables	Internal	External
	Strengths	**Opportunities**
Positive	◆ Existing team of health professionals and midwives who know the mothers ◆ The team feels passionately about this topic	◆ Mothers are aware of the health benefits to babies and themselves ◆ Work is going on to make the city a place where people will be allowed to breastfeed in public
	Weaknesses	**Threats**
Negative	◆ The health visitors are confused about local policy towards formula milk – some believe the current policy states that you are not even allowed to talk to mothers about formula milk ◆ Many of the health visitors feel under pressure and therefore spend little time with the mothers ◆ Some of the health visitors see social marketing as just a tool for the Primary Care Trust to criticize their work	◆ Hospital practices (separation of mother and baby, early discharge) tended to erode positive decisions to breastfeed ◆ Aggressive advertising for infant formula in media and other outlets that effectively reach expecting and new mothers (television, parenting magazines, mail, etc.)

- used behavioural theory to understand what influences people's behaviour;
- learned about previous efforts to address the issue (what worked and just importantly what did not);
- identified and developed a strategy for dealing with key stakeholders;
- conducted a SWOT analysis; and
- written a Phase 1 scoping review, summarizing findings, making informed recommendations, and suggesting areas where further research is required.

Phase 2

In Phase 2 of the scoping process, you will conduct new research to better understand your audience and refine the definition you have already created based on secondary data and your own experience. Your aim in this phase should be to:

- fill in any gaps in the information collected in Phase 1;
- confirm key findings or amend assumptions from Phase 1; and
- gather practical information to inform your social marketing strategy.

Conduct primary research

There may be gaps in the knowledge provided by your secondary research from Phase 1 of scoping, or you may be unclear as how it applies to your target audience. You may, therefore, decide to conduct primary research, which 'consists of information collected for the specific purpose at hand, for the first time' (Kotler and Lee, 2008, p. 77). This means that you can tailor it specifically to answer any questions and get a clearer picture of the knowledge, behaviour and needs of your target audience(s).

Primary research can be more expensive and time-consuming than secondary research, so before commissioning any research explore your in-house options. Consider whether:

- you have sufficient in-house expertise to undertake robust research;
- the proposed in-house researchers have the necessary training and experience to conduct research; and
- there are sufficient analytical skills in-house to collate and interpret data.

If you can say 'yes' to all of the above considerations, you can proceed with in-house research. If not, you will need to commission an external agency to conduct the research.

Defining your research needs

There are important questions you will need to ask before defining your research needs.

- What do you need to know about the issue and its causes which was not revealed by the secondary research?
- What do you want to clarify or confirm about why people behave as they do?
- What questions do you have about applying a possible intervention to your specific target audience? (e.g. how might it be received? What issues might it raise? Are there other options which might be more effective?)

During Phase 2 of scoping, you will also aim to learn as much as possible about the customer. Important areas to explore include:

- the barriers and benefits of the recommended behaviour and anything that acts in competition;
- the aspirations of audience members;
- factors that would make the desired behaviour more fun, easy, and popular to adopt;
- how, where, and when the problematic behaviour takes place;
- who helps to create these opportunities and who has influence on this audience; and
- the media channels that the audience uses to get its information.

You may also need to clarify:

- the size of potential segments;
- differences between segments;
- those segments it is most important to target (perhaps those most at risk);
- those segments that are most reachable; and
- those segments that are most ready for change.

Once you have considered all these options, list the research questions that need to be answered in order for your project to move forwards.

Example: Drawing up a list of research questions

These are possible research questions for an initiative to increase fruit and vegetable intake amongst a specific target audience.

- Where do you get your food from? (Probe: is it prepared at home or bought?)
- At what times of day to you buy things to eat? Are these scheduled times, or do you shop when you feel like it?

- What types of food do you eat at these different times? (Probe: why are some foods eaten at different times and occasions? What role do convenience and cost play?)
- What kind of foods do you buy when you are in different moods?
- Thinking about your 'main shopping trips', how frequently would you say these are? What kind of things do you get at these shopping trips?
- Take us through what kind of things go through your mind when selecting what you are buying? Who are you thinking of?
- Identify all the shops you buy food from. (Probe: local shops, machines, markets, supermarkets?)
- How frequently do you shop at (specific venue)? (Probe: frequently (once a week or more), moderately (1–2 times a month), infrequently (less than once a month), never?)
- Thinking about the different shops, what type of food do you buy from each? (Probe: Where would you get snacks from? Where would you buy fruit and vegetables from?)
- How does transport impact on the shops that you use?
- Which fruit and vegetables would you say you eat on an average day? (Probe: why do you eat these types of fruit and vegetables? How many fruit and vegetables do you eat in an average day? How many fruit and vegetables do you think you should eat a day?)
- What is a portion of fruit or vegetable?
- Do you think you should be eating more fruit and vegetables? (Probe: why?)
- What kind of things could make it easier for you to eat more fruit and vegetables? (Probe: access, cost, taste, time, family, choice, quality, appearance, cooking skills, and food knowledge?)
- What kind of people do you think eat the recommended amount of fruit and vegetables? (Probe: are they similar to you? What is their routine like? What makes it easier for them to do this? What role do character type, wealth and access play?)
- What do you think are the positive aspects if any, of eating fruit and vegetables? (Probe: health benefits and the value placed on this – e.g. what does healthy mean to you?)
- What kind of things get in the way when considering the positive aspects? (Probe: how could you get over these obstacles/barriers?)
- What do you think are the negative aspects, if any, of eating fruit and vegetables?
- How can you overcome these types of aspects?
- Thinking about getting people to eat more fruit and vegetables, what kind of organizations do you think can help with this and how? (Probe: supermarkets, local shops, schools, health services, and local community?)

Qualitative or quantitative research?

You will need to decide whether you want your research to be quantitative (research providing measurable data) or qualitative (research into the processes influencing your audience's knowledge, behaviour, or needs). Whichever method you are conducting, it is important to have a clear sense of what it is that you are trying to discover before embarking on research.

Qualitative research methods *consist of semi-structured, open-ended questioning techniques, in which the responses are subject to varying degrees of interpretation* (Donovan and Henley, 2003, p. 122). It produces rich, descriptive information and is exploratory in nature, seeking to clarify issues raised in Phase 1 scoping via word-of-mouth accounts of personal experience. Qualitative research will not provide you with accurate statistics, but will allow you to identify key themes and recurring issues. It will usually be conducted until a point of 'data saturation' is reached. This is the point when the researcher no longer sees or hears any new information. If you are already working from fairly comprehensive secondary data, this saturation point may be reached relatively quickly.

Quantitative research methods *consist mostly of structured, closed-ended questioning techniques, in which there is little variation in degrees of interpretation* (Donovan and Henley, 2003, p. 122). It uses controlled data-collection methods to generate numerical data and statistics. This will allow you to assess the scope of the issue overall and within various subgroups.

Table 11.8 sets out examples of techniques used for qualitative and quantitative research.

When deciding on a research approach, remember that 'all research methods involve compromises with reality. Researchers prefer more than one method whenever possible, because human thought and behaviour are too complex for any one method to capture fully' (Zaltman, 2003, pp. 73–4).

Write a research plan

Once you have identified the types of primary research you will carry out, create a research plan that sets out clear timescales for research planning, preparation, and delivery. Possible components of the primary research process will include:

- putting together a research team;
- developing questionnaires and other research tools;
- testing and finalizing research tools;
- training or recruiting people who will be conducting research;
- recruiting people to participate in the research;
- conducting the research;
- organizing the feedback;
- analysing the feedback; and
- creating a final research report.

Table 11.8 Types of qualitative and quantitative research

Qualitative	Quantitative
◆ In-depth interviews with individuals ◆ Focus groups with around 6 to 10 participants ◆ Casual observation ◆ Informal information gathering ◆ Meetings with internal and external groups to discuss issues	◆ Knowledge, attitude, and behaviour surveys ◆ Telephone surveys ◆ Mail surveys ◆ Online surveys ◆ Intercept interviews at relevant sites (e.g. shopping centres, leisure centres, youth centres)

Example: Defining the need for primary research

Secondary research for an initiative to increase uptake of school meals identified that a wealth of information existed concerning the school meal service and reasons why meals were or were not popular with children. It also revealed that parents and head teachers were key influencers of uptake.

However, while there was some secondary data on parents and head-teachers, no detailed research had been done with the target audiences themselves.

As a result, a need for primary qualitative research with the two target groups was identified. In-depth, one-to-one interviews with head teachers were conducted, across a range of schools with high, medium, and low uptake. Focus groups were also conducted with parents with children at these schools.

This primary research allowed a number of recurrent themes to be identified:

- the importance of head teachers eating meals with the children;
- a lack of understanding about the head teacher's management of and control over kitchen staff;
- a need for professional training for school cooks;
- a reluctance amongst staff to take school meals, due to the high price for adults; and
- the inability of parents to afford school emails if trying to provide for more than one child.

These primary research findings will be analysed and used to guide intervention options and design.

Analyse your primary data

Once you have collected your primary data, you need to know what to do with it.

If you have carried out quantitative research, such as surveys and questionnaires with a set range of answer options, you should have a good set of tangible results. These can be analysed by hand or by computer software, depending on the sample size, number of questions asked, and the complexity of your analysis.

If you have carried out qualitative data, such as focus groups or interviews with open-ended questions, you should have a range of 'themes' which have been produced. One way to analyse these themes is to follow these four steps:

1. Read through the transcripts of the interview/conversation
2. Identify the major themes in answers to each question
3. Support themes with anonymous quotes (followed by a brief description of the speaker which doesn't identify them – e.g. 'a London GP')
4. Summarize 'top-line' findings

There are special computer programmes that help to manage lengthy transcripts and analyse qualitative data. However, 'human' analysis of qualitative data is a must, as it can uncover unexpected themes or complexities that software really cannot capture or weigh up.

Summarize research results

As in Phase 1, it is important to capture the learning from Phase 2 scoping and present your findings in a clear and concise research report. This will help you to develop your social marketing strategy and to write your scoping report in Phase 3.

This research report should include the following sections:

Executive Summary

- States title of project
- Tells who was responsible for project
- Gives overview of research activities conducted
- Summarizes main findings and lessons
- Makes recommendations

Introduction

- Provides background about the issue and context for research

Methodology

- Describes research and sampling design and data-collection methods

Results

- Presents data organized by research question, highlighting:
  - key audience segments;
  - key differences and similarities among segments;
  - how segments perceive the problematic behaviour, especially its benefits and barriers;
  - how segments perceive its competition;
  - the segments that are likely or ready to change; and
  - channels of influence and information for each segment.

Conclusions

- Provides detailed explanations for findings
- Explains how far findings can be generalized
- Describes overall lessons
- Suggests ways to use findings to inform social marketing strategy
- Points out what questions could not be answered, explains why and suggests further research

Analyse the competition

In the commercial world, competition is defined as other organizations offering similar goods or services. In social marketing competition is defined as the current or preferred behaviour of the target segment (Kotler et al., 2002). For instance, with regards to school meals, the main competition may be packed lunches, and 'trendy' commercial products such as snack packs or lunchbox items.

Competition can be internal or external. When considering competition, it is important to think of it not as individual competitors (e.g. McDonald's), but in terms of what the competition gives the target audience (e.g. a place to take children with no worry about their table manners or noise level, cheap and filling food which children like, a toy in the kids meal to entertain them – the whole experience).

You will also need to know what is being done locally to combat the problem you are tackling and what other local services exist. This will help you to identify gaps or avoid duplicating effort and resources. For example, you may unwittingly be competing with a national campaign, or another service in the local area, which is trying to target the same behaviour. If there are already local, regional, or national interventions focussing on the same issue, or if there are programmes aimed at the same target audience, you may be able to join forces with those organizations and complement or expand their efforts. Alternatively, you may wish to approach the issue from a different angle or to target a different audience. Therefore, linking your competition analysis to your resource map (see below) is important.

Review your assets

Financially, it might be better to improve an existing product or service than to develop one from scratch (which can be very costly). Assets mapping forms an important part of scoping and helps you make the most of existing resources. It enables you to:

- identify what services are currently available for the target audience(s);
- find out what services the target audience(s) currently access;
- identify if the project crosses over with any other, and if resources could be drawn from other budgets; and
- assess and consider the potential of commercial sector partnerships/sponsorship.

There are various ways to present your mapping work, several examples are given in Table 11.9. However, it is the information that is collected and that the findings are action which is key, not the presentation.

Table 11.9 contains an example taken from a Brinnington-based project to increase use of smoking-cessation services, particularly among men and young mothers. The actual assets map contains additional columns, with information with regards to contact details, opening times, and operating area for each service, as well as details of who was interviewed for information. For confidentiality reasons, these columns have been removed, and the list abbreviated, but the table gives a good example of the range of existing activities that might be used to inform a project's development and delivery.

Summarizing Phase 2

To sum up, by the end of Phase 2 you should have:

- conducted primary research to fill in any knowledge gaps from scoping Phase 1;
- analysed this research and confirmed key findings or amended assumptions from Phase 1;
- summarized research findings in a written report;
- conducted a competition analysis for your project; and
- completed an assets map for your area.

Phase 3

With your research done, it is time to make the big decisions that will shape your social marketing project. These decisions can be tough to make and to justify to stakeholders, because they involve narrowing your focus to particular audience segments and a limited number of activities.

Table 11.9 Example assets map

Group or service	Possible partnership output
Brinnington Health Centre	Further advertising and promotion. Health days. Upstream social marketing with health professionals.
Quit for Life Smoking Support Group	Improve access by extending hours. Improve promotion. Welcome couples – promote further. Various activities. Include anger management for men. Copy model for other venues and times. Use past attendees for word of mouth. Train past attendees for to deliver.
Brinnington Walking Group	Align time to be just after one of the smoking-cessation-group meetings (e.g. Quit for Life) so that it can be an extension of the group to make the most of self-efficacy and confidence produced during the group.
Fit and Fun	No smoking agenda. Employees trained to deliver smoking-cessation advice.
Family Info link	They have two outreach workers who go to events across Stockport handing out fliers etc. Also go to libraries, children's centres etc promoting the service. They rarely talk about smoking cessation, although they know what services are available. This could be an opportunity for simple upstream social marketing to raise the profile.
Yoga Class	This would be a great partnership venture. Yoga is good stress management. It could be part of the quit-smoking package. A Stop Smoking group could be adjoined to the yoga class, either before or after.
Play time 4 Tots	Could be ideal for upstream social marketing to care workers (to encourage signposting) and to promote the Smoke Free Homes message.
Keep It Off For Good	Ideal for partnership working. Mothers are concerned about putting weight on when they give up smoking so this, or another model, could be used in conjunction with a cessation group to encourage quitting, healthy eating, and exercise without an increase in weight.
	Smoking group could be adjoined and meet at the centre just after or just before the community group.

The more firmly the decisions are grounded in the research from Phases 1 and 2 the better everyone is likely to feel about the decisions, and the more effective your intervention(s) will be.

At the end of this phase, you will have a clear idea of your chosen social marketing strategy, including specific target-audience segments and desired behaviours, and possible interventions to be taken forwards into the developmental stage. There are three clear steps to reaching this point.

- Select your target audience segment(s).
- Define current and desired behaviour for each segment.
- Write a scoping report to share your findings, your decisions, and the interventional options you will recommend.

Define your target audience segment(s)

Audience segmentation is one of the most important features of social marketing. A segment is a homogeneous group of people who share similar beliefs, attitudes, and behaviours (Wind and Cardozo, 1974). In commercial marketing, firms either:

- identify a target segment and then tailor the marketing mix for that segment; or
- use mass marketing, through which a single product is offered to the entire market.

Traditional awareness-raising campaigns often rely on a whitewash approach: they give one message to everybody in the hope that some of those who need to change their behaviour will do so. Opting for this approach may increase brand recognition. However, it is costly and may fail to reach any segment at all. Marketers use an aerosol analogy, sometimes referred to as the 'spray and pray' approach, to communicate the problem: as you spray it on the surface, some of it hits the target: most of it drifts away; and very little of it penetrates (Mendelsohn, 1968).

Social marketing differs from this approach. It understands that one size does not fit all: it is almost impossible to influence all members of a large, diverse population. For interventions to be most effective, they should be tailored to the needs of specific sub-groups or groups of people with common needs or characteristics (Kotler and Armstrong, 2001).

By segmenting your target audience you can:

- increase the effectiveness of your intervention(s) – by understanding and addressing the unique characteristics of a particular segment;
- increase the efficiency of your intervention – by strategically targeting resources towards specific targets, rather than spraying money at an unknown audience; and
- gain in-depth customer understanding – via detailed segment profiles, which will be used to develop strategies that respond to real needs, wants, or abilities.

Prioritization of resources can be based upon the different characteristics of specific segments, including:

- **segment size:** How many people are in this segment? What percentage of the population do they represent?
- **problem incidence:** How many people in this segment are engaged in the problematic behaviour or not engaged in the desired behaviour?
- **problem severity:** How severe are the consequences of the problematic behaviour in this segment?
- **defenselessness:** Can people in this segment take care of themselves or do they need help from others?
- **reachability:** Is this an audience that can be easily identified and reached?
- **general responsiveness:** How 'ready, willing and able' to respond are the people in this segment?
- **incremental costs:** How do estimated costs to reach and influence this segment compare with those for other segments?
- **responsiveness to marketing mix:** How responsive is this market likely to be to a social marketing intervention?
- **organizational capabilities:** How much staff expertise or outside resources do you have to assist in the development and implementation of activities for this segment? (Andreasen, 1995, pp. 177–179)

A full explanation of segmentation and examples of how it can be achieved is given in Chapter 7, but it essentially involves dividing your target population into segments according to a range of characteristics, examples of which are given in Tables 11.10 and 11.11.

There are three steps to follow when identifying which segment(s) you will target.

1. Define the different segments

   Divide your population into smaller sub-groups. Do this by grouping together those people who have something in common (e.g. behavioural patterns, needs, aspirations, motivations,

Table 11.10 Examples of segmentation characteristics

Demographic	Geographic
Age/generation Gender Family size Income Occupation Education Religion Race	Region Population size (city/town/village) County Postcode City Density – urban/rural Climate
Behavioural	**Psychographic**
Occasions – regular, social Benefits – quality, service, convenience User status – non-user, ex-user, potential user Usage rate Loyalty status Readiness to change stage Attitude towards product/service	Attitudes Values Beliefs Personality Lifestyle Social class

Source: Adapted from Kotler, Roberto, Lee, 2002.

Table 11.11 Example of segmentation for NHS Stop Smoking Services (SSS)

Target audience	Cigarette smokers
Segmented by region	Smokers in London
Segmented by geographic characteristics	Smokers in Lewisham
Segmented by demographic characteristics	Adults who smoke and have children (under 12 years old) in Lewisham
Segmented by behavioural characteristics	Have thought about giving up smoking, but not made a serious attempt Strong entrenched resisters – do not want to give up smoking Have actively attempted to give up smoking
Segmented by current knowledge	Know about the SSS Don't know about the SSS
Segmented by attitude	Think SSS could help and would be happy to go Think SSS could help but would not want to go Think SSS could not help them
Segmented by past quit attempts	Have tried going cold turkey Have attended an SSS Have used another method to quit (for example the Allan Carr technique)
Segmented by past behaviour	Successfully set a quit date Failed to set a quit date Successfully quit at the 4-week target, then restarted smoking within the year

lifestyles, or social groups). The people in each group will probably require similar prompts or support in order to change their behaviour. For example, new mothers might be segmented according to whether they are currently breastfeeding, started to breastfeed but then stopped, want to breastfeed but feel unable, or do not want to breastfeed.

2. Assess each segment

   Look at each segment individually and try to prioritize the ones which you might target (e.g. breastfeeding mothers might be rated according to their willingness to breastfeed and their past experience of breastfeeding).

3. Select the segment(s) you will target

   When you have assessed the segments, you will probably decide that it will be most beneficial to target one or two segments. It may be that there are certain groups that are most likely to change their current behaviour or that you think most urgently require change.

Review the information you gathered when defining the issue and considering its causes, and then ask yourself which of your segments is:

- most affected by the issue (e.g. the largest segment size, highest incidence, most severe or prevalent risk factors);
- most likely to change its behaviour;
- most feasible to reach; and
- a key secondary audience.

A social marketing project does not have to target one segment alone. However, if you choose to target more than one, it is likely that you will need to design different interventions for each of the segments. For example, a project that encourages mothers to breastfeed might target women who have tried breastfeeding but who have switched to bottle feeding. However, it may also target a key secondary audience: those mothers who want to breastfeed but feel unable to because their partner wants to be involved in the feeding of his child at night. The needs of each group will be very different, as will the intervention(s) required.

Example: Segmentation and intervention targeting

Worcester has received government funding to help it set the trend for transport policy across the UK. Its 'Choose How You Move' initiative aims to tackle traffic congestion and reduce the environmental impact of personal travel by developing a package of measures to promote walking, cycling, public transport, and car sharing. Three audience segments have been identified: schools, residents, and employers. The project team works with these target audiences to tailor services and information to meet their different needs.

Schools

Produced in conjunction with Worcestershire County Council, School Travel Plans encompass all the issues relevant to journeys to and from school, including concerns about health and safety and proposals for improvements. There are now 30 active School Travel Plans in Worcester, involving almost three-quarters of the city's schools. Working groups at each school are working with the local community to encourage more cycling, walking, car sharing, and use of public transport.

Example: Segmentation and intervention targeting *(continued)*

Residents

Between 2005 and 2007, travel experts contacted residents across Worcester to invite them to participate in a programme of Individualized Travel Marketing. Those who expressed an interest received information relevant to their personal needs, including information on walking, cycling, public transport and car sharing. Residents could also request a Personalized Journey Plan, a home visit and incentive gifts to encourage them to try new ways of moving about the city. In total almost 21 000 households were contacted, 50% of which were interested in receiving information, support, and incentives, and 26% of which reported that they already regularly use sustainable travel modes.

Employers

An Employer Travel Plan is a package of measures designed to encourage staff to consider alternatives to single-occupancy car use. A dedicated member of staff works with an employer to assess the transport needs of the site, employees, and visitors before discussing how to resolve these needs. These discussions feed into an action plan which forms the basis of the Travel Plan. Worcestershire County Council then supports the employer to implement the plan and monitor progress.

Behavioural research conducted after the first and second phases of the Individualized Travel Marketing programme (2005–06) found that, compared with residents who were not involved in the programme, walking had increased by 19%, cycling had increased by 32%, public transport had increased by 16%, and single-occupancy car usage had decreased by 12%. A repeat of the 2004 baseline behavioural research will be repeated in 2008 to investigate modal shift across the city.

For a full write up of this case study, please visit the National Social Marketing Centre's 'ShowCase' resource, at: http://www.nsmcentre.org.uk/public/CSView.aspx?casestudy=68

Defining behaviours for each audience segment

For your chosen segments, you will now need to clarify the behaviour they are currently doing and identify the behaviour you want them to do. Ask yourself:

- what behaviour could be changed in the short term;
- is it likely to change with a little more incentive; and
- if audience members take the desired action, will it make a tangible difference in achieving my overall project goal?

Be sure the behaviour you are linking to each audience segment makes sense.

- Are the selected behaviours supported by your market research findings?
- How did audience members view the behaviour and did they express a desire to change it?
- Is the behavioural objective different from what they are already doing?
- Is the given behaviour under an individual's control?

Try also to clarify what the required behavioural change actually requires of the individual. For example, does it consist of:

- a one-off action (easiest to bring about) such as signing up to be an organ donor;
- repeated or daily actions that are simple and take little effort (e.g. using a seat-belt);

- repeated actions within a finite time period (e.g. having children fully immunized by the time they start school);
- situational actions (e.g. administering oral rehydration therapy when a child has diarrhoea); or
- a permanent lifestyle change (hardest to bring about) such as exercising regularly.

If the ultimate behavioural objective is not feasible, consider intermediary behaviours as objectives, which will allow the end-result to be reached via a series of smaller, more achievable steps.

For target segment(s), you can now list a selection of current behaviours and a selection of desired behaviours, as in the example in Table 11.12.

Write a scoping report

You are now ready to write your scoping report, which is where you summarize the rationale for the intervention option(s) selected, and which serves as the blueprint for the following development stage. In it, you will outline the research findings from Phases 1 and 2 and draw together the conclusions you have made with regards to your chosen target audience(s) and the behavioural change(s) you will aim to effect. Box 11.2 contains a list of suggested content for your report.

Table 11.12 Current and desired behaviour for segments for a breastfeeding campaign

Audience segment	Current behaviour	Desired behaviour
Pregnant women who had not made a decision to breast/bottle feed and who expressed these barriers to breastfeeding: ◆ embarrassment; ◆ fear of being tied to the baby and conflict with work, school, or an active social life; ◆ fear of not being able to nourish or nurse adequately; ◆ fear of jeopardizing relationships with the grandmother/father of the baby/other network ties; ◆ lack of support or encouragement from family and friends Pregnant women from lowest socio-economic group	◆ Lower rates of breastfeeding initiation than national average for women at higher socioeconomic levels ◆ Lower rates of breastfeeding duration than national average for women at higher socio-economic levels	◆ Increase initiation of breastfeeding ◆ Increase duration of breastfeeding
Family and friends	◆ Criticism and lack of support for breastfeeding	◆ Provide support for breastfeeding ◆ Increase referrals to breastfeeding support service
Professionals and health service providers	◆ Not encouraging breastfeeding during patient contact due to lack of time, training, and resources	◆ Encourage breastfeeding during patient contact ◆ Use campaign materials and resources
General public		◆ Increase general knowledge and support of breastfeeding

Source: adapted from CDC, http://www.cdc.gov/healthmarketing/cdcynergy/, Accessed January 2009.

Box 11.2 Suggested contents for a scoping report

- Statement on selection of the intervention option(s) with summary rationale
- Problem statement
- Provisional aims
- Initial customer/audience analysis, and segmentation
- Potential behavioural focus
- Initial behavioural goals
- Possible interventional options
- Potential ethical issues
- Working proposition outlining ideas of how to achieve and maintain desired behaviour
- Initial literature review of evidence and social marketing case-studies relevant to presenting issue
- Research findings to support customer insights
- List of stakeholders

When you have finished a draft scoping report, distribute it to stakeholders and other decision-makers, inviting them to comment on, amend, or verify any of your conclusions. You should then make necessary adjustments distribute the finished report to your steering group, your solution group (see below), and all major stakeholders. It will enable all those involved to understand the research informing your initiative, and to see clearly which options have been selected to go forwards into the development stage. It will also serve as a practical planning tool in the development stage.

Conclusion

Whilst the scoping stage might seem daunting, it is a vital part of the social marketing process. The key task is to consider and select an appropriate intervention (or mix) that is thought most likely to achieve the desired behaviour, and to set out clearly the rationale for this, as a foundation on which the rest of the work, and evaluation, can be based.

There is often an impatience to 'just do something' when faced with a pressing health or social issue. In a target-driven world, where quick wins are valuable, it can be tempting to bypass or rush through research and to jump ahead to development and implementation. However, as Jon Haber commented, 'The laziest thing people do is go right to tactics' (Fenton Communications, 2001, p. 9). In spite of the urge to act quickly, proper investment in a project's front-end is crucial. The scoping stage sets the foundations for a well-targeted, sustainable intervention, based on real insights and customer understanding. By investing time and effort here, you will be well set to reap future dividends in terms of impact and effectiveness. Remember: there is no point hurtling off at full speed, if you are heading in the wrong direction!

Review exercise

Think of a social marketing project that you are about to start, or a hypothetical one:

- What is the problem you are looking to address?
- Whom would you invite to be on the project's steering group?

- Who are the key stakeholders you need to engage with?
- Who are your primary and secondary target audiences?

Limit yourself to no more than five bullet points for each response.

References

Ajzen, I. and Fishbein, M. (1980). *Understanding Attitudes and Predicting Social Behaviour.* Englewood Cliffs: Prentice Hall.

Andreasen, A.R. (1995). *Marketing Social Change: Changing Behaviour to Promote Health, Social Development and the Environment.* San Francisco: Jossey-Bass.

CDC (Centers for Disease Control and Prevention) CDCynergy: social marketing edition, CD-ROM. Available at: http://www.cdc.gov/healthmarketing/cdcynergy/ (Accessed January 2009).

Dixon-Woods, M., Fitzpatrick, R., and Roberts, K. (2001). Including qualitative research in systematic reviews: opportunities and problems. *Journal of Evaluation in Clinical Practices*, 7: 125–133.

Donovan, R. and Henley, N. (2003). *Social Marketing: Principles and Practice.* Melbourne: IP Communications.

East, R. (1997). *Consumer Behaviour.* Sydney: Prentice Hall.

Sheeran, P. et al. (2006). *End of Award Report: Does Changing Attitudes, Norms or self-efficacy change intentions and behaviour?* Swindon: Economic and Social Research Council (ESRC). Available at: http://www.esrcsocietytoday.ac.uk/ESRCInfoCentre/ViewAwardPage.aspx?AwardId=3544 (Accessed February 2009).

Fenton Communications (2001). *Now Hear This: The Nine Laws of Successful Advocacy Communications, With Words of Wisdom from more than 25 leading experts, p. 9*

Ferguson, J. et al. (2005). The English smoking treatment services: one year outcomes, *Addiction*, April, 100 (Suppl. 2): 59–69.

Gardner, J.R., Rachlin, R., and Sweeny, H.W.A. (1986). *Handbook of Strategic Planning.* New York: John Wiley & Sons Inc.

Kessing, L., Hansen, H., Demyttenaere, K., et al. (2005). Depressive and bipolar disorders: patients' attitudes and beliefs towards depression and antidepressants. *Psychologie Medicale*, 35: 1205–1213.

Kotler, P. and Armstrong, G. (2001). *Principles in Marketing.* Upper Saddle River, NJ: Prentice Hall.

Kotler, P. and Lee, N. (2008). *Social Marketing: Influencing Behaviours for Good*, Third Edition. California: Sage Publications.

Kotler, et al. (2002). *Social Marketing: Improving the Quality of Life*, Second Edition. California: Sage Publications.

Mendelsohn, H. (1968). Which shall it be: mass education or mass persuasion for health? *AJPH*, 58: 131–137.

West, R. et al. (2000). National smoking cessation guidelines for health professionals: an update. *Thorax*, 55: 987–999.

Wind, Y. and Cardozo, R. (1974). Industrial market segmentation. *Industrial Marketing Management*, 3: 153–166.

Zaltman, G. (2003). *How Customers Think: Essential Insights into the Mind of the Market*, Boston: Harvard Business School Press. 73–74.

Chapter 12

Development

Rowena Merritt

All great achievements require time.
Maya Angelou

Learning points

This chapter

- Introduces the concept of the marketing mix;
- Describes the importance of each component of the marketing mix to the success of the development of your intervention(s); and
- Stresses the importance of pre-testing interventions and suggests possible methods for doing so.

Chapter overview

The second stage of the Total Process Planning (TPP) framework is 'development'. As set out in Chapter 11, by the time you reach the development stage you should have:

- an understanding of your target audience – the environment in which they live, what is important to them and what moves and motivates them;
- engaged with key stakeholders;
- completed a competition analysis; and
- produced a scoping report.

During the developmental stage, you will use the findings set out in your scoping report to shape your social marketing intervention(s). As many of the most successful interventions take a multi-pronged approach, it is likely that the scoping report will point towards a variety of interventions.

Aim of developing stage

- To develop a tailored programme, campaign or other intervention (product or service)

Objective of the developing stage

- To build on initial behavioural goals and insights to develop the intervention (or programme/campaign)
- To pre-test ideas with relevant audience, and then refine work as required

Primary output

- A marketing plan for the development stage

Introduction

Up until now the work you have carried out may have seemed like an academic exercise, and although time intensive, simple to conduct and manage. The developmental stage is slightly more complicated, how do you turn all the data collected during the scoping stage into interventional tactics and activities that will have an actual impact on your target audience's behaviour? This chapter aims to answer this question, informed by the marketing mix.

The chapter sets out the four elements of the marketing mix (product, price, place, and promotion) sequentially. But it is important to note that the marketing mix refers to the blending of the four components. By concentrating on just one element of the mix, failure is likely.

The marketing mix

'The marketing mix' is probably the most famous phrase in marketing, and is also known as the 4Ps. Identified by Jerome McCarthy in 1960, the 4Ps are the four principal marketing 'tactics' used to achieve marketing objectives: product, price, place and promotion. To meet objectives successfully, it is important to balance all four Ps. For example, if uptake of a newly priced service is poor, the answer could be to change the service, or to deliver it in a way that is more convenient to the user, or to improve the quality of the promotion (rather than to cut the price). Box 12.1 shows how the 4Ps can be applied to social marketing initiatives.

The 4Ps are not without their critics, and it has been suggested that we should not try to force fit commercial marketing's 4Ps into social marketing (Peattie and Peattie, 2003). Some critics have suggested alternatives to the 4Ps to reflect a more client-oriented marketing philosophy: 4Cs – convenience, cost to the user, communication and customer needs and wants (Lauterborn, 1990); and 4As – appealing, affordable, available, and appreciated (Hastings, 2007). However, most marketing texts still tend to prefer to use the 4Ps when describing the elements of the mix.

Product

Your 'product' is what you are selling: the desired behaviour and the associated benefits of that behaviour. Products are often intangible, i.e. they are about feeling different or doing different things rather than a hard physical product. It also includes any tangible objects and services developed to support and facilitate the target audience's behavioural change. The product platform has three levels: the core product, the actual product, and the augmented product (Kotler, 1988). These levels are explained in Box 12.2.

The 'augmented product' is important, as often a simple product or service (e.g. a larger recycling bin) can be the vital ingredient in helping the target audience achieve the desired behaviour. During the scoping stage, research with the target audience should tease out if they feel a certain product or service would help them achieve the promoted behaviour.

In the UK there are already a large range of services developed to address a variety of public health issues. However, these services are often underused. Your research at the scoping stage should have identified existing services and provided some insight into why they are not currently used to capacity. It is far more economical to improve an existing service than develop a new one.

Box 12.1 The marketing mix for social marketing initiatives

Element of the marketing mix	Definition
Product	Product refers to the desired behaviour you are asking of the audience, associated benefits of doing the desired behaviour and any tangible objects or services that support or facilitate the desired behaviour. Included in this are the characteristics of the product or service, such as features, product design, quality, and branding.
Price	This is the cost and barriers the target audience faces when changing to the promoted behaviour. Non-monetary costs, such as physical, emotional, time, and/or psychological costs, should also be considered. The benefits of changing to the promoted behaviour must be greater than the costs.
Place	This is where the target audience will perform the desired behaviour, or where the product or service is made available to the target audience. It is important to consider where the target audience should receive the product or service and to make this as convenient and pleasant as possible.
Promotion	This is how the product or service is made known to the target segment. Promotion includes advertising, personal selling, sales promotions, and atmospherics. Promotion leads you to consider the type of media your target audience attends to, where and when they will attend to your message, and the style of the communication.

Source: adapted from McCarthy (1960)

Box 12.2 The three levels of a product platform

	Explanation	Example: stopping smoking
Core product	The core product is the underlying Benefit/s that the consumer obtains by 'buying' the product or service	Improvements in health outcomes (e.g. reduced risk of heart disease and lung cancer), as well as sense of personal achievement, and financial saving
Actual product	The product or service you develop to deliver the core product benefits	A stop smoking clinic
Augmented product	The features that encourage and support uptake of the actual product or service	A stop smoking clinic with flexible opening times, accessible locations and features such as: free nicotine replacement therapy, counselling and a buddy to help

It can be debated that, if by improving existing products, instead of developing new ones, social marketers are in fact doing 'sales' as opposed to 'marketing' (Merritt et al., 2009). However, with the financial constraints that operate in the public sector, developing a new product or service is often not feasible. Therefore, improving an existing product or service is frequently the most pragmatic approach (and one regularly employed by successful commercial companies (see Box 12.3)).

Box 12.3 Adapting existing products to meet changing consumer trends

Example: Coca-Cola

Many commercial companies also focus on sales, and look to develop changes to their augmented product and line extensions, rather than developing completely new products. An example of a company which has successfully made changes to their augmented product to maintain market share and change with trends is Coca-Cola. Originally intended as a medicine in the late nineteenth century, Coca-Cola was bought out by a businessman, whose marketing strategy led Coke to become the world leader in the soft drinks market.

Since the original Coca-Cola was launched, various modifications of the original brand have been developed. These changes have been made, based on customer insights and consumer trends, in an attempt to retain market share and to appeal to new audiences. These include:

- **Coke Zero** (developed to appeal to men conscious of their weight (Tungate, 2008));
- **Diet Coke** (developed to appeal to people conscious of their weight (mainly women));
- **Caffeine-free Coke**; and
- **Cherry Coke** (which is popular in the US and Japan, but was unsuccessful in Australasian countries, where it was subsequently withdrawn)

Special editions of Coke – such as coke with lemon and coke with lime – are also marketed a certain times of the year and in certain countries.

Price

The price of a social marketing product is the cost that the target audience associates with adopting the new behaviour. Costs may be monetary or non-monetary in nature, and may be associated with the target audience's exiting the current behaviour as well as entering the promoted behaviour. In the UK many products and services are provided free of charge, therefore price may not be seen as an issue. However, when thinking about price, it is important not to overlook the non-monetary costs, such as physical and/or psychological costs (Roselius, 1971). Often the costs may be perceived by the target audience and may not be actual costs associated with the promoted behaviour. However, perceived costs are 'real' to the target audience and therefore should be regarded as a very real cost by the marketer.

Is free the best pricing strategy?

There is extensive literature that tries to answer whether providing a health product for free is really the best way to ensure positive behaviour change. For example, by giving away free condoms, does that make people use them more, or do people think they must be of poor quality as they are free? Findings from the research on the ideal cost of health products and services are often polarized: it appears to depend very much on who your target audience is and what product or service you are offering. For example, a study conducted in the UK showed that those young people accessing free condoms through the health services were more likely to use condoms when having sex (Parkes et al., 2005), while another study conducted in Nigeria found that only 1% of men and 2% of women reported that they would take a voluntary HIV test if it were offered free

Box 12.4 Potential costs

Example: NHS Stop Smoking Services

NHS Stop Smoking Services (SSS) began in 2000 and have continued to be funded on a yearly or three yearly basis (Health Education Authority, 2000 and 1998). There are now over 150 SSS across England. The service is run free of charge and offers smokers a range of services including 6 weeks of support by trained specialists with knowledge about behavioural change and pharmacological product suitability and prescription drugs to help with smoking cessation.

Research conducted by the Department of Health (DH) in England, shows that the biggest competition to the SSS is people going 'cold turkey'. So, what are the possible costs of attending the SSS?

Fear of failing	The more people who know you are trying to quit the worse it feels when you fail. By attending a SSS this is a very obvious quit attempt, compared with just going it alone.
Fear of not knowing what to expect at the clinics	Some smokers think that the clinics are 'not for people like them'.
Fear of what life would be like without smoking	Some smokers fear their life will be worse when they give up smoking.
Time/effort	Some smokers cannot attend the clinics, because they are run during working hours or at locations with poor access by public transport.

The DH stop smoking advert, launched in January 2008 (shown again in January 2009), tries to address some of these costs.

Source: based on discussions with the National Support Team and a member of the DH England tobacco policy team, March 2008.

(Sunmola et al., 2007). Therefore, when developing a social marketing intervention, it is important not to simply assume that because you are offering a product or service for free, that there are no costs involved.

Exchange theory

An important concept to consider when thinking about price is that of exchange. Exchange has been defined as 'the exchange of resources or values between two or more parties with the expectation of some benefits' (MacFadyen et al., 1999). The concept of exchange is illustrated by the following commercial example of purchasing a chocolate bar. For the exchange of 60p customers not only receive a product, they also get a range of other benefits too. The benefits are often intangible and are developed and communicated by the promotional element of the marketing mix.

Whether consciously or subconsciously, people go through a cost–benefit analysis at some level before they decide to act. The marketer's task is to ensure that the offering to the target market (benefits) is equal to or greater than what they will have to give up (costs). However, this is a rather simplistic notion and some have suggested that the benefits have to outweigh the costs (Homans, 1974). It is also important to stress that all costs and benefits will not be perceived

Box 12.5 Exchange for customers

Example: Cadbury's 'Crunchie' chocolate bar

You pay	You get
◆ 60p	◆ A bar of chocolate
	◆ A sugar-level boost
	◆ Something to stop/reduce your hunger
	◆ Good taste
	◆ 'That Friday feeling'
	◆ Fun/enjoyment

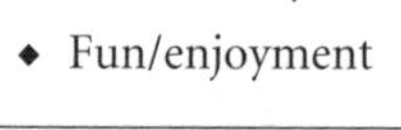

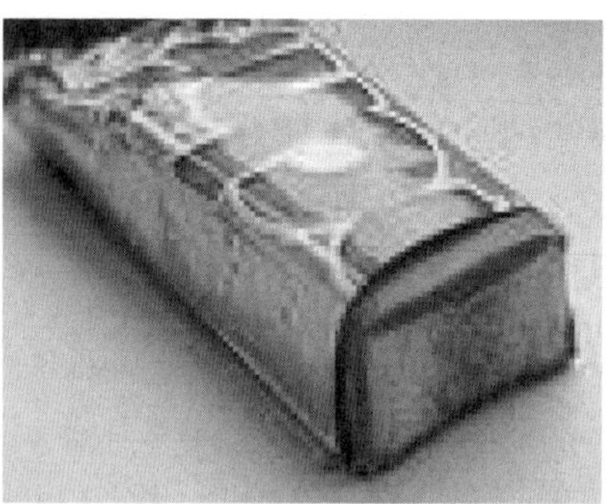

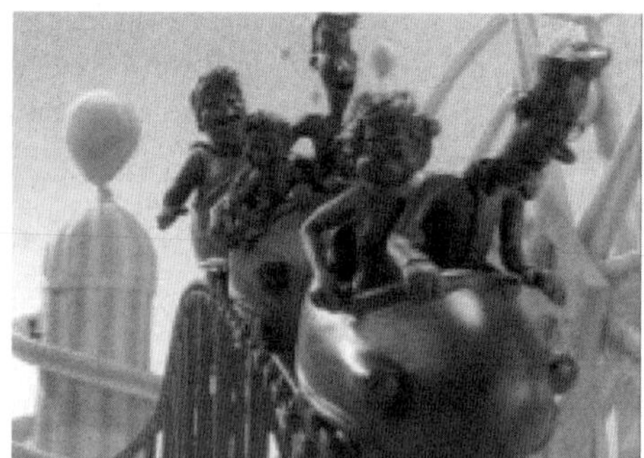

Source: adapted from Turning Point (2008). Cadbury's 'Crunchie' images reproduced with permissions

as equal. Good qualitative research undertaken in the scoping phase should have explored the weighting of the 'costs' identified by the target audience. If you did not conduct such research during the scoping stage, you must conduct it now.

Place

In social marketing, 'place' is where and when the target audience will perform the desired behaviour, acquire any related tangible objects, and receive any associated services (Kotler et al, 2002). We live in a world where time is in short supply and a valuable commodity – so convenience is a key element to success. In the commercial world, it is those companies who know the importance of convenience that have thrived (see Box 12.6).

Public health-care services often expect the customer to come to them; the successful commercial companies know that in a very competitive market, they have to go to the customer. If we compare the efforts of Tesco to many of the NHS services offered in the UK, the difference is often staggering. For example, family planning clinics are often held at inconvenient times, at places difficult to get to using public transport, and there are often inadequate parking spaces at many hospitals, making attending appointments problematic. Despite these examples of poor practice in the NHS, there are many cases where convenience and a consumer-focussed approach are integral to the services success (see Box 12.7). A marketer's objective is therefore to make access as convenient and pleasant as possible for the target audience.

Box 12.6 The importance of convenience

Example: Tesco

Tesco plc is a British-based international grocery and general merchandizing retail chain. It is the largest British retailer by both global sales and domestic market share. The supermarket retail business is highly competitive, and to retain its competitive advantage Tesco must constantly develop new ways to better serve its customers. Below are just a few of the ways in which the company has made its stores and products convenient for its customers.

- Originally specializing in food, Tesco has diversified into areas such as clothing, electronics, consumer financial services, garden furniture, and selling and renting DVDs and compact discs. This means customers can go to just one shop to buy all their essentials.
- Tesco metros (smaller stores) are mainly located in city centres and on the high streets of small towns.
- Tesco Express neighbourhood convenience shops (stocking mainly higher-margin food products and everyday essentials) are found in busy city-centre districts, small shopping precincts in residential areas, and on petrol-station forecourts.
- In some areas, the company has a minibus service for people who do not have transport to get to a store.
- Larger stores have ample parking.
- Online shopping with home delivery is available 24 h a day.

Box 12.7 Making public health-care services convenient

Example: Chlamydia screening

Chlamydia is a sexually transmitted infection that is spreading fast among young people aged between 16 and 25 (one in 10 of this age group screened in England has the infection). Responding to the increased prevalence of the condition, DH England has set screening targets for local areas, which poses a problem as this age group is often not engaged with health services. However, some areas are trying to make screening services more convenient, so that young people do not need to come to the already existing sexual health/family-planning clinics.

In 2007, North Tyneside Primary Care Trust launched its new screening service for this target age group. It distributed home testing kits, which required users to provide a urine sample and send it off to a laboratory free of charge. They also designed a website that explained the kits and also gave information on chlamydia. The results were either posted, texted, or telephoned through to the young people, depending on which method they had selected. As well as the home testing kits, health professionals held special events at local universities and youth clubs, encouraging the young people to use the kit there and then.

Source: North Tyneside Primary Care Trust press release: 30 January 2007.

Promotion

'Promotion' is the component of the marketing mix that many people often jump to first, ignoring the other three Ps or only considering them retrospectively. By concentrating solely on promotion, whilst knowledge and awareness can be increased, behavioural objectives are frequently not met (See Box 12.9). However, promotion is the last element of the marketing mix that should be considered. Promotion is used to communicate the product benefits, the value of the product/service in relation to the competitors and the place where the product/service is available. The communications job is to make sure that the target audience knows about the offer, believes it will experience the stated benefits and is inspired to act (Kotler et al., 2002, p. 264).

There are a range of techniques that can be included in the promotional mix:

- advertising;
- public relations;
- sponsorship;
- sales promotion;
- publicity; and
- personal selling (Donovan and Henley, 2003).

You will need to decide what your message should be, how it should be presented, and where and when the message will appear. These are decisions that should be made in the context of the competition's positioning. The competition for a target audience's attention can be great: research shows that we are bombarded by hundreds, if not thousands, of advertising messages everyday (Brower and Leon, 1999). So how can we ensure our message is received and translated into action instead of being lost in all the noise (the confusion caused by too many messages being delivered at once)?

This is where research into the target audience at the scoping stage and the pre-testing conducted in the development stage (discussed later in this chapter) will assist. Insight generated from research with the target audience can help the marketer to select the correct media channels and determine timings for the launch and airing of communications. Pre-testing will confirm or refute your ideas.

When developing the promotional element of your intervention, ask yourself the following questions:

- What do we want them to know?
- What do we want them to believe?
- What do we want them to do? (Kotler et al., 2002)

You should also ask: How do we want them to do it?

If we look at past governmental work in England, it is often difficult to work out what people are in fact being asked to do. By just communicating a health message, e.g. 'Do not smoke' or 'Have safer sex', we will fail to achieve the behavioural promotion we desire. More recent governmental communications have moved away from simply communicating a 'don't' message to give their target audience a clear message of what they want them to do and how they can help them do it. However, despite these recent improvements, the government still needs to work harder to let people know what they are being asked to do and how they are supposed to do it.

Ways to improve your promotional work

In the early 1950s the American Alex Osborne drew up a checklist of ways to stimulate new ideas. Osborne's checklist was originally conceived as an aid to the improvement and development of products. Since then, the checklist has been refined to be used by advertising teams (Priken, 2002). Box 12.8 contains questions from the checklist that your creative team can ask when developing the promotion mix. You can also ask your target audience the same questions during pre-testing of the promotional approach.

Re-branding of communication campaigns is not social marketing!

In response to the positive climate to social marketing, it is becoming common practice to re-brand traditional communications campaigns as social marketing. This is justified by tacking an element of market research onto the development stage of the campaign. While this represents an improvement to a degree (any research is better than none!), these campaigns neglect to consider the rest of the marketing mix. In the commercial world a successful company would not apply one of the elements of the marketing mix in isolation. For example, money would not be spent promoting a message if the right product was not in the right place, and at a price the target audience would value.

More Ps to consider

Some marketers believe that the 4Ps are too restrictive and therefore add extra Ps. Amongst the many included in the marketing literature are policy, physical environment, people, process, performance, profit, and packaging. Type 'Ps of marketing' into the search engine

Box 12.8 Sample questions from Osborne's checklist

How can the size or proportions be altered?
Make it bigger, longer, inflatable, foldable, narrower, thinner?

How can the shape or function be altered?
Make it more complicated, spherical, simpler, reusable, amorphous?

How many ways are there to construct it?
Could it have more parts, more variables, fewer parts? Can you fold it, roll it, stick bits together?

Can the user do something different with it?
Is there a puzzle to solve? Is the something to cut out, assemble?

How can the information be put across better?
Make it more obvious, scandalous, concealed, incisive?

What style could be used?
Conservative, traditional, futuristic?

What character should it have?
Friendlier, cuddlier, funnier, cooler, grander?

What about colour?
Brighter, multicoloured, plain, transparent, black and white?

What sounds or noises can be used?
Softer, muffled, singing, more musical?

Source: Pricken, 2002.

Box 12.9 The danger of neglecting some of the 4Ps

Example: Got Milk?

By the 1990s, sales of milk in California had been on a 20-year decline. In 1993, the Californian Milk Processing Board (CMPB) decided to tackle the decline and respond to several identified barriers:

- *Competition.* People were drinking soft drinks instead of milk, because they associated sweet, carbonated drinks with youthful lifestyles and fun.
- *Packaging.* Whilst soft drinks came in colourful, easy to open, and convenient to use containers, milk still came in litre bottles or cardboard boxes which were fiddly to open and could not be easily resealed.
- *Product image.* Milk was boring. Compared with the proliferation of brightly coloured beverages in myriad, imaginative packages, milk had an image problem (Holt, 2002).

However, around 94% of people still believed that milk was good for you, and 70% of Californians claimed to drink milk frequently. It was decided that the marketing strategy would target those who already consume milk rather than try and convert new users (Holt, 2002).

Qualitative research found that many consumers linked milk with sweet, sticky snacks. When asked how they felt when they ate food that demanded milk to wash it down but they did not have milk in the house, respondents were able to convey the feeling of having a brownie or cookie remnants stuck in their throat, calling out for a gulp of milk to cleanse the palette (Holt, 2002).

Based on this insight, a duel advertising strategy was subsequently developed:

- *The deprivation strategy.* To encourage people to drink milk when they ate complementary foods, adverts were developed depicting cookies and sandwiches with a bite out of them and cats with sad looks on their faces.
- *Making milk cool and interesting.* Adverts with the slogan 'Where's your moustache' showed celebrities and fictional characters with a milk moustache.

Although the campaign achieved over 90% awareness, when it was first launched sales of milk did not increase. Why? It has been argued that it was the failure to consider other elements of the marketing mix, such as the product and distribution channels. Since then, a huge variety of milk products have been developed (e.g. chocolate milk) and milk has been sold in packaging resembling soft drink packaging, allowing it to be distributed in fridges alongside its major competitors. By 2002, milk sales in California had increased to their highest levels since 1992 (Source: http://www.gotmilk.com/ Accessed March 2008).

Google and you will be presented with a whole range of Ps: the 10 Ps, the 7 Ps, the 6 Ps, and the 9 Ps!

However, although you will not want to ignore the extra Ps, there is no need to get bogged down with them. Consider which are most relevant to your project and focus on them. The physical environment and policy are often more relevant to social marketing projects than some of the others. For example, if we want more people to go outdoors to exercise, we must consider the physical environment and make sure that there are paths on housing estates and lighting on public footpaths.

Branding

We live in a branded world and the word 'branding' is commonly referred to by those working in health promotion. But what does it actually mean? How can you get it? And, most importantly, how will it benefit your social marketing intervention?

Brands are often mistaken as being just the name and logo of a product or service. However, a brand is far more than a label of ownership: a brand reflects the image the company wants its product or service to have, engages with the target audience and influences where the product 'fits' in relations to competitors. Branding is an important intangible product attribute, and powerful brands can drive success in competitive markets, and indeed become an organization's most valuable asset.

The public health arena often has to compete against some of the biggest, well-known, and successful brands in the world, e.g. cigarette and confectionary brands (see Box 12.10). So, how can we create brands in the public sector to take on such strong competition?

Developing a brand

The brand is developed using the whole of the marketing mix – not just by promotion. The marketing mix is used to develop the brand's 'personality', known as the 'brand attributes'. Brand attributes are the basic elements for establishing a brand identity and are the functional and emotional associations that are assigned to a brand by its customers. Brand attributes can be either negative or positive and can have different degrees of relevance and importance to different customer segments, markets and cultures.

It is important to mention that brands need to be refined and developed over time. As with any social marketing intervention, once you have succeeded in creating the correct intervention, you must monitor the situation to meet the changing needs of consumers through continuous innovation and improvement. In the same way, brands need to be refined and developed over time.

Should you use a government logo?

In the UK public sector, we have some of the best known and most powerful brands (e.g. the NHS). However, there is often much debate over whether the relevant government department's logo should be used. If they have funded the project, most government departments require their logo to be used. However, this can sometimes discredit the intervention (Perman and Henley, 2001). Therefore, it is advisable to pre-test any intervention materials with and without the funder's logo before launching the intervention.

Box 12.10 The power of branding

Research conducted by the National Consumer Council has shown that the average British child today is familiar with up to 400 brand names by the time they reach the age of 10. Researchers report that our children are more likely to recognize Ronald McDonald and the Nike swoosh than Jesus. One study found that 69% of all 3-year-olds could identify the McDonald's golden arches – while half of all 4-year-olds did not know their own surname.

Source: The Guardian, Tuesday 25th October 2005 – http://www.guardian.co.uk/media/2005/oct/25/advertising.food.

Getting buy-in from the 'deliverers'

After developing your marketing mix, and before pre-testing it with your target audience, it is useful to set up what is sometimes termed a 'solutions group'.

The solution group is made up of key stakeholders, usually the people who will actually have to implement the marketing mix you design. However, unlike the steering group, which meets regularly and is responsible for the project's entire delivery, the solution group may only meet a couple of times in the whole life span of the project.

The solution group has two main purposes:

- it is there to provide you with a steer from experts in the field – a 'sense check' on your findings; and
- it is an important tool for gaining stakeholder buy-in.

By sharing the project's planning process, and asking for input from those affected, you will reassure individuals that the process is participative and open to suggestion, as well as pre-empting any problems or oppositions that are likely to occur later down the line in the implementation phase (described in Chapter 13).

Ask yourself which groups, community leaders, or other individuals, might oppose your programme and whether you might turn them into allies by inviting them onto the solution group and securing their buy-in.

Pre-testing interventional strategies

The consumer is always at the centre of the social marketing process, so you should pre-test your intervention thoroughly with the target audience. During the pre-testing period, a number of intervention strategies are usually tested to see which ones are most effective and well received by the target audience. The feedback from the pre-testing is then used to fine-tune the intervention. This is an iterative process and it may take several refinements of the intervention before it is ready to be launched.

It is not only materials which should be pre-tested. You should also pre-test, revise, pilot test, and monitor:

- new or improved services;
- new or adapted products;
- policies;
- concepts;
- messages;
- settings; and
- distribution channels.

Pre-testing and piloting may be difficult with some interventions, e.g. when the intervention requires the purchase of an expensive product (i.e. a fleet of buses, etc.). In this instance the concept can be pre-tested instead. However, some form of pre-testing will always be possible and so it should always be done. Different methods may be more appropriate, depending on the intervention to be pre-tested.

Two frequently used pre-testing methods are focus groups and individual interviews:

Focus groups

Focus groups are commonly used to pre-test more often than is advisable (Sigel and Doner, 2004). However, they can be useful when pre-testing new product or service concepts or lengthy materials, in particular if it is useful to hear an interactive discussion about the materials, how they are interpreted, and how they might be distributed. Despite their advantages, focus groups can be costly and take time.

Individual interviews

As with focus groups, individual interviews can be useful when pre-testing new product and service concepts or promotional materials. In particular, they are useful when it is difficult to get the target audience to a central site (this might occur, for example, with GPs or policy-makers). However, as with focus groups, individual interviews cost money and take time. Despite this, they are often worth investing in as they can provide an opportunity to discover why participants react in a certain way as well as how well they react.

Other methods of pre-testing are presented in Boxes 12.11 and 12.12.

Evaluation

As mentioned previously (see Chapter 11), evaluation is not something that should be considered only once the intervention is in place: it is integral to every stage of the process. Evaluation during

Box 12.11 Different pre-testing methods for products and services

Pre-testing method	When to use it
Product/service prototype tests	Product prototype tests examine consumer reactions to an actual early version of the product. This early prototype should have been developed based on earlier consumer research. The product in this case is given to consumers to use for a couple of weeks and then follow-up interviews are conducted. The purpose of these interviews is to find out what consumers like and dislike about the product and the likelihood of usage.
Product/service pricing research	As previously stated, giving the product or service away for free may not be the best pricing strategy. But how much should you charge? The amount can be tested and determined using product pricing research. The goal of many pricing studies is to measure consumer sensitivity to different prices. In the commercial world, this is often done using scanner-based research.
Packaging tests	Packaging has two roles: to protect the products and make the product desirable to the target audience. You may wish use street surveys or focus groups to test reactions to the packaging's: ◆ colour; ◆ delivery approach (e.g. screw-off cap, glass or plastic bottle); and ◆ shape.
Product/service concept test	This is a popular type of product research. A product concept is an idea for a new product or a significant modification of an existing product or service. The product development process usually begins with the generation of ideas or concepts for new products. Normally, this process generates many more ideas for new products than could ever be developed. It is, therefore, the researcher's job to work out which ideas to explore further. In order to test out these ideas, focus groups and individual interviews are often used.

Source: McDaniel and Gates (1999); Sigel and Doner (2004).

Box 12.12 Different pre-testing methods for promotional materials

Pre-testing method	When to use it
Ad positioning statement testing	The objective of this testing is to obtain consumer reactions to positioning statements such as 'Condom. Essential Wear', which was used by DH in 2008 to promote condom use or 'It's not for girls', which Nestlé used to promote its Yorkie bar in the same year. In the process of designing major advertising campaigns, it is important that statements are received positively by the target audience and actually initiate the desired behaviour.
Ad concept testing	This usually follows positioning statement testing. At this point, preliminary versions of the printed materials have been developed and you may be testing concepts for print work, radio, or television adverts. A variety of methods can be used, but face-to-face data collection procedures (usually focus groups) are the norm.
Readability testing	Readability is an attempt to match the reading level of written material to the 'reading with understanding' level of the reader. Readability tests are designed to give a statistical analysis of the difficulty of a text. While any attempt to reduce language use, which is inherently creative, to statistics can be criticized, readability tests can be used to give an approximate indication.
Expert and field review	This will enable you to obtain 'buy-in' from key stakeholders. Expert and field reviews can be done either by sending experts/key stakeholders information on the intervention and a self-administered questionnaire or by setting up a focus group or individual interviews. Whilst this method is mostly employed for pre-testing promotional materials, it can also be used for the pre-testing of new products and services.

Source: McDaniel and Gates (1999); Sigel and Doner (2004).

the development stage includes the pre-testing of the proposed intervention(s). This allows you to identify any gaps or discrepancies between what people say they want and what they actually want. People will often tell you what they think you want to hear or what they know they should say (see Box 12.13). At this stage, it is also important to determine appropriate indicators of success and develop your evaluation design.

Ethical considerations

We have already discussed ethical considerations for social marketing in Chapter 9. However, it is important to reconsider ethical issues during the developmental stage. At this point you must continually ask yourself if the marketing mix developed is ethically acceptable. The following questions can assist in this:

- Does the intervention mix meet normal ethical standards?
- Will people be hurt or damaged by the intervention(s)?
- Are you being entirely truthful?
- Are you inadvertently perpetuating inappropriate or harmful stereotypes? (Source: Smith, 2001)

Box 12.13 Do people want what they say they want?

Example: McDonalds

When the fast-food chain McDonald's introduced salads onto its menu, it had some short-term success. Sales of salads and other healthier options such as bags of fruit and deli sandwiches reached about £160 million (10% of sales) but have since remained static. In an all-day survey of six branches only three customers asked for a salad. The manager of a McDonald's in Bristol was quoted as saying: 'People will always go for chips over lettuce'. (Evening Standard, 8th November 2006).

The slump in McDonald's sales and the poor reception of its healthier product range has led to bosses allegedly ordering a 'back-to-basics' focus on McDonald's traditional range of burgers, fries, and fizzy drinks. Other fast-food restaurants have reported similar findings. A Wendy's spokesperson said: 'We listened to consumers who said they wanted to eat fresh fruit – but apparently they lied'. (The Guardian, 23rd August 2006 – www.guardian.co.uk/society/2006/aug/23/health.food).

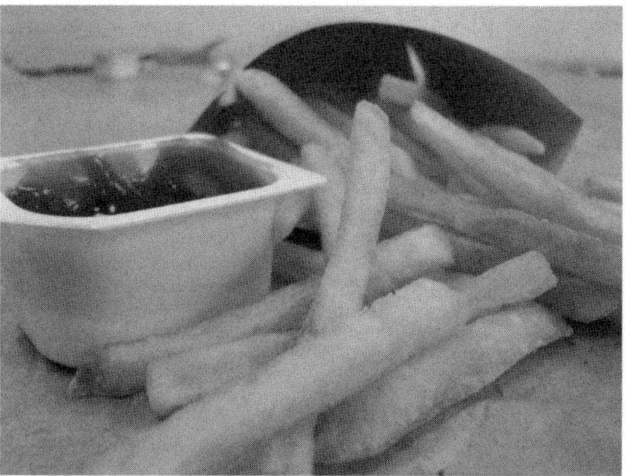

Conclusion

In many respects social marketing is much harder than commercial marketing, as the social marketer is often trying to get people to do something unpleasant (e.g. going for a smear test), frightening (e.g. going for a mammogram), or uncomfortable (e.g. giving blood). Therefore, in social marketing, having the right product or service, in the right place, at a price which can be seen to clearly add value for the target audience, and a creative promotional strategy is invaluable.

Review exercise

Think of a commercial company.

- What is their marketing mix?
- What are their brand's attributes?

Now think of a social marketing intervention you either have worked on or know of.

- What is their marketing mix?
- What are their brand's attributes?

When developing the marketing mix, sometimes leaflets and posters are regarded as the Augmented Product. Do you think they are the Augmented Product? If so why/why not?

References

Brower, M. and Leon, W. (1999). *The Consumer's Guide to Effective Environmental Choices: Practical Advice from the Union of Concerned Scientists.* New York, NY: Three Rivers Press.

Conference 2001 Proceedings, In Donovan R and Henley N (2003) *Social Marketing: Principles and Practice.* Melbourne: IP Communications.

Donovan, R. and Henley, N. (2003). *Social Marketing: Principles and Practice.* Melbourne: IP Communications.

Goodchild, J. and Callow, C. (2001). *Brands: Visions and Values.* New York, NY: John Wiley & Sons.

Hastings, G. (2007). *The Potential of Social Marketing: Why Should the Devil have all the Best Tunes?* Oxford: Butterworth-Heinemann.

Health Education Authority (1998). *Smoking cessation guidelines for health professionals,* published as a supplement to the December issue of the Thorax Guidelines 1998, Vol 53, Suppl 5, part 1.

Health Education Authority (2000). Updated thorax guidelines, again updated by the HEA and published in *Thorax Journal,* 2000, 55: 987–999.

Holt, D.B. (2002). *Got Milk*? Available at: http://www.aef.com/on_campus/classroom/case_histories/3000 (Accessed February 2009).

Homans, G.C. (1974). *Social Behaviour: its Elementary Forms.* Orlando, Fl: Harcourt Brace.

Kotler, P. (1988). *Marketing Management: Analysis, Planning, Implementation and Control.* Englewood Cliffs: Prentice-Hall.

Kotler, P. et al. (2002). *Social Marketing: Improving the Quality of Life.* Thousand Oaks, CA: Sage Publications.

Lauterborn, B. (1990). New Marketing Litany: Four Ps Passe: C-Words Take Over. Advert, *Age,* 61, 26.

MacFadyen, L. et al. (1999). *A synopsis of social marketing.* Available at: http://www.ism.stir.ac.uk/pdf_docs/social_marketing.pdf (Accessed March 2008).

McCarthy, J. (1960). *Basic Marketing: a Managerial Approach.* Homewood Il: Irwin.

McDaniel, C.D. and Gates, R.H. (1999). *Contemporary Marketing Research.* Ohio: South-Western College Publishing.

Merritt, R.K., Christopoulos, A., and Thorpe, A. (2009). *Social Marketing Quarterly.* In print.

Parkes, et al. (2005). Do sexual health services encourage teenagers to use condoms? A longitudinal study. *The Journal of Family Planning and Reproductive Health Care,* October, 31 (4): 271–280.

Peattie, S. and Peattie, K.J. (2003). Ready to fly solo? Reducing Social Marketing's Dependence on Commercial Marketing Theory. *Marketing Theory,* 2003 (Sept) (3)3: 365–385.

Perman, F. and Henley, N. (2001). Marketing the anti-drug message: source credibility varies by use/non-use of marijuana, Australia and New Zealand Marketing Academy.

Pricken, M. (2002). *Creative Advertising: Ideas and Techniques from the World's Best Campaigns.* New York, NY: Thames and Hudson.

Roselius, T. (1971). Consumer rankings of risk reduction methods. *Journal of Mental Health,* 35: 56–61.

Siegel, M. and Doner, L. (2004). *Marketing Public Health: Strategies to Promote Social Change.* Massachusetts: Jones and Bartlett Publishers.

Smith, W.A. (2001). Ethics and the social marketer: a framework for practitioners. In A. Andreasen (ed.) *Ethics in Social Marketing,* 1–16. Washington DC: Georgetown University Press.

Sunmola, A.M. et al. (2007). Predictors of condom use among sexually active persons involved in compulsory national service in Ibadam, Nigeria, *Health Education Research,* August, 22(4): 459–472.

Tungate, M. (2008). *Branded Male: Marketing to Men.* London and Philadelphia: Kogan Page Limited.

Chapter 13

Implementation

Rowena Merritt

When it is obvious that the goals cannot be reached, don't adjust the goals, adjust the action steps.
Confucius

Learning points

This chapter

- Examines ways of ensuring effective implementation of a social marketing intervention;
- Highlights the concept of live monitoring and adjustment; and
- Provides an understanding of how to ensure active 'opportunity spotting' and 'early problem tackling' are incorporated into the implementation phase.

Chapter overview

The third stage of the Total Process Planning framework is 'implementation'. By the time the implementation phase is reached, you should have completed the scoping report, used the marketing mix to develop your marketing strategy, pre-tested your interventions, and refined them accordingly.

During the implementation phase you will monitor your intervention(s) closely, ensuring that any potential opportunities are seized and problems swiftly dealt with. This chapter discusses ways of ensuring effective implementation and methods of monitoring a social marketing project.

Aim of the implementation stage

To carry out and actively manage marketing actions defined in the development stage.

Objective of the implementation stage

To launch and monitor the marketing activities and ensure efforts stay on target, on time, and on budget. As you execute your plans, you will use the mechanisms you have set in place to anticipate, identify, and address potential threats to your project efforts. In this stage, you will:

- plan the intervention launch;
- execute intervention plans;

- monitor progress;
- identify and act upon any opportunities arising; and
- modify project components based on feedback.

Output from the implementation stage

Intervention activities and documentation of any feedback and lessons learned, which may take the form of the reports you produce in Stage 4: Evaluation.

Introduction

Once each element of the marketing mix has been considered and the proposed intervention(s) are pre-tested and refined accordingly, the full intervention is ready to be launched. It is vital that you have systems in place to ensure close monitoring of the intervention. Such systems allow you act on any feedback highlighting problems or opportunities.

This chapter divides the implementation stage into three phases, discussed in turn:

1. Internal launch preparations.
2. Spotting opportunities and dealing with problems.
3. Monitoring plans and modification of interventional activities.

Moving from the 'Development' to 'Implementation' stage of the Total Process Planning (TPP) model

Often, people ask, 'how do you know it is time to move from the development to implementation stage?'

Although marketing is a discipline, it is not an exact science. We sometimes look too scientifically at the social marketing process; if we do A and B, then X will occur. In the commercial world, a company may launch a product which has been successfully pre-tested, and it will still be a flop. Sometimes you have to take a 'leap of faith' and just move onto the implementation phase. If it fails, then cut your losses quickly. That is why close monitoring and clear evaluation is needed (as discussed further in this chapter and Chapter 14).

However, if you have a clear marketing plan, in which all 4Ps have been accounted for, the eight-benchmark criteria considered (and acted upon!), the intervention(s) have been pre-tested and refined, and stakeholders have been engaged, then you are ready as you will ever be! So go for it.

Phase 1

Preparing for your launch

By now, you should have pre-tested and refined, if necessary, your selected marketing mix. It is now time to prepare for the launch. Before the launch you should:

1. receive organizational clearance for the proposed intervention(s) and gain stakeholder buy-in;
2. inform staff about the intervention and, if necessary, train them to deliver it;
3. distribute materials and resources; and
4. decide upon launch timings.

Ensuring stakeholder buy-in and getting organizational clearance

You need to get organizational clearance for the marketing mix you have developed, pre-tested, and refined in the development stage. You should get clearance from your senior managers and the staff who will be implementing the intervention.

Colleagues are a common barrier at this stage: they may have preconceived ideas of what they want the intervention to be, and therefore may not accept the interventions which have been developed based on consumer insight and pre-tested with the target audience. If this occurs, it is important to stress that the intervention has not been developed for your colleagues and that they are very unlikely to be part of the target audience. If they insist on blocking the intervention, and revert to their preconceived ideas of what it should be, they are no longer following a social marketing approach. By involving key stakeholders (which should include colleagues and managers) during the scoping and development stages, and by sharing the findings from the research with them, any potential problems can hopefully be addressed before this stage.

Staff training

One criticism faced by some of the past national governmental campaigns is that frontline staff (those working at the local level) often know nothing about the campaign before they see it on the television. You must have all your staff on board and ready to launch the intervention if it is to be successful. Staff should be trained to prepare them for the intervention activities. If any changes have been made, you should make sure that all staff understand the rationale for these changes or the new direction. Roles and responsibilities should also be defined and agreed upon, and if there are several interventions, you should explain how they are integrated.

Finally, it is important that one person has overall responsibility for the entire project, and that everyone knows who this person is.

Resource allocation

You must source resources before the launch, so that checks can be done to ensure adequate resources are in place. Any key stakeholders who may be affected by the intervention also have to be informed, trained, and checks done to ensure that they also have sufficient resources. For example, if you have developed an intervention designed to increase the number of women self-checking their breast for signs of cancer:

- have the nurses and doctors at the local surgeries been informed; and
- does the local hospital have sufficient resources to cope with the possible increase in the numbers needing mammograms?

Deciding on the timings of the launch

When launching the developed intervention, it is important to select an appropriate date for announcing (and publicizing, if appropriate) the intervention's official start. Consideration of staff holiday periods and existing patterns in the behaviour of the target audience must be considered. During the scoping phase, information collected on the target audience can help to ensure the correct timing of a launch. For example, campaigns encouraging people to give up smoking are usually launched on 1st January, in time for peoples New Year resolutions. Box 13.1 provides an example where timing was key.

Before you move onto Phase 2 and launch your intervention, the following checklist maybe useful:

- Have tasks been assigned to frontline staff?
- Has any necessary training been delivered to the staff?
- Have the programme objectives and implementation plans been shared?

Box 13.1 Increasing school meal uptake in a deprived region in England

School meals in primary schools make a vital contribution to the dietary intake of school children in England (Nelson et al., 2005). However, in recent years the number of school meals purchased has fallen in 75% of schools (Ofsted, 2007). In March 2007, a social marketing project was initiated in North East England. The project aimed to increase the uptake of school meals by children in three particularly deprived areas.

When looking at the existing data surrounding the update of school meals during the scoping phase, clear seasonal patterns were observed. Autumn and winter terms had the highest uptake. However the number of school meals taken during the warmer summer months dropped significantly. Some schools had tried to reverse this trend by making school lunches similar to pack lunches (the main competition for school meals); however, any increases in uptake by such initiatives were often short lived.

The project's steering group took into the account the decline in meal uptake in summer and decided not to launch their intervention in the summer months as previously planned. Instead the pilots were held in the winter months, when the competition was less desirable. Evaluation is currently ongoing as the pilot is being run on a long-term basis. Nevertheless, early results are positive. Further information on the project can be found at www.nsmcentre.org.uk.

- Have roles and responsibilities been discussed and agreed upon?
- Has one person been made responsible for the overall programme?
- Has feedback been sought from staff and stakeholders before the launch to avoid any problems/challenges they may see?

Phase 2

Spotting opportunities

Opportunities often arise when a new intervention is in place, and it may be tempting for staff and key stakeholders to move away from the core project and start a new one. While it is important to recognize and act upon such opportunities, discussions must be held with the relevant managers and stakeholders to determine how to take advantage of opportunities without causing the core intervention to suffer.

During the discussion, you should try to determine whether an opportunity really is worth acting upon. Opportunities such as new funding to reach a different audience or invitations to join coalitions that work on related issues may or may not improve your intervention. Make sure that any opportunities you embrace do not alter the direction of the project or dilute resources for reaching the set objectives.

Dealing with problems

Unexpected problems will almost certainly arise during the implementation stage. In significant matters:

- decide how to address the problem;
- take the necessary corrective steps; and

- make staff and other stakeholders aware that adjustments are being made to original plans and why they are being made.

Keeping on track of budgets and resources

Many social marketing interventions have to operate on limited funding. Therefore, budgets must be managed carefully to ensure that the intervention is implemented within the planned budget. Predict expenses on budget timelines and regularly review expenditures against the timelines. If you have an unanticipated and uncontrollable expense in one area, adjust other budget items downwards, always with the project's objectives foremost in mind.

Phase 3

Monitoring plans and modification of the intervention

Marketers view evaluation as a tool to improve their interventions. Consequently, they place enormous emphasis on formative, process, and outcome evaluation (Siegel and Doner, 2004). Building process-evaluation measures into an initiative's tactics provides an important set of management tools. By using process-evaluation data to monitor regularly an intervention's success, timely refinements can be made. Chapter 14 discusses formative, process, and outcome evaluation. However, process evaluation should be started in the implementation stage. With this in mind, details on process evaluation are presented in this chapter also.

Process-evaluation methods

The monitoring of information provided by evaluation can serve as a powerful management device. As Andreasen noted:

> Commercial sector marketers crave data ... they want to correct things before it is too late ... a cybernetic self-correcting system that constantly looks at what is happening, diagnoses why it is happening, and takes corrective action as needed.
>
> (Andreasen, 1995, p. 128)

Process evaluation should document actual implementation, compare it to planned implementation, and allow for adjustments to be made (Siegel and Doner, 2004).

For multi-pronged interventions, process evaluation is often piecemeal, as the data is collected separately for each part of the intervention. Process evaluation works when it draws together the results of all the interventions and provides an opportunity to systematically evaluate overall performance. This will allow an overall picture to emerge of the effort, and also reveal which part of the intervention needs refinement.

As soon as the intervention is launched, activities should be documented and spot-checked for fidelity to the plan. You should also have in place a system for recording target-audience feedback on the interventional activities, communication materials, services, and products.

Evaluation methods

When developing your process plan, you need to think carefully about what data will best help you identify how your intervention is doing and what refinements are needed. For example, tracking the number of leaflets distributed may be meaningless if they are picked up by people and then never read, or they are read but fail to change behaviour (Carré et al., 2008; Wicke et al., 1994). Some common process-evaluation methods are listed in Table 13.1.

Table 13.1 Process-evaluation methods

Evaluation method	Application in social marketing
Mass media monitoring	The most effective way to discover media coverage is by subscribing to a clippings service. Such services scan hundreds of newspapers and listen to news programmes daily. Once these clippings have been received, the next step is to analyse the clips' findings. Analysis of the clips is best done qualitatively. It is important that the clips are checked for accuracy and desirability.
Event monitoring	Monitoring of events can be done inexpensively. For example, after each event a simple questionnaire will allow feedback to be recorded and acted upon if necessary. The numbers attending the events should always be recorded. If the event is being held more than once, evaluation allows for revision and improvement.
Bounceback cards	These are short questionnaires on the back of a postcard. They can be sent to the target audience, just asking a few questions about the intervention (e.g. how much of the leaflet did you read? Do you think it was too long?) Bounceback cards are a relatively inexpensive method; however, response rates are often low.
Inventory tracking	This helps to ensure that adequate numbers of the products/materials are in stock as well as tracking what items are the most popular. There are a variety of computer programmes which will assist in inventory tracking, or you can set up a simple database to log what is being distributed, in what quantity, at what date, and to which geographical locations.
Client satisfaction	Ways of measuring client satisfaction include: ◆ unsolicited client responses (for example suggestion or comment boxes); ◆ observations (e.g. observe those attending a newly opened Stop Smoking Service); ◆ questionnaires; and ◆ qualitative studies (which can shed light on the reasons underlying service usage and satisfaction or dissatisfaction (CDC, 1993)).
Telephone helpline	Both automated and live-operated helplines can provide a wealth of knowledge. Analysis of call volume by date can indicate which promotional tools people are responding to. If live operators are in post, questions can be asked as to where the respondent saw the telephone number. Basic demographic data can also be collected to check whether the correct target audience is responding.
Coupons	If you are offering a new product (e.g. a compost bin) and distribute coupons in a number of printed materials or on a website, you can determine where people received the coupons and, therefore, which communication channels are most effective.
Website evaluations	Websites offering information support, online discussion forums, and online health checks are becoming a staple feature of social marketing interventions. Web tools that record the quantity and quality of customer interaction are readily available and help build up comprehensive databases on customers and provide samples for future interventions or evaluation surveys.
Quantitative tracking services	These often take the form of public opinion polls. They provide a means of monitoring knowledge levels, current attitudes, and self-reported behaviour. However, this method can be costly, especially if it is commissioned through one of the large market-research companies.

Source: Adapted from Siegel and Doner (2004); Weinreich (2006)

Feedback from staff and stakeholders

Feedback from staff on the progress of your intervention activities should be collected in one-on-one sessions or formal meetings. It is also important to receive feedback from your key stakeholders as well as other ground staff, who may not work for your organization, but who are affected by the intervention (e.g. general practitioners (GPs) at the local surgery and hospital staff conducting mammograms). It is important to make sure they are receiving the target audience and not simply the 'worried well' (By 'worried well' we mean people who are receptive to health messages, but often misjudge the relevance of the message to their personal circumstances and likely health outcomes) (see Box 13.2).

With complex, multifaceted interventions involving many players, an analysis of stakeholder views at several points in an intervention's lifetime will be an essential component of formative, process, and outcome evaluations. Stakeholders may include:

- intervention mangers (e.g. campaign managers, press officers, advertising agencies, research agencies, public relations (PR) agency, communication and research managers);
- service managers and people working on the ground (e.g. teachers, doctors, health and clinic staff, local authority workers, outreach staff and police);
- local commissioners;
- local leaders (e.g. politicians, pressure group leaders and faith leaders) and
- voluntary and NGO (non-governmental organization) sector players.

Understanding the stakeholders' perceptions and expectations of the project and their views as to what has contributed to success or failure will produce key findings for any process evaluation.

Document analysis

Projects generate a lot of paperwork: minutes of meetings, project plans, advertising briefs, strengths, weaknesses, opportunities, and threats (SWOT) analyses – to name but a few. These documents provide insight into the thinking, debates, the level of buy-in from stakeholders, the delays, the success, and the degree to which the intervention is delivered as planned. Commissioning an external person to analyse these documents as part of the process evaluation is often a worthwhile investment.

Disseminating findings

When reviewing the process and the intervention, it is important to examine both positive and negative outcomes to learn what worked and what did not. These findings, whether positive or negative, must be shared as widely as possible. Showing your efforts in a realistic light and sharing challenges and successes can be beneficial to other managers, who can learn from your work. When disseminating the findings, try to use the channels and venues that best suit the needs and interests of key stakeholders. Whilst publishing negative or neutral findings in academic literature can be difficult (Rothstein et al., 2005; Dickersin, 1990), they can be published on your organization's website, presented at conferences and added to databases which reference grey literature, such as System for Information on Grey Literature in Europe Archive (SIGLE). The important thing is to make sure the information is in the public domain.

Developments in the wider environment

To make sure the intervention stays up-to-date and consistent with trends and developments in the area, you need to monitor the wider environment. For example, this may include monitoring

Box 13.2 Checking your intervention is appealing to your target audience

Example: 'AIDS – Don't Die of Ignorance'

In the mid-1980s, a nationwide educational campaign was launched with the aim of educating the public about human immunodeficiency virus/acquired immune deficiency syndrome (HIV/AIDS). 'I remember it just as an issue which was of fundamental importance,' says Lord Fowler (former Health Secretary). 'We didn't know a great deal ... nothing like what we know today about HIV/AIDS. There was no cure and literally, public education, advertisement, publicity, they were the only weapons that we actually had.' Television adverts, which have now become iconic, were shown. An astonishing voice-over from the actor John Hurt, which began, 'There is now a dreadful disease ...' electrified the UK.

A leaflet was sent to every household in the country. There was a week of educational programming at peak time. Whilst some critics of the campaign now say that the government was guilty of scaremongering, the campaign had a profound effect not only on HIV rates (new diagnoses of HIV, which were over 3000 in 1985, dropped by a third in 3 years), but also on all sexually transmitted infections. Following the campaign, the number of diagnoses of gonorrhoea in England and Wales dropped from around 50 000 in 1985 to just 18 000 in 1988 – and had dropped to a twentieth-century low by the mid-1990s.

Despite the campaign's obvious success, some unforeseen circumstances arose. The campaign put a huge strain on the existing screening services, and these services were often being used by the 'worried well'.

Source: BBC News, 16 October 2005

Box 13.3 Reacting to unforeseen negative effects

Example: Smoking in pregnancy

It is important to correct unintended intervention effects that monitoring and evaluation reveal. It is well documented in medical literature that smoking during pregnancy leads to smaller babies. We know that smaller babies have more problems: they need to eat more, they sleep less, and they often require more frequent hospitalization. They are also more likely to have intrauterine growth retardation (IUGR). However, for young, first-time mothers fearing childbirth, finding out that if they smoke they will have a smaller baby may encourage them to smoke, with the hope that the childbirth is less painful.

other media coverage, policy changes, and changes in treatment guidelines. By using this data, your intervention will remain fresh and responsive. This may involve using new communication channels to reach your audience or responding to new trends.

Ethical considerations

As with all stages of the Total Process Planning framework, you must consider ethical issues during the implementation stage. As some interventions developed to promote positive behavioural change may inadvertently lead to negative outcomes, the social marketing process allows safeguards to be put into place to ensure that such negative effects do not occur and if they do occur, they are swiftly rectified (see Box 13.3). Safeguards such as thorough pre-testing of the intervention with the target audience, and consulting and including key stakeholders and delivery staff throughout the process, help to identify negative effects before the launch. However, by incorporating robust evaluation during the implementation stage, if negative effects are subsequently revealed and reported, these can be dealt with immediately.

Conclusion

During the implementation stage, your intervention must be monitored closely. Process evaluation can assist in this, and the methods of the evaluation must be considered and put into place before the intervention is launched. Determine whether changes in your community, the target audience, or the environment (e.g. policy changes) can help you reach your objectives, and take advantage of these opportunities. Use audience feedback, intervention monitoring, and evaluation data to revise your intervention(s) if your assumptions are proved to be incorrect. Or use the data to tweak activities to better serve your target audience.

Review exercise

Consider a social marketing intervention that you have either worked on or a project you know about. When the project was in the intervention phase:

- What opportunities did you spot?
- Did any problems arise? How did you deal with these?
- What would you do differently in future projects?

Limit yourself to no more than five bullet points for each response.

References

Andreasen, A.R. (1995). *Marketing Social Change: Changing Behaviour to Promote Health, Social, Development, and the Environment.* San Francisco, CA: Jossey-Bass Publications.

Carré, P.C. Roche, N., Neukirch, F. et al. (2008). The effect of an information leaflet upon knowledge and awareness of COPD in potential sufferers: a randomized controlled study, *Respiration*, Feb 2008.

Centres for Disease Control and Prevention Academy for Educational Development. (1993). Planning and evaluating HIV/AIDS prevention programs in state and local health departments: a companion to program announcement # 300. Washington, DC: Academy for Educational Development.

Dickersin, K. (1990). The existence of publication bias and risk factors for its occurrence, *Journal of the American Medical Association*, 263(10):1385–1389.

Nelson, M., Nicholas, J., Suleiman, S., et al. (2005). School Meals in Primary Schools in England. *Research Report RR753.* London: Department for Education and Skills.

Ofsted (2007, October). *Food in Schools: Encouraging Healthier Eating.* Available at: http://www.ofsted.gov.uk/Ofsted-home/Publications-and-research/Browse-all-by/Education/Curriculum/Food-technology/Food-in-schools-encouraging-healthier-eating (Accessed March 2009)>

Rothstein, H. et al. (2005). Publication Bias in Meta-Analysis, In Rothstein, H. et al. (eds.) *Publication Bias in Meta-Analysis, Prevention, Assessment and Adjustments.* Chichester: Wiley.

Siegel, M. and Doner, L. (2004). *Marketing Public Health: Strategies to Promote Social Change.* Massachusetts: Jones & Bartlett Publishers.

Chapter 14

Evaluation

Dominic McVey, Adam Crosier, and Alex Christopoulos

I know of no more encouraging fact than the unquestioning ability of man to evaluate his life by a conscious endeavor.
Henry David Thoreau

Learning points

This chapter

- Explains why evaluation is important to social marketing;
- Outlines the different research methods;
- Explains the different stages of evaluation that can be carried out on social marketing projects; and
- Provides case studies of evaluation in practice.

Chapter overview

The main purpose of this chapter is to describe the common approaches to evaluation, which is the fourth step in the Total Process Planning (TPP) framework. As well as setting out the theory behind designing and conducting evaluation research, this chapter provides case studies that show how evaluation works in practice. By the time the evaluation phase is reached, you should have completed the scoping report, and developed and implemented your marketing strategy. However, as mentioned previously, evaluation is not a distinct stage, which only needs to be addressed when you have implemented your intervention. It must be considered from the scoping stage onwards.

Aim of the evaluation stage

To identify the strengths and weaknesses of your intervention and to determine if it is making a difference.

Objective of the evaluation stage

To produce detailed information about:

- what your project has achieved;
- how well it has contributed to your aim, and met your objectives;
- what worked well and what did not, and why;
- whether there were any unintended outcomes; and
- what can be learned from this project to improve practice and inform other projects

Output from the evaluation stage

A report detailing the findings of the evaluation work. Ideally this report should be made available in the public domain, or the findings should be published in an academic journal.

Introduction

Evaluation is about assessing the value or worth of something. Without being cynical, it is clear that some people use evaluation as a 'rubber stamp' – to justify spend on a project or to please stakeholders and funders, some treat it as a quest for the holy grail of 'best practice', whilst others include it as an essential part of all work they undertake.

Evaluation is a vital tool for:

- checking how well your intervention is going;
- seeing whether the intervention is making a difference;
- identifying its strengths and weaknesses;
- getting ideas on how to improve the intervention;
- supporting advocacy for the continuation or extension of the project; and
- being accountable to funders and stakeholders.

In their influential book *Realistic Evaluation* (1997) Pawson and Tilley attributed the inexorable rise of evaluation to the information and knowledge revolution of the post-industrial age. In a world where information and knowledge are prized above almost every other commodity, evaluation has acquired a 'guru' status, because it promises to sort and sift the valuable from the valueless and guides management decisions to create effective policy.

The debates about assessing value and effectiveness that have raged in the field of health promotion for decades are as relevant today and apply just as much to social marketing as they do to health promotion. These debates – which call into question the quality of evidence used to assess effectiveness of social interventions, including social marketing – lay it open to criticism and make such interventions vulnerable to cuts in funding (Speller et al., 1998).

To get out of this downward spiral, social marketers must demonstrate evidence of the effectiveness of evaluation by establishing a robust evidence base.

What do we mean by evaluation?

Evaluation is a complex subject and there is a great deal of literature dedicated to its merits and how it can be done effectively. To begin with, it is important to outline what we mean by 'evaluation'. The following definition is taken from the World Health organization (WHO) in 1981:

> Evaluation is a systematic way of learning from experience and using lessons learnt to improve current activities and to promote better planning by careful selection of alternatives for future actions
>
> WHO

Evidence in government

When evaluating social marketing projects, it is important to set the standard of evidence as high as possible, and aim for an objective assessment of impact. The quality of research required to evaluate the effectiveness of publicly funded projects tends to have greater rigour than research applied to commercially funded projects. However, the type and quality of the evidence required to make policy decisions does vary across government and the public sector. For example, a broader definition of evidence is generally used by government than by academics. As discussed in the report *Is Evidence Based Government Possible*? (Davies, 2004), many sources of evidence are used by government, some of which are more reliable that others. For example, papers written by opinion leaders and 'think-tanks' can be given precedence over systematic reviews of evidence. When considering how to evaluate your social marketing project, it is important to consider who will use the evidence and what evidence your key stakeholders (in particular, your funders) require.

Why do we evaluate?

Without any robust evaluation of projects there is no proof that what you are doing works or is effective. There are ineffective projects which continue to be funded because a flawed evaluation has judged them to be effective. Alternatively, many good programmes and ideas have been discarded because of poor or inappropriate evaluations. When an evaluation of a population health intervention is lacking or insufficient, the tendency has been to label the intervention ineffective when in reality it is the evaluation that is flawed. Lessons from the field of health promotion on the need for evidence can be taken from the debate which has occurred over the last two decades.

The need to evaluate social marketing interventions: lessons from health promotion

Health promotion, and the need to evaluate its activities thoroughly, sparked a somewhat frenzied debate in the 1990s. One of the leading proponents of the need for robust evaluation was Ann Oakley, who followed up criticism of the AIDS-prevention campaigns in the early 1990s with a series of articles that drew attention to the importance of research and evaluation in social interventions (Oakley, 1988).

Oakley's criticisms were that the prevention campaigns and other responses of governmental agencies to the emerging pandemic were untested and unproven, were probably wasteful, and possibly harmful. Oakley's contention was that health-education and -promotion campaigns were just as capable as medical interventions to do harm as well as good. Her recommendation was that social interventions of this type should be subjected to the same standards of assessment as clinical interventions. These included, where appropriate, the use of randomized controlled trials (RCTs), and certainly the systematic review of good-quality evidence to inform policy.

Health promoters responded to these criticisms of the research methods used to evaluate health-promotion interventions. They argued that there were both practical and philosophical differences between health promotion and clinical interventions that made clinical-style evaluation procedures inappropriate for health promotion. They pointed to the time and complexity of these multidimensional programmes (in which the unit of intervention is rarely the individual but often whole populations) and argued that they may make them inappropriate for assessment by a conventional clinical experimental design. They also argued that whereas medical practices were mainly concerned with achieving a predetermined objective, health promotion often relied on the emergence and 'ownership' of aims by people among whom the intervention takes place (Nutbeam, 1999). Furthermore, health-promotion initiatives trend to have more complex casual chains than clinical intervention – and many go beyond individual behavioural change to tackle the social determinants of health (Victora, 2004). Tones (1997) put forward alternative models of assessing effectiveness, moving away from what he described as a 'politically motivated' pursuit at all costs of experimental evidence. For example, he suggested that a test should be developed based on the idea that evidence should be sufficient to satisfy a jury of relevant experts.

Evidence-based decision making in the UK health-care sector – based on systematic reviews – are being applied further field and call into question the quality of evidence used to assess effectiveness of social interventions including social marketing. As evaluations of social interventions can never compete with the rigour that can be successfully applied to medical interventions, the evidence will always favour investment in medical rather than social programmes. Social interventions must establish their own robust criteria by which studies are accepted or rejected. These must be firmly rooted in the real world and built on appropriate methodologies to meet these needs. This is not to say that evaluation should not be systematic and rigorous – it should – but it is to recognize that the real world is not a laboratory. Humans rarely behave like a collection of viruses or lab animals, and while we can take knowledge from the clinical sciences, we should not pretend that evaluation in the real world is of the same order. For example, the distal outcomes associated with many social marketing interventions result in long causal chains between a social intervention and the effect on behaviour. This makes the attribution of observed change to particular interventions a challenge.

One clear lesson from the evidence debate is the importance of ensuring that the appropriate research design and research methods are used to answer the specific research questions.

Benefits of evaluating

Apart from merely seeing whether your social marketing project has achieved the set aims and objectives, evaluating your intervention can also:

- help you remain accountable to funders and to provide them with evidence of effectiveness;
- check that your intervention is being accessed by the right people (or if it is just being accessed by the 'worried-well');
- inform the revision and/or development of materials, methods, and services;
- ensure ethical practice is being undertaken;
- optimize utilization of resources – where are there stresses and slack in the system?
- inform practice and contribute to the evidence base – without shared learning projects may keep reinventing the wheel and duplicating ineffective procedures;
- provide feedback for those involved;
- inform programme planning; and
- identify any unintended effects of your intervention.

Hierarchies of evidence

As part of the debate about the quality of the evidence that should be used to determine effectiveness, researchers have developed the notion of 'hierarchies of evidence'. While the detail between the different hierarchies varies, the aim is clear: to establish that evidence derived from certain kinds of research design are better than others. The hierarchy of evidence (Petticrew & Roberts, 2003) applied to studies of health and well-being are summarized below in Table 14.1.

Clinical drug trials provide the most robust forms of evidence using RCTs which feed into systematic reviews and meta-analyses. However, applying RCT designs to complex multifaceted interventions such as social marketing and health promotion can be difficult and so methodologies that are lower down on the evidence hierarchy tend to be employed.

Table 14.2 sets out some of the differences between clinical trials and social marketing/health-promotion interventions. This helps to explain why research designs that are appropriate for assessing clinical interventions may be inappropriate for assessing social marketing interventions.

One of the main problems with using RCTs to evaluate social marketing interventions is the issue of controlling extraneous 'noise'. Sometimes, one of the main objectives for a social marketing intervention may be to 'create' noise and awareness about an issue to help change individual and organizational behaviour. Conversely, one of the primary objectives of RCTs is to 'control' such extraneous noise. Applying this research methodology can, therefore, work against the objectives of your intervention.

Table 14.1 Rank and definition of evidence type

Rank	Methodology	Description
1	Systematic reviews and meta-analyses	A 'systematic review' is a review of a body of data that uses explicit methods to locate primary studies, and explicit criteria to assess their quality.
		Meta-analysis is a statistical analysis that combines or integrates the results of several independent trials. The appeal of meta-analysis is that it, in effect, combines all the research on one topic into one large study with many participants.
2	Randomized controlled trials	Individuals are randomly allocated to a 'test' group and receive a specific intervention or a 'control' group who receive no intervention. Both groups are interviewed before and after the test intervention.
3	Cohort studies	Groups of people are selected on the basis of their exposure to a particular agent and followed up for specific outcomes.
4	Case-control studies	'Cases' with the condition are matched with 'controls' without, and a retrospective analysis used to look for differences between the two groups.
5	Cross sectional surveys	Quantitative survey of a sample of the population of interest conducted before an intervention and a similar sample interviewed after the intervention.
6	Case reports	A report based on a few patients or subjects; sometimes collected together into a short series.
7	Expert opinion	Opinions from respected authorities and experts, based on clinical evidence, descriptive studies or reports from committees.

Table 14.2 Differences between clinical trials and social marketing interventions

Clinical trials	Social marketing / health promotion interventions
Participants are usually seeking a cure.	Participants are currently well and may not perceive themselves as needing help. Also the interventions are often preventative, not curing.
Clinical trials often have a simpler biological basis (e.g. drugs, surgery) and are easier to control.	Social marketing interventions are generally multifaceted, which diffuse into the population to achieve behavioural change at the individual or societal level. There is a lot of extraneous 'noise' to control.
The unit of randomization is usually individual, or clusters.	The unit of randomization can be individual, community or nation. Individual randomization can be difficult.
Internal validity (a measure of the extent to which the findings are real and not the result of bias). This is not a problem with RCTs, as this can be achieved using control groups who receive a placebo. Double blind (neither the individuals nor the researchers know who belongs to the control group and the experimental group) and triple blind (multiple investigators are all blinded to the protocol) is also possible.	It is often very difficult to devise a placebo for a community development intervention and to blind people to the fact they have received the intervention.
The exposure of control group to the intervention is more easily controlled.	There is a high risk that the control group (e.g. a neighbouring community) is exposed to intervention.

What does evaluation involve?

In a world of limitless budget and timescales, evaluation plans can be designed to give evidence beyond reasonable doubt that proves the effectiveness of an intervention. However, in reality we do not live in such a world. We need to be practical about what evaluation we can actually do. In order to provide value, evaluation activities should be:

- **Useful** – Does the evaluation serve a purpose? Will it be responsive to stakeholder information needs?
- **Feasible** – What time, resources, and expertise are available to you?
- **Accurate** – What information do you need to make your decisions?
- **Ethical** – Will the evaluation cause harm or distress to your target audience?

It is important that the original objectives are the starting point of the evaluation. This sentiment is echoed by Hastings (2007) *It is not possible to measure achievements without clear original intentions.* Once the objectives are set, the evaluation process should look to gather data that measures or indicates success or failure in meeting them.

When designing the evaluation of a project, you need to be pragmatic as you will always have to limit the number of variables measured. It is important to prioritize the aspects of your intervention(s) that are most important to evaluate.

Maintain objectivity

There is always a political dimension to any evaluation. Whilst there is a desire to demonstrate effectiveness it is important for evaluators to remain objective and have in place governance procedures to ensure the independence of the research, which may reveal that projects were not as effective as the programme managers expected them to be. Managing the intervention and the evaluation can create conflicts of interest and compromise the objectivity of the evaluator. Employing external evaluators can create distance and engender some objectivity between the intervention and the evaluation. At the very least, you should build a small advisory group of a few social science academics from the local university or college to check over your evaluation plans and help with the interpretation of the results.

It is worth noting that poor results can also be very useful. The identification of what has gone wrong, and why, can be as useful to an organization as the identification of what has gone well. Early identification of an ineffective service may save an organization from rolling it out on a wider scale and therefore save money and resources. In addition, if the project has an adverse unintended effect on users, this can be alleviated.

Types of research

There are various methods which can be used to collect the data to evaluate your social marketing intervention. Data collection techniques usually fall under one of two broad methodologies: *Quantitative Research* (such as questionnaire-based face to face in-home interviews, street surveys, telephone interviews, or web-based surveys) and *Qualitative Research* (such as focus groups and individual in-depth interviews).

Both these methods provide different but valuable data and are often most valuable when combined. Despite the advantage of combining the methods, they are frequently used independently. Sometimes, those researchers that advocate one method do not value the other. This has lead to debates about the relative merits of the approaches being often polarized (MacNaughton, 1996). However, as Britten and Fisher (1993) pointed out, each research approach had advantages and disadvantages.

> There is some truth in the quip that quantitative methods are reliable but not valid and that qualitative methods are valid but not reliable.
>
> (Britten and Fisher, 1993, p. 271)

Whilst quantitative research produces 'hard' and reliable evidence, which is invaluable in scientific and medical studies, qualitative research allows individuals to 'speak' for themselves, and is useful in the exploration of complex and interrelated issues, such as patients' attitudes (Bryman, 1988). Definitions for qualitative and quantitative research are given in Box 14.1.

Tools and methods

An evaluator should use a number of different research methods to produce a quantitative and qualitative analysis of the intervention. Some of the research methodologies that generate valuable evaluation data for the social marketer include:

- media analysis
- event monitoring
- inventory tracking
- client-satisfaction studies
- telephone helpline analysis
- customer/patient journey mapping
- website evaluations

Box 14.1 Qualitative and quantitative research methods defined

Qualitative research can be defined as follows:

> By the term qualitative research we mean any kind of research that produces findings not arrived at by means of statistical procedures or other means of quantification. It can refer to research about persons' lives, stories, behaviour, but also about organisational functioning, social movements, or interactional relationships.
>
> Strauss and Corbin, 1990. p. 17

Qualitative research techniques, which are commonly used, include focus groups and individual or paired in-depth interviews. Although used less often, participant and non-participant observation techniques can be very useful for generating subtle insights into health related behaviour.

Quantitative research can be more simply defined as techniques that are used to gather quantitative data (information dealing with numbers and anything that is measurable).

Quantitative research techniques, which are commonly used, include structured questionnaires, administered by face-to-face in-home surveys, web based surveys, telephone surveys, and postal surveys. Many large scale face-to-face surveys are now administered using laptop computers whereby the interviewer inputs the respondents responses directly into the computer and in some cases, for the more sensitive questions, allows the respondents to input data themselves..

- qualitative and quantitative monitoring
- controlled and quasi-controlled trials
- stakeholder research
- document analysis

Most of these methods will be discussed in this chapter and Chapter 13.

Stages of evaluation

There are a number of different stages of evaluation that can be carried out on a social marketing project; this chapter discusses three of these:

(1) Formative evaluation is used to help develop a programme and its implementation.

(2) Process evaluation looks at whether interventions are working as planned.

(3) Outcome evaluations look at whether the project worked in relation to its objectives.

Typically, the evaluation of a project entails monitoring on a continual basis *and* conducting one or more time-limited outcome-evaluation studies. The three stages of evaluation are now discussed in more detail.

Formative evaluation

Formative evaluation is especially useful in the development of social marketing, but in our experience, is rarely given the time or resources it requires to demonstrate its true value. In fact, formative evaluation is one of the areas of social marketing that is most often performed poorly, or not done at all.

The term relates to the 'front-end' evaluation – finding out what is likely to be effective in motivating the target audience (for more information about gaining insight into your target group to shape your intervention see Chapters 11 and 7) – and ensuring that the intervention will be accessible and understandable. It is particularly useful to test whether the exchange and propositions are likely to work with the target audience.

Formative evaluation involves a number of steps. The following steps were developed with a media campaign in mind, but have application to other forms of social marketing interventions.

- Finding out the needs of your target group;
- Testing out elements of your intervention prior its implementation;
- Helping you to establish and clarify your aims and objectives;
- Identifying barriers to implementation;
- Establishing baseline data.

Qualitative research methods (focus groups and in-depth interviews) tend to predominate in formative research particularly in the testing phase, e.g.

- generating intervention ideas;
- testing concepts;
- testing the proposition or positioning statement;
- testing 'copy' (the actual words you will use to elicit behaviour change); and
- testing the marketing

There are a wide range of qualitative research methods to employ. Focus groups are the most widely understood but other methods include, paired depth interviews, participant observation, non-participant observation, ethnography, etc.

Establishing a baseline and setting realistic objectives

One of the elements of the formative stage is the establishment of baseline data of knowledge, attitudes, and behaviour. This provides an assessment of the magnitude of the task ahead and informs the design of the intervention. The baseline will help with setting realistic objectives and the outcome measures which will be assessed following the intervention.

Process evaluation

A process evaluation is concerned with how the intervention was implemented and functioned. It is a vital element of the programme because without it social marketers could measure outcomes without knowing how and why they were achieved.

Many evaluations do not include an adequate process evaluation, and some do not have one at all, making it very difficult to understand why an intervention has succeeded or failed.

Hamilton et al. (1977), in their book *Beyond the Numbers Game*, make the case for process evaluation.

> It's rather like a critic who reviews a production on the basis of the script and the applause meter readings, having missed the performance.
>
> (Hamilton et al., 1977)

Below, are the key components of a process evaluation:

Context

An intervention can be affected positively or negatively by the wider social, cultural, political, and economic environment in which it operates. For example, in England, the smoking prevalence among all adults is approximately 25% (General Household Survey, 2006), but the societal norm is non-smoking. However, in certain areas of the UK the smoking prevalence is 60%, so the norm in these areas is clearly to smoke. The effectiveness of a smoking intervention in such communities will clearly be influenced by the social context, and this should be taken into account in the planning of interventions and the interpretation of the evaluation findings.

Reach

Although awareness should not be your primary measure of effectiveness, it is important to measure it. If your target group is not aware of your initiative then there is not much hope of anything else changing.

Dose delivered and dose received

There needs to be some estimate of the amount and intensity of the intervention you expect the target groups to receive. For example, if as part of your campaign you expect to deliver a mass media component, you should have a clear idea of how many times you expect the target group to see your campaign over a specified period of time (known as the 'opportunities to see' or OTS figure). This is media space you have paid for, and is an estimate of the dose delivered. The dose received (the number of times the target groups claim they saw your campaigns) should tally approximately with the dose delivered. If they are very different, this indicates that there are problems with the delivery of the campaign. This could be due to an inappropriate mix of marketing channels; e.g. using press advertisements when radio would be more appropriate or using radio but placing the ads in the wrong radio programmes with poor listening figures for your target audience. Learning from marketing-mix errors can help get it right next time. Another reason for a low-dose response could be that the audience are not responding to a poorly constructed message, one that has no resonance with them and hence is easily forgotten.

Was the intervention delivered as planned?

Social marketing interventions are built on the work of a wide range of professional stakeholders; researchers, programme managers, advertising agencies, press officers, outreach workers, and medical professionals. These people work at different speeds and to their own professional standards, which means that strong project management is essential to keep the original objectives on course and to minimize 'project drift'. With complex interventions involving many players, projects will drift from the agreed objectives to some degree. Implementation plans based on robust scoping research may drift off course and look very different in terms of the exchange, the propositions and the marketing mix. As an evaluator, it is important that you assess this. Many good ideas are judged to be ineffective and discarded when in effect the evaluation has assessed something which drifted considerably from the original good idea.

For example, an intervention may aim to provide a customer-friendly and accessible advice service to teenagers looking for advice on matters such as sexual health or drugs. The service should open at appropriate times and provide a safe, enjoyable space to which teenagers feel they can return if they need to. In this typical example, numerous agencies become involved and tinker with the original idea until the project drifts off course. The resulting service will not resemble the original vision and, unsurprisingly, evaluate poorly. If the process evaluation makes the distinction between the planned and actual intervention, it will ensure that the ambitions of the original idea are not discarded nor deemed a failure.

Even when projects remain on course it is important to assess which elements have worked well and explain which have not worked so well.

Box 14.2 Evaluating a health intervention in young-offender institutions

'*Music4Messages*' was a campaign that sought to prevent Hepatitis C infection in young offenders in custodial settings in England. Introduced by the Department of Health (DH), and aimed at all new arrivals in English young-offender institutions (YOIs), the campaign provided inmates with a CD containing a series of rap and hip-hop tracks interspersed with interviews with guest artists, who aimed to reduce the stigma associated with Hepatitis C infection by discussing its impact on their lives.

The CD was developed following qualitative research amongst the target group to ensure its form and content were relevant to those it sought to reach. A key consideration in its design was the poor level of literacy among young offenders: this prompted the designers to ensure that important information was communicated by voice and sound rather than text.

DH sought to conduct an evaluation of the CD's implementation and its impact on the knowledge, attitudes, and behaviours of young offenders. A quasi-experimental design (i.e. respondents were not randomly assigned to test and control groups) was proposed, involving a total of eight YOIs: four 'intervention' and four 'control' establishments. It conducted 50 quantitative interviews in each establishment before and after the intervention. The design also included qualitative research among prison officers, to assess matters of process, particularly to assess how the project was implemented on the ground. It also included qualitative research among young offenders, to assess their views of the CD and its distribution processes.

There were practical difficulties in conducting the quantitative parts of the evaluation, due to the high rate of turnover of young offenders in institutions and the problem of gaining access to inmates. The scale of the task (400 interviews before and 200 interviews after the intervention) proved wildly optimistic.

In several establishments there were an insufficient number of suitable respondents. Only people with at least three months to serve at the time of the first interview were eligible, as they would need to be re-interviewed after exposure to the CD. However, sentence length for detainees varied between institutions and young offenders moved prisons during the course of their sentence.

There were other problems. Inmates had to be escorted to and from interviews, and this change in prison routine relied on the goodwill of prison staff. Sometimes disturbances and miscounted roll calls meant that prisoners were prevented from moving around the prison. All this had an inevitable impact on the numbers of interviews that could be conducted. In the end, the study fell short of the intended number of interviews, achieving 250 interviews before and 150 interviews after the intervention.

However, although sample sizes were smaller than had been expected, the evaluation was able to give an indication of what the intervention had achieved: it showed that project managers had underestimated the change in offenders' knowledge that could be achieved with this approach and provided valuable information for developing the intervention further.

Source: McVey D, Crosier A, and Wellings K (2006) 'An Evaluation of Music4Messages: Hepatitis C prevention project'. Report to Department of Health. London School of Hygiene and Tropical Medicine. Unpublished

Some of the areas for investigation include:

- failure to take account of the context within which the intervention operates;
- an inability to fulfil the implementation objectives and deliver the correct mix of approaches;
- management and leadership problems;
- an inability to achieve enough stakeholder buy-in;
- poor translation into practice of the theories underpinning the intervention;
- poor use of the scoping research, resulting in poor project design and prioritization of target groups; and
- unforeseen positive and negative consequences of the intervention.

As discussed previously in this chapter, there are many research methods which can be employed to build a good process evaluation and a rich description of what has occurred.

Outcome evaluation

The outcome evaluation is dedicated to examining and reviewing the overall impact of the intervention. At this stage an assessment is made of the achievement of aims and objectives using a range of short-, medium-, and long-term indicators:

- Short-term outcomes – e.g. who was aware of a programme during its evaluation period;
- Mid-term outcomes – e.g. which determinants of behaviour were changed; and
- Long-term outcomes – e.g. the intended (and unintended) affects on behaviour and health outcomes.

As highlighted previously, it is vital that clear and measurable behavioural goals are set from the outset so that evaluation can assess whether they have been satisfied. A key role of outcome evaluation is to determine the actual impact on these specific behavioural goals. While factors such as 'levels of awareness' and 'audience views' are important; they are secondary considerations to what actually happens in terms of the targeted behaviours.

It may be that the timescale or budget does not enable you to evaluate longer-term outcomes, which may mean you cannot look fully at the impact on behaviour. If so, it is important that your evaluation is tied into a behavioural change model. For example, using Prochaska's Stages of Change (1984) model to illustrate, it may be that a survey looks to measure the level of the population in the 'preparation' stage based on the assumption that in the long term they will move into the 'action' stage.

Theoretical perspectives

Social marketing operates to large degree on the social-psychological elements of behavioural models. The essential factor in most social-psychological models is attitudes, which tend to be conceived as the product of a deliberative calculation weighing an individual's beliefs about behaviour with the value they attach to those characteristics. According to Darnton (GSRU, 2008) in his review of behavioural models, the constructs have developed further – building in additional factors to explain behavioural outcomes. These in turn diminish the primacy of attitudes in determining behaviour.

While attitudes, norms, and agency are common to most models, habit and emotion only appear in some (GSRU, 2008). Similarly, contextual factors beyond an individual's control including access to services, levels of deprivation, and other environmental indicators – which clearly can mitigate the effectiveness of any intervention – are seldom taken into account when designing programmes.

Influencing social norms can play a significant part in mass media communication when trying to stimulate behavioural change at the population level. If mass media campaigns are effective, it is likely that they activate a complex process of change in social norms rather than because they directly affect the behaviour of individuals. For example, when asked, children always significantly overestimate the proportion of their classmates who smoke (Clemens et al., 2008). They are operating in a false social norm, and normative education debunking the myths about smoking prevalence can contribute to maintaining non-smoker status in this group. In this example a model which did not include norms would miss a fundamental explanatory factor.

The inherent assumption in many mass media interventions is that changing attitudes and convincing people that they can change will lead to a behavioural change. There is evidence that this assumption can hold true when applied to purchasing products or switching to a different brand. However, when applied to more complicated health behaviours, this assertion is rightly questioned. Sheeran (2006) examined more than 200 studies and confirmed that changing attitudes, norms, or self-efficacy had a casual impact on people's intentions and behaviour and showed that interventions that succeed in generating significant changes in these factors engendered changes in intentions and behaviour. The theories which tended to give rise to the large changes in behaviour were social cognitive-behaviour theory and learning theory.

Using large 'logic models', i.e. graphic depictions of the relationship between a programme's activities and its intended short-, medium-, and long-term outcomes, can help identify evaluation opportunities. Based on your chosen theory of behavioural change the model serves as an 'outcomes roadmap' that shows the underlying logic behind the programme and how it should work. Logic models convey not only the activities that comprise the programme and the interrelationship of those activities, but the link between those components and outcomes. Over time, evaluation, research, and day-to-day experience will deepen the understanding of what does and does not work, and the model will change and develop further (CDC, 2006).

The existing evidence base in public health is very sparse on large tracts of logic models. Furthermore, key points in the logic model involve evidence of a type that has never been near an evidence hierarchy (Kelly, 2008)

Chapter 4 discusses some of the different behavioural models in more detail. An example of an intervention which considered a behavioural model is given in Box 14.4.

Box 14.3 Realistic expectations: lessons from governmental campaigns

In a review of government campaigns, conducted by the National Social Marketing Centre (Wellings et al., 2006), it was clear that a number of governmental campaigns had not clearly articulated the level of knowledge, attitude, or behavioural change expected from the intervention. Moreover, the sample sizes put in place to assess change would have been capable of measuring only large changes (between 5% and 10%) over a typical campaign period of 3–6 months. If a national smoking campaign were judged to have resulted in a real change in population prevalence of 1–2% in a year, above what was expected given the prevailing downwards trend, this should be considered a success. However, the evaluation designs in place were not sensitive enough to detect these small but significant changes. Small changes to behaviour over the course of a year of intervention are the most that can be expected from well run national interventions. A 1% change in national prevalence equates to hundreds of thousands of smokers quitting. For smaller, focussed, higher-intensity interventions, with more one-to-one personal support available to the target group, larger behaviour changes should be expected. Larger changes in knowledge and attitude measures would also be expected as these are easier to shift in the short term to medium term.

Triangulation

Using other data sources to cross-validate study findings provides another objective measure of performance and lends more rigour to the research conclusions.

Rather than relying solely on the reported impact on the intended beneficiaries, an evaluation study may seek evidence of impact on those involved in delivering the intervention and evidence of impact on the social and physical environment, as well as checking for any unintended consequences. In these situations, a multi-method approach is employed to capture what has happened.

Reported changes in a knowledge, attitude, belief, and practice survey (KABP) can be triangulated with increases in helpline calls and changes in media coverage with each independent measure validating the other – or not.

Reported behaviours can be triangulated with industry sales data. For example, trends in reported condom use can be compared to industry data on condom sales to see if peaks in reported condom use coincide with peaks in sales (Goodrich et al., 1998). Similarly, reports of eating more fruit can be compared with food sales at a local or national level. Reports of increases in physical activity can be triangulated with increased sales in sport clothes and equipment and membership of health clubs and exercise classes. Likewise, trends in sexual health clinic attendance and test data can be compared with behavioural trend data. Cigarette sales data were once a good source of data to triangulate with claimed behavioural survey estimates. Today, however, significant proportions of cigarettes are now smuggled and sold cheaply and are not captured by retail audit data.

Other sources of data

There are many sources of commercial and government data which you can access to help shape your evaluation and triangulate or cross-validate your findings.

Health and social research funded by government is readily available for free or for a small charge. Although the sample sizes for some of these studies can be as large as 20 000 respondents, they may include only a small sample within your local area. The National Centre for Social Research has taken The Health Survey for England and attempted to model the national data to produce 'synthetic estimates' at ward level for some of the key health indicators. You will find more information on this online at: www.dh.gov.uk/en/Publicationsandstatistics/Statistics/StatisticalWorkAreas/Statisticalworkareaneighbourhood/

There are numerous national and local surveys which provide baseline data and tested questions for use on your own surveys. The National Social Marketing Centre has produced a resource guide which provides a description and access details for more than 80 social surveys and market-research studies covering a range of topics. It is available at: http://www.nsms.org.uk/images/CoreFiles/NSMC-R11_compendium.pdf

Another useful resource is the Economic and Social Research Council (ESRC) question bank of attitudinal and behavioural questions available at: www.surveynet.essex.ac.uk/sqb/qb

Both resources are a good starting point for developing a questionnaire.

Sales data from industry can be a useful additional indicator of success. The sales figures for fast food, healthy food, use of gyms, purchase of sports equipment, and condom sales, e.g. can help assess changes in people's behaviour or intentions to change behaviour. Getting access to this data can be difficult, as it is privately owned and companies do not want to give it away, fearing they would lose some commercial advantage. However, there are some established useful sources of industry data that are available in market research compendia (Advertising Association, 2009).

Box 14.4 Evaluating a national smoking-cessation initiative

The Health Education Authority[1] (HEA) conducted a national intervention to reduce smoking prevalence in the general population. The target audience was adults (in particular, parents) of social grade C2DE who were at the 'contemplation stage' of giving up smoking, according to the Prochaska and Di Clemente theoretical model which underpinned the intervention.

The research conducted during the scoping stage revealed that the intervention should:

- provide telephone helpline support for smokers' efforts to quit and stay a non-smoker;
- display an understanding of the difficulties of stopping;
- build smokers' confidence in their ability to quit; and
- have a tone that is anti-smoking not anti-smoker.

The proposition for smokers was that it is 'easier than you think to give up smoking'. The exchange offered to smokers was that if they gave up they would feel some short-term health benefits and would be around to see their kids grow up. Furthermore, there would be help and support available via telephone support lines and other resources to help them quit.

Research design to assess attitudinal and behavioural outcomes

A control trial was conducted to assess the effects of the intervention. There were three test areas which received the mass media interventions. One of these areas was also exposed to a local activity-network of health professionals and campaigners who organized activity in workplaces and social settings and ran local interventions to encourage quitting.

It was not possible to randomize the population to test and control groups as would be the case in a clinical trial. This was a real-world intervention where people are exposed to the mass media all the time. There was no way of selectively targeting individuals within each television region. However, it was possible to define the control group to be a whole region i.e. a television region that did not receive anti-smoking messages in the advertisement break. This would not result in the gold standard RCT design but would provide an opportunity to control for some of the background 'noise' on smoking that would be present in test and control regions, and assess the added benefit of the intervention. Furthermore, the level of media buying was varied across the test regions to permit an analysis of the 'dose response'.

A sample of at least 5000 people spread across the test and control samples would be interviewed before the intervention began, then re-interviewed after the first wave of the campaign and then re-interviewed again after the second wave of the campaigning to assess their smoking status.

Methods

The survey questionnaire which was administered to stratified random samples of respondents in the test and control areas contained many questions including:

- smoking status;
- motivations to quit;

Box 14.4 Evaluating a national smoking-cessation initiative *(continued)*

- how often people had tried to quit;
- attitudes towards smoking;
- whether people had been exposed to other stop smoking interventions in the workplace or the GP surgery;
- whether any other family members smoked; and
- whether they had seen the campaign or phoned the helpline.

Awareness of the intervention was also monitored in the control region to see if any of the campaign leaked from the test into the control region.

The smoking helpline was an important source of support to smokers and was evaluated by interviewing samples of callers to assess their opinion of the quality of the helpline counselling service. The volume of calls and the average length of calls were automatically collected by the call centre software.

Monitoring the competition

As with all social marketing, there was competition to this initiative. During the course of the intervention the tobacco industry invested more than £200 million in advertising and sponsorship to promote their products – almost a hundred times the budget of the HEA intervention. On the positive side, nicotine replacement therapy (NRT) was launched into the market only a few months before the HEA campaign. When conducting a controlled trial, trying to control for this negative and positive extraneous 'noise' around the intervention is a big challenge. If, for example, the NRT manufactures had invested considerably more in advertising in the test regions compared to the control region, this would present difficulties for the analysis in terms of attributing any effect to the intervention. The same can be said for disproportionate tobacco industry expenditure. Data on NRT advertising expenditure was readily available, whereas data from tobacco companies' advertising and sponsorship expenditure was more difficult to assess. Fortunately for the evaluation, the tobacco companies and the NRT manufacturers had spent their money evenly across the country, so the test and control regions received the same dose of their interventions.

Triangulation with other data sources

National surveys of smoking prevalence are conducted almost every year in England. It was possible to re-analyse this data and examine changes in smoking prevalence in the test and control regions during pre- and post-campaign periods. The data was compared with the quantitative surveys to see if the same trends were emerging.

Governance and analysis

The research tasks were spread out over a number of external suppliers: qualitative research agencies, quantitative agencies, media-buying auditors, media analysts, and academic departments specializing in process evaluators. The analysis and interpretation was conducted by research specialists at the HEA and by external academics and was verified by external academic statisticians.

Results

The results suggested that over an 18-month period, the intervention would reduce smoking prevalence by about 1.2% (McVey and Stapleton, 2000).This may not seem a large change, but in population terms it equates to hundreds of thousands of smokers giving up. Applying a very basic return on investment analysis to the amount of money put into the campaign and the effects observed indicated that the intervention was more cost-effective that NRT.

Note:[1]The HEA is now dissolved. In 2000, the HEA was replaced by the Health Development Agency (HDA). The HDA is now part of NICE (National Institute for Health and Clinical Excellence).

Cost-effectiveness analysis

Another action that can be done at the outcome-evaluation stage is the calculation of the cost-effectiveness of the intervention.

As health-care resources are finite, information about cost-effectiveness is essential to make evidence-based decisions about competing health-care interventions. In the White Paper *The New NHS: Modern, Dependable*, (Department of Health, 1997), the government made a commitment to ensure that every penny of taxpayers' money received by the NHS would be spent in the most efficient way possible. However, this commitment is highly dependent upon studies providing a synthesis of comparative costs and effectiveness in the form of economic evaluations.

There are various ways to calculate the cost-effectiveness of an intervention: (i) cost–benefit analysis; (ii) cost-effectives analysis; and (iii) cost–utility analysis. The NHS Centre for Reviews and Dissemination provides detailed definition of these methods. (The NHS Centre for Reviews and Dissemination 2002).

Despite the importance and value of such data, cost-effectiveness analyses are rarely done in the social marketing field. This could be because they are difficult and can be costly to carry out. However, it is important that the true costs of an intervention are calculated so that it's true impact can be measured. Producing data relating to the cost-effectiveness of interventions and providing some estimate of the return on investment (ROI) can make a compelling case for continued funding.

Types of evaluation data

There are a wide range of different types of data that can be collected for the evaluation of a social marketing project. As mentioned previously, the type of data you collect depends on its use; e.g. robust quantitative data may be needed for the final outcome evaluation; however, qualitative research looking at the mechanisms of the work could be used for the process evaluation. Examples are given below.

Direct indicators – these are data sources that can be used for outcome evaluations:

- Prevalence statistics – e.g. changes in the number of people smoking.
- Self-reported behavioural change.
- Increased uptake of a particular product or service.
- Changes in footfall in an area – e.g. are more people walking into a smoking-cessation clinic?

Intermediary indicators – these are indicators that can be precursors to behavioural change:

- Measuring changes in awareness, knowledge, beliefs, and attitudes.
- Media analysis – e.g. column inches, quality of coverage, campaign mentions in the media.
- Analysing helpline data, such as number and quality of calls.
- Stakeholder analysis – looking at the views of people delivering work on the ground.
- Service Data – who is using the service and what do they think?

Indirect indicators – these may not be a direct objective of your intervention. However, they can prove to be important indicators of its impact:

- Looking at indirect sales data. For example, is the consequence of a safe-sex intervention an increase in condom sales?
- The quality of materials and services provided.
- Looking at impact on policy decisions or the law.
- The affect on opinion formers.
- Changes in the social climate – e.g. this would be important when assessing a campaign to reduce stigma against people with human immunodeficiency virus (HIV).
- Looking at the skills acquisition and increasing levels of empowerment of the team delivering the intervention.

Conclusion

Determining the effectiveness of a social marketing intervention is always a challenge for evaluators. Attributing effects to complex multifaceted interventions requires the use of a range of qualitative and quantitative techniques which, where possible, should be triangulated with existing data sources.

Using the model of behavioural change adopted by the intervention can help construct and focus the evaluation effort on the key indicators of effectiveness. However, as well as measuring the hard quantitative outcomes, it is essential to conduct a process evaluation to build up a rich description of what has occurred during the intervention; scanning the environment for unforeseen negative and positive events and looking to see what the competition is doing. Using some of the emerging insights from the process evaluation can keep the key stakeholders and user groups involved and stimulated by the research and ensure findings are used to fine-tune the intervention. Stakeholders' involvement should, however, be balanced by having in place adequate research governance to ensure that the evaluators maintain a degree of independence and objectivity in the design, collection, and reporting of the findings.

Policy and programme planners learn from interventions that succeed and interventions that fail. Good-quality data on the effectiveness of an intervention should be shared, so publish the findings, or at least make them available in the public domain.

References

Advertising Association (2009). *Marketing Pocketbook*. London: Advertising Association.

Britten, N. and Fisher, B. (1993). Qualitative research and general practice. *The British Journal of General Practice*, 43(372): 270–271.

Bryman, A. (1988). *Quantity and Quality in Social Research*. London, New York: Routledge.

Centre for Disease Control and Prevention (2006). *Get Smart Program Planners Evaluation Manual*. Atlanta, USA: Centre for Disease Control and Prevention.

Clemens, S., Jotangia, D., Lynch, S., et al. (2008). *Drug Use, Smoking and Drinking Among Young People in England in 2007*: A survey carried out for the NHS Information Centre by the National Centre for Social Research and the National Foundation for Educational Research. [Online] NHS Information Centre. Available at: http://www.ic.nhs.uk/pubs/sdd07fullreport (Accessed January 2009).

Darnton, A. (2008). *An Overview of Behaviour Change Models and Their Uses; a Report to the Government Social Research Unit.* Government Social Research Unit, London. Available at: http://www.gsr.gov.uk/downloads/resources/behaviour_change_review/reference_report.pdf (Accessed January 2009).

Davies, P. (2004). *Is Evidence-Based Government Possible?* Jerry Lee Lecture 2004; Presented at the 4th Annual Campbell Collaboration Colloquium. Washington Feb 2004. Available at: http://www.nationalschool.gov.uk/policyhub/downloads/JerryLeeLecture1202041.pdf (Accessed January 2009).

Department of Health (1997). *The New NHS: Modern, Dependable.* London: Department of Health. Available at: http://www.dh.gov.uk/en/Publicationsandstatistics/Publications/PublicationsPolicyAndGuidance/DH_4008869 (Accessed February 2009).

General Household Survey (2005). *Smoking and Drinking Among Adults 2005.* UK: Office of National Statistics 2006.

Goodrich, J., Wellings, K., and McVey, D. (1998). Using condom data to assess the impact of HIV/AIDS preventive interventions. *Health Educ Res*, 13(2): 267–74.

Hamilton, D., Jenkins, D., King, C., et al. (eds.) (1977). *Beyond the Numbers Game: a Reader in Educational Evaluation.* Basingstoke: Macmillan.

Hastings, G. (2007). *Social Marketing. Why Should the Devil Have All the Best Tunes?* Oxford: Butterworth-Heinemann.

Kelly, M. (2008). The Centre for Public Health Excellence, NICE. The NICE Guidance on Attitude and Behaviour Change. *Brighton, September 2008: First World Social Marketing Conference.*

Macnaughton, R.J. (1996). Numbers, scales, and qualitative research. *Lancet*, 347: 1099–2000.

McVey, D. and Stapleton, J. (2000). Can anti-smoking television advertising affect smoking behaviour? A controlled trial of the Health Education Authority for England's anti-smoking TV campaign. *Tob Control*, 9(3): 273–282.

NHS Centre for Reviews and Dissemination (2002). Cost-effectiveness matters: Available at: http://www.york.ac.uk/inst/crd/EM/em61.pdf (Accessed January 2009).

Nutbeam, D. (1999). Oakley's case for using randomised controlled trials is misleading. *British Medical Journal*, 318: 944b.

Oakley, A. (1988). Experimentation and social interventions: a forgotten but important history. *British Medical Journal*, 317: 1239–1242.

Pawson, R. and Tilley, N. (1997). *Realistic Evaluation.* London: Sage.

Petticrew, M. and Roberts, H. (2003). Evidence, hierarchies, and typologies: horses for course. *Journal of Epidemiology and Community Health*, 57: 527–529.

Prochaska, J.O. and DiClemente, C.C. (1984). Self-change processes, self-efficacy and decisional balance across five stages of smoking cessation. In *Advances in Cancer Control, 1983.* New York, NY: Alan R. Liss, Inc.

Sheeran, P. (2006). *Does Changing Attitudes, Norms or Self-Efficacy Change Intentions and Behaviour?* End of project report. Swindon: The Economic and Social Research Council.

Speller, V., Learmonth, A., and Harrison, D. (1998). Evaluating health promotion is complex. *British Medical Journal*, May 9, 316(7142):1463.

Strauss, A. and Corbin, J. (1990). *Basics of Qualitative Research: Grounded Theory Procedures and Techniques.* Newbury Park, CA: Sage Publications.

Tones, K. (1997). Beyond the randomized controlled trial: a case for 'judicial review'. *Health Education Research*; 12(2): i–iv.

Victora, C.G., Habicht, J.P., and Bryce, J. (2004). Evidence-based public health: moving beyond randomized trials. *American Journal of Public Health*, 94(3): 400–405.

Wellings, K., Crosier, A., McVey, D., Jennings, T. (2006). *The National Health-related Campaigns Review; A review of 11 national campaigns.* National Social Marketing Centre, London. Available at: http://www.nsms.org.uk/images/CoreFiles/NSMC-R7_health_related_campaigns.pdf (Accessed January 2009).

World Health Organization (1981). *Health Programme Evaluation – Guiding Principles.* Geneva: World Health Organization.

Chapter 15

Follow-up

Alex Christopoulos, Clive Blair-Stevens, and Jeff French

The important thing is not to stop questioning.
Albert Einstein

Learning points

This chapter

- Stresses the importance of conducting a follow-up stage;
- Recognizes that it is vital to actively feed back, discuss findings, and thank stakeholders; and
- Promotes a reflective, learning culture in which understanding of work that has been less successful can be of critical value in future developments.

Chapter overview

The fifth and final stage of the Total Process Planning (TPP) framework is 'follow-up'. By the time you reach the follow-up stage you should have:

- scoped and developed your intervention(s);
- pre-tested and developed your interventions;
- implemented your programme; and
- evaluated your programme.

The importance of moving beyond communicating information to ensure a clear focus on behaviour when seeking to address different behavioural challenges has already been discussed previously. The need to raise the aim beyond the simple notion of 'behavioural change' (i.e. moving from a problem behaviour to a desired behaviour) to focus instead on the greater challenge of both establishing and sustaining behaviour over time is also vital.

This chapter demonstrates why a reflective 'follow-up' stage plays an important role in developing effective behavioural interventions that have long-term impact not just within your project or local area but also by adding the accumulated understanding of what works, what does not, and under what conditions.

Aim of the follow-up stage

To share and use the findings of monitoring and evaluation so that future developments and interventions can build on successes and failures that have been learnt.

Objectives of the follow-up stage

To provide:

- a shared understanding of what has been achieved, what remains to be achieved and what worked and what did not;
- commissioners or funders with information about the kinds of processes they should expect from providers and mangers of social marketing interventions about what has been done, what has been achieved, and also a realistic understanding and appreciation of the constraints and challenges in the process and what can be learnt from this; and
- project and/or programme staff with time to reflect on learning to date and how they can further improve the intervention.

Output from the follow-up stage

A clear action-plan for next phases of work, including:

- specific follow-up actions to address key findings from the evaluation;
- clarity on next stages in addressing the relevant behaviours and, specifically, how to further establish and maintain them; and
- published information on learning from work completed to provide access to the findings to others who could benefit, via appropriate channels and mechanisms.

Introduction

The evaluation phase of a social marketing programme or project is often seen as its end-point. The intervention has been completed and reviewed, there has either been an impact on the target behaviour or there has not. It is, therefore, only natural at this time for team members to start thinking about their next initiative. However, it is essential not to rest on your laurels and to recognize the importance of maintaining and sustaining what you have achieved. The follow-up stage of the Total Process Planning (TPP) framework helps ensure you do this successfully. Box 15.1 contains a checklist for the follow-up stage, but we have set out the important steps in more detail below.

The follow-up stage

If you end your intervention immediately after evaluation, you may miss the lessons learnt from the intervention, and fail to strengthen the relationships you have built throughout the course of the initiative with your stakeholders. Evaluating the intervention, whilst very important, is usually not sufficient to get all those people who could benefit from what you have learnt to appreciate how this new knowledge can be used in the future. The marketing of your results so that others not only understand them but also reflect on what they mean for their own practice and programmes is a key responsibility for all social marketers.

Box 15.1 Follow-up stage checklist

Have I …	Comments/notes
Captured the learning and made this more readily available to others in the form of a report?	
Reported back the results and implications to managers and funders?	
Distributed the report to all the people who helped deliver the intervention	
Fed back the results to the target group (e.g. via meetings, the media, etc.)?	
Provided opportunities to brief other interested parties and stakeholders on the work to date? (e.g. professional associations, academics, etc.)	
Distributed the evaluation report to all interested stakeholders?	
Considered the intended and unintended consequences of the intervention?	
Considered ways to further extend or roll out the intervention to increase its impact?	
Directly thanked and showed appreciation to (personally and/or in writing) all those stakeholders who have contributed?	

Having a dedicated 'follow-up' stage gives you the opportunity to understand:

- the relevance of your findings;
- where they fit in;
- who they affect and are useful to; and
- how they can be used by others to influence their programmes.

Even when an intervention appears to have had little or no measurable effect on the target behaviour(s), you can still use the follow-up stage to build on stakeholder involvement, learn lessons from the findings, and revise plans accordingly. The publication of negative results and the learning about why something did not work is very helpful to other practitioners and researchers as it can obviously help them avoid similar mistakes or traps.

You can also use evaluation findings to go beyond short-term thinking to explore impact on the medium and long term and what your evaluation might mean for other programmes of action. For example, finding that the provision of an interpreter boosts the uptake of an immunization service by mothers who speak English as a second language could be used to inform the development of other health projects aimed at this target group.

The follow-up stage ensures that the 'footprint of the project', is clear and helps to ensure that you have left something behind upon which others can build, locally and or further afield or possibly at some point in the future. It is also important that the follow-up stage leads to some kind of action. For example, if evaluation reveals that a project is succeeding, you will need to decide how to maintain or expand the intervention and share good practice. Conversely, if the evaluation shows a project has not met its objectives, you will need to decide whether to adapt it, change the targets, or stop the project.

You will need to consider how your intervention has impacted on the wider world as well as on an individual's behaviour. Your project may have successfully achieved its behavioural goal, but remember that a core component of social marketing interventions is that that they focus on 'social good'. So you may need to ask yourself other questions based on the evaluation: questions such as: 'even though the behavioural goals of the programme were met, were their any unforeseen negative consequences to the intervention or any unforeseen additional benefits to the intervention.

Building on stakeholder engagement

Whatever an intervention's impact, it is essential that the follow-up stage helps sustain and develop stakeholder engagement, as stakeholders are arguably the most important resource available to you. This is one of the most important aspects of the follow-up stage and will be central to any future intervention work. It is, therefore, important that learning gained from the earlier evaluation stage is fully utilized and does not join the tomes of literature gathering dust on a shelf. Without regards to how favourable or unfavourable the evaluation of a project has been, its application is still beneficial for a wide range of different stakeholders.

The process of meeting with stakeholders and following up on the evaluation gives concerned parties the opportunity to see how effective the evaluation was. The 'follow-up' can look at whether it covered the correct indicators and if the research was conducted robustly and with the correct target audience. Some stakeholders may disagree with elements of the evaluation, and it is important to address this to ensure its validity. In addition, this review can identify where there are any gaps in the evaluation and if any further analysis is required.

Encouraging a learning culture

A key role of the follow-up stage is to reflect on the whole process and the evaluatory findings, with everyone involved being encouraged to ask 'What does this really mean – for the target audience and relevant stakeholders?' The answer to this question can be shared by all concerned and used to inform future developments.

For learning to be shared, intervention teams need to be open, transparent, and generous with the evaluatory findings to avoid constant reinvention of the wheel or repeated bad practice. It can be tempting to 'guard' the evaluation and treat it as a judgement of your, or your team's, ability or performance. However, you should bear in mind how useful this information will be to others. It is vital that both the evaluation and the follow-up stages take place in a learning culture as opposed to one where blame is expected. Learning from projects that have not been as successful as expected is just as valuable as the learning derived from more successful projects. Both can be of equal importance when feeding into the development of new projects.

Thanking stakeholders

The 'follow-up' is also a phase for recognition. It is important to value and respect the contribution of project members and stakeholders. This should happen whether a project has met its targets or not. Irrespective of the outcome, it is valuable to recognize, support, and develop members of your project team and to strengthen relationships.

Deciding the next steps

The follow-up stage plays a key role in looking to the future and determining next steps for delivery partners, stakeholders, the target audience, and the intervention itself.

You should look to the medium and long term to ask what will happen to the target audience and how you (and the partners you brought on board at scoping stage) can ensure sustainability of behavioural change. For example, if your intervention aimed to help people to stop smoking over a 4-week period, you need to ensure that further services are provided to help the target audience sustain that behaviour. It is a waste of resources to concentrate on helping the target audience during the first stage of behavioural change only to subsequently cut them adrift because your intervention has reached the extent of its remit (or you have reached your target set by your funders). If you stop your intervention abruptly without sufficient support mechanisms, you could disengage your target audience and create a barrier to the success of future interventions. This is especially the case if you are using participatory techniques, be careful not to make those involved feel as though they were 'used' in your work and then discarded.

Communicating the findings

Communicating the results of the evaluation and other aspects of your review is one of the most important elements of the follow-up. After the effort expended in designing, running, and evaluating an intervention, it is easy to forget to communicate the results of this process to others. This may be spreading the good word. For example, letting people know about an intervention designed to increase physical activity among people aged between 30 and 55 which has shown that they also have reduced their alcohol intake. This information would be useful to those working in the alcohol sphere and could help them explain changes in their own evaluations and can be used to develop services. However, 'follow-up' might also have to prepare organizations for the negative consequence of an intervention that was not identified during scoping and development. For example, if an intervention banning smoking in public places has shown that parents are now more likely to smoke in the home and around their children; relevant organizations need to understand this situation and react to it.

Without effectively communicating impact, initiatives may miss out on funding or recognition, even if they have been successful. Often, once funding decisions have been made it is difficult to reverse them. It is therefore vital to let funders and potential funders know, as early as possible, the results of your programme and how successful you have been. Again, communicate not only your achievements but also what has not worked as well as expected and what you would recommend as a result. Do not assume that sharing data on what has not gone well will only result in negative consequences. For example, stakeholders may see solutions to the issues raised or at least recognize factors that may have had an impact on the success of the project.

However, it is not just funders and stakeholders who may be interested in the findings. Think about whether your target audience would benefit from understanding more about your intervention. In addition, consider who else might benefit from this knowledge.

Before communicating your results, it is important to remember that the follow-up stage is not a one-way process. Communicating your results is also an opportunity to get feedback on what you have learnt and the conclusions you have reached about what this means and what to do next. Therefore, when communicating the results of your intervention, you must ensure there are sufficient mechanisms in place for feedback to occur. You can generate feedback via mechanisms that you use to disseminate results such as meetings and seminars but you can also set up additional mechanisms such as dedicated feedback events, questionnaires, and website-based comments pages.

When planning how you will communicate the results of your evaluation, think about your audience and the most appropriate channels to use to get this information to them. For example, what would be the best way to influence decision-makers?

Some common routes used are:

- face-to-face meeting with stakeholders;
- distributing reports;
- attempting to get the results of your intervention on local or national news;

- writing up evaluation in relevant journals, read by your audience;
- contributing to existing knowledge-sharing systems, such as the professional case-study database;
- oral reports to internal groups;
- one-to-one briefings for key stakeholders;
- external oral report to community groups;
- non-technical written report for external use;
- newsletter features;
- press release;
- web cast/news item;
- press feature;
- radio/television interviews;
- seminar or conference presentation, workshops, or posters;
- news item form professional journal;
- article for professional journal; and
- case-study write-up and publication.

Communicating the findings does not have to follow a formal process. For example, calling up stakeholders or sending a letter to those who participated in the intervention can be an effective route. It is vital to use some form of communication, as it can help to nurture and develop the relationships created at the scoping phase which may also be valuable in the future.

Contributing to wider learning

Have you ever experienced the frustration of searching for information that you know should exist but you cannot find? Or have you ever looked for reviews of projects that have never been written-up? It is a common occurrence. When scoping an intervention, it can be disappointing to find that there is little evidence and background information in areas where you know work has been undertaken this can especially be the case with smaller, localized projects. Without this evidence we run the risk of reinventing the wheel or taking actions that have been proved to be ineffective. The follow-up stage is your opportunity to add to the evidence-base; to create a legacy for the project outside your own area and beyond the life cycle of the programme.

There can be a tendency to think that you or your colleagues will stay in your job for a long time and therefore can share learning with interested parties when needed. However, this tends to ignore the reality that more and more people change jobs frequently. It also fails to cater to the needs of people and organizations that may not be in direct contact with you but are the target audience of key stakeholders in a programme. Therefore, it is important that the learning and intelligence gained from your evaluation enters the public arena and is as accessible as possible.

One obvious way is to write a formal paper on your intervention and submit it for publication in a relevant, recognized professional journal. Recording results in this way is helpful for others tackling similar issues or using similar interventional techniques. Publication of your findings can also, from a personal or project team point of view, give recognition to those involved and help increase the awareness of your intervention.

By making the results of your intervention available, you provide a starting point for others addressing similar interventions in the future. For example, other project teams can base their performance targets on findings from your intervention to ensure that they are realistic and achievable. Others can also learn form any mistakes that you made and seek to avoid similar errors.

Conclusion

Maintaining and sustaining behaviour over time is a difficult challenge. The dynamic nature of behaviour means that it is subject to different influences and contexts over time, and what might work now may not work in the future. However, it is vital to plan and secure funding so that the intervention can be sustained in the medium and long term. Thanking and feeding back the findings from the initial evaluatory work, can help to secure future buy-in, and importantly, future funding.

Chapter 16

Social marketing on a shoestring budget

Jeff French

Success is neither magical nor mysterious. Success is the natural consequence of consistently applying the basic fundamentals.
Jim Rohn

Learning points

This chapter

- Provides an understanding of how social marketing principles can be applied to all behavioural change programmes;
- Explains how social marketing can be applied without a large budget for research, development, or implementation; and
- Explains how to get help in your own area from social and professional networks, and internationally.

Chapter overview

The key to effective social marketing on a shoestring is to start by thinking like a marketer. This means thinking of the customer and being systematic in your planning. It does not mean worrying about not having enough money to run a big, flashy campaign on television or the newspapers. It is often assumed that social marketing can only be conducted by large organizations with large budgets and lots of accumulated expertise and experience. This chapter makes the case that one of the real strengths of the social marketing approach is that it can be adapted and used by almost anyone who wants to help people to change some form of behaviour that will help the individual or their wider community.

The chapter gives examples of how people with limited or no budgets can still apply a social marketing mindset and procedures to the issues they are concerned with. It also gives details of sources of free help and support for anyone who has access to the Internet.

A key message of this chapter is that low-cost or shoestring social marketing does not make poor-quality work acceptable. If you are working with little or no budget, you still have the most important resource at your disposal for any social marketing programme: the social marketing mindset.

Introduction

The title of this chapter implies that it is possible to conduct social marketing with little or no resources. Whilst 'no resources' is a fairly clear statement, the word 'little' needs clarification. For the purposes of this chapter, it is assumed that we are talking about a situation in which a practitioner or concerned individual has only their own time or, in the case of an employed worker, no more than 10% or less of their employed time, to allocate to a social marketing initiative.

Lots of people think that effective social marketing programmes require a lot of investment and the application of expensive market research techniques and the support of specialist agencies that charge a lot for their services. It is true that for large-scale, regional or national social marketing programmes it is wise to invest in building up a very accurate picture of the population through market research and research into the behavioural challenges to be tackled. It is also wise to take time to develop and test interventions and to employ specialist agencies and consultants to help develop, deliver, and evaluate interventions. However, many of the essential approaches of social marketing set out in Chapters 10–15 can be applied without access to the kinds of funding or human resources needed for large-scale programmes.

Can you do social marketing on a shoestring budget?

The short answer to the above question is a definite yes. The essential 'must have' is the application of a social marketing mindset, a way of thinking that embodies:

- the key principles of social marketing and the social marketing benchmark-criteria (set out in Chapter 3).

The essential elements of this kind of thinking are:

- absolute clarity about the particular behavioural challenge to be addressed;
- an understanding of the target audience you are trying to help; and
- a systematic set of processes to investigate develop, implement evaluate, and share what has been learnt.

It is also very important to be realistic about the scope of what can be achieved with little or no resources. However, this important consideration is also true for social marketers who have access to large budgets. Priorities always need to be decided, and the limits or focus of a particular programme invariably need to be spelled out clearly. On a shoestring budget, the need for clarity of purpose and the scope of what can reasonably be expected are even more important if we are not to set ourselves up for failure.

There are three things to constantly hold in your mind when you are developing social marketing interventions. These can be set out as four simple questions:

1. What explicitly are you trying to achieve?
2. Who precisely are you trying to help?
3. How can you develop interventions that will help these people and that they will want to participate in?
4. How will you measure and report what happens?

With regards to the third of these questions, Bill Smith (2007) has advised 'We need to make social marketing fun, easy and popular'. By this, Smith means that the task is not to develop sophisticated media campaigns that will somehow mysteriously manipulate people into changing what they do. As social marketers, our job is to create goods and services that people say help them, that they think are great and they think are easy to take up and use. If we are successful, we will see lots of people taking up these goods and services – and in many instances we will also see them promoting uptake and helping to further refine interventions, so that they are even better at helping them and people like them.

Scoping on a shoestring

This section sets out how to follow the first stage of the Total Planning Process (TPP) framework (see Chapter 10) with a small or non-existent budget. For more information about the scoping stage, see Chapter 11, which provides a more in-depth discussion of the most important scoping issues.

Making the most of all your assets

If you think like a social marketer, you will start to constantly spot opportunities for progressing your programme. One of the best ways to start this process is 'asset mapping'. As Chapter 11 explains, in the scoping stage you need to discover as much as you can about the audience and issue that you are trying to address. This process should, however, not focus purely on the problem but also on the solution and the assets that exist to tackle the issue. Assets mapping is a process of identifying all the resources that exist in a community to deal with a community issues such as obesity, crime, and poor education attainment. It is also a process guided by the view that issues are best tackled by community-led action and engagement.

Asset mapping can be a costly business, but it can be done on a very low budget. A good way to start is by drawing up a list of local communities, organizations, people, companies, and not-for-profit organizations that may be interested in or are already seeking to deal with the issue you are trying to tackle.

In the first instance, you should target those organizations and communities that have a deep concern about the issue or the potential to have a big impact. Meetings and discussions with these organizations and groups should be an early priority in your programme.

Low-cost research

Libraries

One of the big costs in large-scale social marketing programmes is that of gathering market research data. There are resources in most communities, however, that can help reduce or even eliminate the need for this expenditure. Local or regional libraries can be of tremendous help in researching what is known about the issues you are trying to tackle and the audience you are trying to reach. Librarians and, increasingly, information scientists are employed by libraries to assist students and researchers. Get to know your local library and what services it offers.

Public sector information services

Many local public and civic institutions (including planning, economic, housing, police, education, fire and rescue, water, power, telecommunications, and media organizations) employ information scientists, researchers, statisticians and geographers, and epidemiologists. As part of your asset mapping, create a map or list of such services. Arrange to visit the organizations or departments and discuss:

- how they may be able to help you;
- whether they have already undertaken mapping or research projects that may be of help to you; and
- whether any data they have is free and of use to you.

Local private sector companies

Local private sector companies and corporations routinely collect data on market research, sales, and service uptake. Obviously some of this data is highly sensitive, and companies will not want to share it with you. However, companies are increasingly making such data available, especially in areas of pubic concern such as health and the environment. Sales data of items such as energy-efficient light bulbs, fruit and vegetables, and service data such as the number of plastic bags given away are being shared for free with the public sector as part of companies' corporate social responsibility agenda. Discuss your issue with local companies and ask how they can help you build a picture of the people and issues you re trying to tackle using their data. Remember also to think about what is in it for the company: setting up a photo call and a news feature with local media can be a good way of persuading and rewarding such cooperation. Clearly, you need to be aware that private sector organizations may have a biased way of presenting their data that you need to bear in mind.

Local universities, colleges, and schools

Learning institutions are assets in terms of knowledge management and research. Many institutions have students and staff who are looking for research topics that will form part of their academic work and count towards exam or qualifications. Many students are also looking for socially relevant research projects. These institutions often have highly skilled staff that can help with research design and analysis as well as desk-based searches of existing research. When approaching such institutions, it is worth stressing the contribution of your project to the local community and the benefits, to the institution, of being seen as partner. It is also important to understand the time cycles of such institutions. There will be certain times of the year when decisions are being made by students and staff who may be looking for research projects. Also bear in mind exam timetables and coursework-submission deadlines.

The third sector

International, national, and local non-government groups (NGOs), foundations, charities, and other third sector organizations are a great source of research and intelligence data. Many have well-developed, searchable websites dealing with specific issues. Many also employ information specialists and researchers who are willing to help you for free. A call or email to these specialists is worthwhile, but make sure you are as clear as possible about what you are asking for, as this will help them help you. Obviously you need to be aware of any possible bias that the organization may have.

Example: Health on Tap

Project overview:

- 'Health on Tap' is a health campaign for anyone working with, or caring for, older people in the UK.
- Following results from a 7-week pilot project, it encourages care-providers to sign up to the Good Hydration Charter, demonstrating how a proactive policy of increasing drinking water consumption in older people in residential care can result in a range of health and well-being benefits.
- The aims were to establish a industry-wide, recognized drinking-water regime, make fresh tap-water freely available, accessible, and attractively presented, and to promote the importance of good hydration to residences and staff.

- Partnership working was crucial to the project, providing expertise, networks, and resources (the research programme was conducted on a budget of less than £6000).

Results summary:

- Pilot participants recorded health improvements, including a 50% reduction in falls and laxative prescription, improved sleeping patterns, more energy, and less urinary tract infections.
- After 6 months, over 100 UK Care Homes signed up to the Good Hydration Charter.
- The project won the National Patient Safety Association's Best Hydration Award 2008 and was shortlisted for the 2008 Utility Awards.

Specialist marketing agencies

If you are working at the local level, as part of your asset mapping you should also locate and record details of any local marketing, market research, campaign, public relations (PR) advertising, and creative agencies. These companies may provide you with insight into the issue you are dealing with, examples of what works, or advice. Some companies have a policy of doing a certain amount of *pro bono* or unbilled work for causes and issues that they believe are important. When approaching specialist agencies, make it clear that you are not a fee-paying customer in the very first meeting. Set out your problem, what you know, who is helping you, and a specific request for support. It is much better to go with a specific request and then be prepared to alter this than go with a vague request for help. Part of any deal for free support work needs to include a clear agreement about how and when the company will be credited for its support. It is an absolute must that you draw up a written and signed agreement of what the company will deliver, over what timeframe, and to what success criteria. Even if no money is changing hands, such an agreement is important for both you and the company to ensure absolute clarity about the nature of the relationship and the support that is being pledged.

Making the most of people and partnerships

Marketing and building partnerships

Perhaps the single most powerful role you have is to convene people. The decision with regards to who to convene and what the agenda ought to be is critical to the success of almost all social marketing efforts. Even those running major national campaigns spend a lot of time, money, and talent on building partnerships. Do not underestimate the importance of this role. Avoid getting bogged down in a process of just building and maintaining good relationships. This can easily become an end in itself, so remember that the point of investing some of your limited time and resources in a relationship is to get a pay back that outstrips the effort you have to put in. Box 16.1 provides a checklist for getting the most out of your partnerships.

A key partner for both promoting your programme and for market research is the media, be it local radio, newspapers, television, or the Internet. The media are normally viewed simply as marketing channels, but they are also a business-sector as well as collections of individuals and are a powerful force in shaping popular societal agendas. It is often worthwhile to invest time in recruiting key editors, writers, or broadcasters as key partners in your delivery coalition.

When building partnerships with the media, it is important to treat them like any other key audience or potential partner. Get to know them. Who are the key influencers? What issues are

Box 16.1 Managing partnerships checklist

1. Anticipate needs and be proactive.
2. Always be 'nice' and 'positive' and with a 'can do'attitude.
3. Be flexible: give to receive.
4. Keep people informed, even if there is nothing to report.
5. Put a lot of effort into marketing your successes and celebrating a launch.
6. Never use 'but'. Always use 'yes and'.
7. Acknowledge and praise people at every opportunity.
8. Take people to lunch or coffee to build personal relationships.
9. Get the critics on the inside.
10. Give people a chance to be praised.
11. Keep it practical, but know the theory. And do not talk theory at people.
12. Put detractors or sceptical people in front of the real people you are trying to help.
13. Use third-party advocates to help you sell in your initiative.
14. Always deliver what you say you will.

they interested in? What kinds of projects or causes have they taken up? What are they against? As with any other partner, trust is important. Many people working in the media rightly view themselves as an important part of democracy. They are used to being lobbied and told half-truths, and they often have an inclination to campaign for particular causes.

Example: Partnering the media

Local media companies are increasingly staffed by very few people, and they are often hungry for copy and ideas to fill their programming schedules. Offer to write, at no cost, a regular feature of an agreed length and to an agreed style on your issues or give some interviews for free to your local radio station.

Generating funds for your programme

If you have little or no funding, a first task may be to secure a small budget to help you research, test, deliver, and evaluate your intervention. There are a number of ways to raise funds that can generate interest and engagement in your project at the same time.

These methods include asking possible donors to give direct funding or to provide goods and services that can then be sold or given away as prizes to promote the issues you are dealing with. For example, a barber shop giving you a voucher for a free haircut can then be used as a prize for people who attend a session about exploring why a community does not come forward for immunization. Often, local business people are more willing to help if they believe that the issue that you are concerned with is something that they would want to be associated with, because it will either give them good publicity or it is something that may adversely affect their business if it is not tackled. Good examples include food hygiene and fire safety. So when planning your project, consider who might be sympathetic, who might have something to gain, and who might see the project as a way of enhancing their reputation or brand.

Kotler and Lee (2007) suggest that when trying to persuade potential funders to support social marketing programmes, the same principles that we apply to understanding and influencing any other type of audience still apply. This means that there is a need to identify and prioritize possible funders and to segment them using criteria appropriate to the issue and sector you are looking at. Next, there is the need to articulate clear and specific requests. Invest in understanding the potential funders and develop a strategy using all elements of the marketing mix to create the best possible chance of the funder deciding to support the progarmme. One key process is to set out the exchange that is on offer to potential funders. When working out the exchange, you should set out both the costs and benefits (see Box 16.2 for examples) in terms that the potential funder will be able to understand and relate to.

Let possible funders know:

- that you understand the issues and have done your research;
- that the proposal meets their priorities as set out in any application criteria;
- about your project with as much real and vivid detail as possible: give examples about what will happen and how you will use the marketing mix;
- the envisaged outcome in hard numerical terms, if possible;
- how you will measure progress;
- key milestones, how budgets will be applied, and what the likely cost of success per person will be; and
- who else is supporting the project and what other pledges of funding you have.

Do not use moral arguments about why a potential funder should support you. Use arguments that demonstrate that a real difference can be achieved; and be realistic: do not over-promise what you can deliver.

If you are approaching funders through a formal application, make sure that you fill in application forms in the way prescribed by the funder and that your request is compatible with the selection criteria set out in the guidance to applicants. If you are unsure about any aspect of a funding

Box 16.2 Possible costs and benefits of partnerships

Possible costs

- Reputation and/or brand damage.
- Time cost: the need for a full scoping and development before impact is observable.
- Resource costs, management time, and programme budget.

Possible Benefits

- Reputation and/or brand enhancement.
- Community engagement and corporate responsibility.
- Market intelligence gained.
- Demonstrable improvement in a cause they care about.

application procedure, it is always best to contact the organization and seek clarity before proceeding with the process, as you may waste a great deal of your – and the funder's – time if you submit applications inappropriately or in a form that does not meet the required specification or timetable.

Making the most of every face-to-face opportunity

Every one-to-one meeting and face-to-face (F2F) encounter you have, and every committee meeting and event you attend, is a free marketing opportunity. F2F communication is the most powerful channel there is, so use these opportunities to the full to gather information and spread your ideas.

To get the most out of these opportunities, you need to think about the people you are meeting (your customer or audience). Consider how you can convey your key messages in a way they will relate to. Think about and write down the key phrases or words that you will need to use. It is a good idea not to talk theory but to give real-life practical examples quoting actual people and how they are affected by the issue to really bring it to life. In addition, do not forget that every F2F is a market-research opportunity. Apply active listening skills and note what is being said. Make a record as soon after the meeting as you can – it is a good idea to carry a small notebook with you to capture these kinds of encounters.

Always be explicit about what counts as success. You need a small number of absolutely clear goals that can be measured preferably in numerical terms. Ensure that every one you are working with also understands the objectives. Remember that internal communication is just as important as external communication.

Development on a shoestring

Here, we set out important information for achieving Stage 2 of the TPP framework if you have a limited or no budget. More comprehensive information, particularly for those with more generous budgets, is included in Chapter 12.

Marketing and market research using target-audience meetings

A good way to gather views and develop a deeper understanding with regards to audience views about a social marketing issues is to invite members of the audience you are trying to help to a meeting to discuss and explore the issue. The setting-up, management, and reporting of these meetings will, however, need careful planning. Inviting in audiences for this kind of meeting can make those responsible for delivering existing services nervous, as they feel they may be exposed to criticism that is sometimes very vocal and even aggressive. When you are planning this kind of 'meet the audience' session, set out answers to the following eight questions:

1. Have I set out clear aims and objectives for the meeting?
2. Have I got a representative sample of the audience I want to learn from?
3. Have I engaged and got the commitment of all relevant officials (who should also be present) and are they happy with the proposed focus of the meeting and the methods that will be used to engage the audience and report on what is discussed?
4. Have I made it easy and attractive for the audience to participate (have I considered issues of time, location, family support such as child care, physical access, and transport)?
5. Are the methods that will be used to engage the audience appropriate, and will they work?
6. How will I handle any conflict or dissent?
7. How will the meeting be facilitated – do I, or whoever will facilitate the meeting, have the skills, personal qualities, and audience respect to succeed?

8. Do I have a way of capturing what comes out of the meeting in a way that is respectful, appropriate, and as accurate as possible?

Treat your target audiences and coalition partners with respect. This means treating information you have gathered as sensitive and confidential and keeping people informed about what you are doing, what you are discovering, and what you plan to do about it.

Promoting a social marketing mindset in your organization

As part of your day-to-day work, you may be required to either review or approve projects, interventions, or strategies. These tasks are opportunities to influence the management culture of you organization and to get it to be more marketing orientated. When reviewing such proposals, you should consider the following three questions:

- Has an understanding of the target audience been used to influence the proposal, and if so, how?
- What is the specific behavioural goal?
- Is there a clearly articulated exchange that the intended audience will value?

You should try to get everyone in your organization to start thinking about the benefits of new services form a user's point of view. Do not be critical for criticism's own sake, and always make constructive recommendations for how proposals or a strategy can be enhanced using social marketing principles. In addition, try to get people to set challenging but realistic goals. Usually the weakest parts of most proposals will concern the evidence for an intervention, the understanding of the audience, and the proposed impact of the proposed intervention. As Chapters 3 and 11 explain, it is vital to ensure that clear, measurable goals are set and that interventions are pretested as thoroughly as possible.

Field testing interventions on a low budget

Before an intervention is fully implemented, it should be tested and refined, if necessary. Whist you may not have sufficient budget to undertake a full pilot and extensive field testing, it is possible to conduct mini-pilots and refine promotional material and/or service changes. The following list of ideas for low-cost testing and refinement is not exhaustive but gives some practical ways that you can refine your intervention prior to full implementation.

- Ask a small number of your target group to read and comment on the written material you produce.
- Ask colleagues to review your plans, intended materials, and approach.
- Stage a role play in which you or a colleague act as a member of the target audience coming into contact with the new service, and note what happens.
- Audio record the reactions of a small number of people to the new service or material.
- Conduct a peer appraisal of the new service or approach, having tried the new system for a week.
- Keep a written record of users' reaction the new service or product.

Implementation on a shoestring

Chapter 13 contains detailed information on implementing social marketing interventions, a process which comprises Stage 3 of the TPP framework. However, if you are working on a low-budget intervention, and the information in that chapter seems daunting, there are still ways to apply social marketing best practice to your initiative. There is no need to cut corners. It is important to remember that large budgets are no guarantee of success: much has been achieved through local interventions that have relied heavily on partnership, e.g. to deliver opportunities to provoke behavioural change.

Creative input for free

For social marketers, creative thinking can be an important and effective marketing tool. Always be on the lookout for innovative and inexpensive ways to promote your campaign or project. Look out for new combinations of marketing methods that are being used nationally and locally, and try to tap into free sources of creative thinking. You can often get great creative ideas by asking local schools or college students to work on ideas as part of design, marketing, art, or social programmes they are studying. Local artists, designers, media-workers, and marketing firms can also be persuaded to help for free. As suggested above, when developing your assets map make a list of all possible creative resources that may be of use to you.

Talks, workshops, and seminars

A great way to gather views from, inform, or influence target audiences is through talks, workshops, and seminars. Presentations are a very low-cost way of interacting with medium-sized groups of people, and they also allow for two-way interaction. If you think like a marketer when planning and organizing presentations, you will ensure that give thought to the people coming to the meeting prior to giving your presentation:

- Who are they?
- What are their views likely to be?
- What troubles them? How can you help them?
- Why are they coming?
- What do they expect to get from the event?
- Are there different sub-groups within the audience?

Next, think about what you want then to understand, know and feel. You should also be clear about what you want to get from them. For example, do you want them to:

- commit to doing something;
- feel that something must be done about the problem you are tackling;
- help with a proposal or research project; or
- better understand an issue or a demonstration?

Set out what success would look like and how you could capture it and measure it. In addition, never make a presentation about data without pinning the data on a real-life story about a real person your target group can understand.

Every meeting with a partner, potential partner, or even somebody representing the competition is a marketing opportunity. Do remember also that marketing is not about selling your ideas and persuading the other person to change against their will, but rather it is about finding an idea or an action that meets your goals and the goals of your target audience. This means active listening and a willingness to modify *your* ideas in the light of what you hear and learn.

Using newsletters

With cheaper and increasing access to computers, low-cost-design software, and the Internet, it need not be an expensive exercise to produce good-quality printed or electronic newsletters, which are a vehicle to communicate highly targeted messages to your target group. Newsletters can also help you generate more supporters and funds for your intervention. You can sell advertising space to people who want to raise their profile or communicate with the same audience as you. Businesses, NGOs, or third-sector organizations may also consider sponsoring you newsletter or buying advertising space.

Swapping advertising space

If you publish a newsletter, blog, or podcast, other publishers may be prepared to give you free or low-cost space if you provide a reciprocal arrangement. If you have a small budget, you can try negotiating with local media (e.g. local newspapers) for discounted advertising space. If the timing or placing of your advertisement is not important, try negotiating a discount for placing an advertisement at the last minute, if the newspaper cannot sell the space at a commercial rate.

If you do work with related partners and organizations to cross-promote interventions or share the cost of advertising, remember that partners represent you and what you are trying to achieve. See also information on making the most of people and partnerships, described above.

Making the most of your content

You can save a lot of time and money by making the content of your communications work as hard as possible for you. For example, you can use articles or news items you have written more than once, editing them if necessary. Make a list of all possible outlets for content you produce, and contact each outlet on a rolling basis to see if they are prepared to carry it.

Prize-draw, lotteries, and contests

Contests, lotteries, and prize-draws are a great way to set up an 'exchange' (see Chapter 3) and to encourage people to participate in your social marketing intervention. For example, children's painting or poster-design competitions that focus on the issue you are tackling are a cheap way to engage large numbers of people and generate media attention. You can also set up competitions or lottery schemes through which people can win prizes if they participate in the scheme. You can even give as a prize something you already own, manufacture, or produce and which others will find valuable (e.g. cakes, food, or new but unwanted gifts). The awarding of a prize also creates a good news story for the local media, again increasing the number of people who will hear about your intervention. Bear in mind that it may be necessary to obtain legal advice before running a competition for a lottery.

Online marketing

As more and more people gain access to the Internet, it becomes an increasingly important marketing, social networking, and communications channel. It is simultaneously a global and a very local tool. Below, we list some ways your social marketing intervention can exploit the Internet with no budget other than that needed for web connection.

Email marketing

Over 40% of all emails are now classed as 'spam' (the online equivalent of junk mail), so email marketing is getting an increasingly bad press. However, a good email can still receive a high response rate and have real impact. The key things to focus on are:

- personalizing the email;
- targeting the recipient;
- keeping it short, interesting, and to the point; and
- providing an easy way to respond and follow-up for those who chose do so.

As with all forms of contact from 'hot prospects' (people who show an interest in your intervention), you need to respond to email responses quickly and effectively. It is a good idea to send out emails in phases, so you have time to deal with responses in a timely and personalized way.

Building your own website

If you have a subscription to an Internet provider, it is easy to set up a website. Many providers even give free software that helps you design your site. A website can be a great marketing tool for providing information about what you are doing, how to contact you, and to gather people's views.

Linking to other websites

Getting other websites to link to yours is not only free, but can also help with your search-engine rankings, as many search engines now factor 'link popularity' into the relevancy of their search results. Site linking is also a good way to build relationships with partner and stakeholder organizations.

Email signature file

Use automated signature files, which can be set up to automatically appear at the bottom of every email you send out. These are like little poster cards, helping you promote your social marketing intervention and its key messages. The signatures can be changed and updated on a regular basis as you develop your intervention.

Discussion groups, forums, message boards, and newsgroups

An excellent way to increase awareness of your intervention is to take part in online discussion groups and message boards and to contribute to newsgroups (these are all websites that allow users to post contributions on a specific topic). You can even set these up to serve specific groups of people you are trying to help or use wider groups to gain support and information that will help you with your programme research and delivery.

Press releases

The press release is a great low-cost way to get media attention. But you have to have some *real* news before you decide to use press releases: your story has to be newsworthy and told in a way that a journalist would find interesting and relevant. If it is not, there is little chance of it getting the desired result.

Make sure your press release is attention grabbing. Try to think creatively about an angle that will interest both the media outlet that will read it and your target group and the organizations they interact with. For example, dressing up in a funny costume and getting photographs taken with a local politician to publicize the issue you are focussed on can be a good way to create a lot of attention. There are also lots of examples of protest movements that have staged peaceful 'sit-ins' to draw attention to their cause.

Other ways of promoting your intervention

- Print some postcards or write letters to your target group, highlighting your intervention. Include links to a follow-up website or telephone number.
- Set up a press conference, rally, picnic, or awareness 'launch meeting' for all the people who have said they will help you
- Set up a public signing of a petition for action, and invite the press and photographers for a photo-shoot of the event. Make sure to think of some memorable images for them.

- The presentation of a petition to an important local person is a great way to get lots of media coverage for free.
- Print up, or hand-make if necessary, business cards that promote your intervention.
- Place signs that publicize your intervention at home, in your workplace, in your car, and at other outlets that will display them for free (e.g. hospitals, schools, libraries, and shops).
- Join professional and social groups to network with other people, and volunteer to speak at local group meetings and seminars.
- Talk with local colleges, schools, and universities to offer workshops on the issue your social marketing intervention is seeking to address.
- Participate in community events (e.g. carnivals, parades, picnics, fairs, fun runs, and walks) to promote your intervention.
- Listen to radio talk-shows, and when the topic is relevant to your issue, call in and offer your opinion.

Evaluation on a shoestring

Chapter 14 provides information about how to evaluate a social marketing intervention (Stage 4 of the TPP framework). It is possible to evaluate social marketing interventions on a low budget but, as with the rest of the advice in this chapter, it is even more important to be very clear and realistic about what can be done. The key tasks are:

- setting aims and objectives;
- identifying evaluation indicators;
- choosing research methods; and
- dissemination of results and follow-up action.

Setting aims and objectives

Although this section does not seek to repeat the information that Chapter 11 provides on setting aims and objectives, it is important to reiterate that without clear and 'smart' objectives, evaluation of programmes becomes very problematic. If clear and precise objectives are set, the method of measuring them becomes much easier. Measurement does not have to be expensive or complicated. For example, you can track response to a feature in a newspaper by asking all the people that contact you what prompted the contact and recording how many say it was the newspaper feature.

When dealing with small or low budgets, some evaluation methods (e.g. extensive longitudinal tracking-studies involving lots of people) are not possible, unless sponsorship can be found. It is also not appropriate to spend a disproportionate amount of your time or resources on evaluating small interventions. A good rule of thumb is that evaluation should take up no more than 10% of your total resources, be that time or funding, and no more that 5% if the total project value is less than £100 000 or $200 000 (providing you are adhering to what professional and research institutes consider to be best practice).

Evaluation methods open to people working with a low budget include:

- short, multiple-choice questionnaires;
- short open-ended questionnaires (of no more than 10 questions);
- reviewing service-utilization data;
- audience interviews;

- group discussions;
- case studies;
- capturing audience stories;
- video, audio, photographic, and art records;
- visual and document analysis;
- observational studies;
- voting records; and
- records of meeting.

You may need specialist help to set these approaches up if you are not experienced, e.g. in developing questionnaires or interpreting numerical or qualitative data.

Example: Co-observation and supportive feedback

Two midwives wanted to evaluate there antenatal education programme. In addition to designing a short questionnaire with the help of a local university researcher (which they gave out to their classes at the end of the sessions), they also set up a process of co-observation and feedback. The co-observation consisted of each of the midwives observing and feeding back to the other on their sessions' educational plan, the conduct of the session and the audience reaction against a pre-agreed set of criteria that included:

- clarity of aims and objectives;
- content, method, and evaluation of the session;
- the conduct of the session;
- verbal and non-verbal communication;
- level of interaction with the class; and
- how questions were dealt with.

The midwives used the observations and the results from the survey to review and modify their programme on an ongoing basis.

Follow-up on a shoestring

As Chapter 14 explains, the usefulness of an evaluation depends on what you do with the results. Evaluations should lead to answering questions such as:

- what worked best;
- what partnerships work well and who else could you work with;
- what should change in the future delivery of the project;
- what improvements to your research methods do you need to make; and
- what further information do you need?

Follow-up is important because it is a way of maintaining a relationship and showing respect for funders, partners, supporters, and the target group(s) of the intervention. You should aim to provide some form of feedback to the target group and anyone who has helped with the intervention, including funders and sponsors. Ideally, you should also give some form of feedback on your intervention to others running, or planning to run, similar projects, so that knowledge about what does and does not work can be disseminated.

Do not delay the dissemination of your findings, as their importance can decrease over time. Set a deadline for getting results published or being put before relevant stakeholders.

It is important not to hide negative findings. Learning that something has not worked is very valuable and will help others not to make similar mistakes. If your intervention has not worked, the key point is not to beat yourself up about it but to understand why or set in train a way to find out why.

Exercise: Develop a micro-social marketing plan

Think of a real-life situation that you think could benefit from the application of social marketing principles but for which you have little or no resources other than your time. Set five headings that relate to the key planning documents needed for each stage of the TPP framework outlined in this chapter and Chapters 10–15. What three to five actions you could take to develop:

- a scoping report;
- a development plan;
- an implementation plan;
- a system to evaluate; and
- a follow-up plan.

Limit yourself to no more than five bullet points for each of these micro-plans.

References

Kotler, P. and Lee, N. (2007). *Social Marketing*. California: Sage Publications.

Smith, W.A. (2007). Social marketing: making it fun, easy & popular. *From Rhetoric to Reality. 2nd National Social Marketing Conference*. Oxford, 24–25th September 2007 Available at: http://www.nsms.org.uk/images/CoreFiles/2ndNSMConf-04BillSmith-MakingItFunEasyPopular-D1P1Sept2007.pdf (accessed 24 January 2009).

Chapter 17

Critical social marketing

Gerard Hastings

To acquire knowledge one must study, but to acquire wisdom one must observe.
Marilyn Vos Savant

Learning points

This chapter

- Introduces the concept of critical marketing;
- Provides a short history of the critical analysis of marketing;
- Explains why critical marketing is important to social marketers; and
- Gives examples of how critical marketing works in practice.

Chapter overview

This chapter introduces critical marketing (the critical analysis of marketing) and explains why it is an invaluable tool for understanding:

- how marketing works;
- how it impacts on behaviour; and
- how it can be turned to social good.

Critical marketing seeks not to just determine what is 'wrong and bad' about commercial marketing, but to reflect on its nature, learn from its successes, and analyse its weaknesses. Reflecting Lazer and Kelly's (1973) definition of the discipline, this chapter argues that *social marketing will flourish by exploiting its twin understanding of the good and the bad that marketing can bring to society* (Hastings and Saren, 2003, p. 305).

The chapter begins by discussing the origins and characteristics of critical marketing, which is a well-trodden path in the academic marketing literature. It then explains how the ideas underpinning critical marketing are as much part of marketing as consumer orientation and market research and, as such, should be adopted by social marketers.

The final part of the chapter presents three critical marketing case studies on food, tobacco, and alcohol marketing, respectively. Amongst them, they illustrate some of the benefits of critical analysis, including healthier public policy, improved insights into effective behavioural change, and the whys and wherefores of collaboration.

Introduction

Origins and principles

Critical marketing has been around a long time. A comprehensive review of the development of marketing thought published in the *Journal of Marketing and Public Policy* (Wilkie and Moore, 2003) demonstrates that, when it began to emerge in the early part of the twentieth century, the discipline was already focussed on a wide and critical agenda. The interest was not just with managerial issues of what works and nurturing the bottom-line, but with much wider concerns about the relationship between business and society, such as whether advertising added value and whether prices were being unfairly manipulated by business. These are major issues that remain as important now as they were then. Case Study 1, e.g. focusses on the current discussion about the role of food advertising in childhood obesity. So, from its earliest days, marketing was clearly focussed on social good as well as shareholder value.

This broader agenda was still much in evidence in the 1970s, when Kotler first coined the term 'social marketing' (Kotler and Zaltman, 1971). Interestingly, although his ideas did not include critical marketing (he concentrated on how marketing precepts could inform social and health behaviour change), they met with resistance. Luck (1969) argued that marketing should be restricted to market transactions and should not cover social marketing activity, which did not, in his view, involve any clear return. Carman (1973) wrote in similar vein.

Luck also argued that broadening the concept of marketing is not in the interests of the discipline, as it confuses its definition and ultimately threatens its identity. Bartels (1976) supported this stance:

> If marketing is to be regarded as so broad as to include both economic and non-economic fields of application, perhaps marketing as originally conceived will ultimately appear under another name.

Others, however, felt that Kotler had not gone far enough. Dawson (1972) felt that the marketing concept was too narrowly defined and should be reframed as the *human concept*, which he felt was *more responsive to human needs in their totality*. Lazer and Kelly (1973, p. *ix*), writing at the same time, also applied this broader thinking to social marketing, seeing it as 'concerned with the application of marketing knowledge, concepts, and techniques to enhance social as well as economic ends ...' and 'also concerned with analysis of the social consequence of marketing policies, decisions and activities'.

Retrospectively, Arnold and Fisher (1996) describe how the emerging discipline was, in this way, flanked on the one hand by marketing 'apologists' – who wanted to keep marketing clearly defined within the firm – and 'reconstructionists', who were pushing for an even broader, macromarketing perspective (see Box 17.1).

Box 17.1 Arnold and Fisher's three strands of marketing thought

- *'Apologists':* Taking a traditional view: marketing is good because it helps the economy. Its domain is, and should be, limited to the firm (e.g. Luck).
- *'Social marketers':* Turning the power of marketing to social good, thereby compensating for its deficiencies with better outcomes (e.g. Kotler, Levy, and Andreasen).
- *'Reconstructionists':* Critical of marketing concept and process, not just its outcomes (e.g. Dawson).

They went on to argue that the apologists had largely won the day and that in most universities it was a case of business as usual.

However, recent developments suggest otherwise. Social marketing is enjoying a renaissance. Business schools and universities in the UK, New Zealand, Australia, and North America now offer courses in it. The idea that skills learnt to push fast-moving consumer goods or financial services can also be used to address pressing social problems such as HIV/AIDS or global warming is extremely appealing to students. The UK government has established the National Social Marketing (NSM) Centre – a collaboration between DH and the Consumer Focus, which has developed the first National Social Marketing Strategy for Health in England. Similarly, the Scottish Executive recently commissioned an investigation into how social marketing can be used to guide health improvement (Stead et al., 2007). Australia, New Zealand, Canada, and the USA all have social marketing facilities embedded high within their health services, or they are in the process of acquiring them. And books have emerged: Kotler (2007) has just produced a new one, Europe has acquired its first text (Hastings, 2007), a Sage *Handbook* is planned, and of course there is the publication you are reading now.

Critical marketers – the successors of Arnold and Fisher's 'reconstructionists' – have also been very active in examining marketing from a number of different perspectives, including sustainability (Fuller, 1999), ethics (Crane, 1997), feminism (Catterall et al., 1999), discourse analysis (Brownlie and Saren, 1997), and postmodernism (Firat and Venkatesh, 1993). In this way they assess both the processes and outcomes of marketing.

Lazer and Kelly's definition brings the two strands together, adding strength and symmetry to social marketing. It also matches much more closely what happens in the commercial sector, where critical marketing is core business. Companies have to consider how they sit with society and have long recognized that economic success is not only dependent on their consumer marketing (getting the right product to the right people in the right place at the right price) but also on the macro-economic environment within which the company operates.

The political and regulatory culture is a crucial element of this environment and so, as David Jobber (2004, p. 145) explains in his core marketing text, *close relationships with politicians are often cultivated by organizations both to monitor political moods and influence them*. By the same token, policy-makers and politicians are used to commercial interests wanting to offer advice and suggestions with regards to the regulation of their industry. It would have been unthinkable, e.g. for recent European Union (EU) consideration of research ethics procedures for the development of new drugs to have taken place without consulting the pharmaceutical companies.

Thus lobbying or 'stakeholder marketing' is as much standard business practice as consumer marketing. As Jobber goes on to note: *the cigarette industry, for example, has a vested interest in maintaining close ties with government to counter proposals from pressure groups such as ASH* (*ibid*). A few years ago, when the European ban on tobacco advertising was being debated, it was estimated that the tobacco industry had no fewer than 200 lobbyists in Brussels (Hastings and Angus, 2004). Acknowledging and engaging with a critical agenda therefore brings business into the mainstream of social change and public policy.

Social marketers should be there too.

Why social marketing should go critical

It would be rude not to

It has been noted many times that social marketing takes learning from commercial marketing. The fact that critical analysis is an integral part of business is therefore reason enough to take it seriously.

It is also clear from Jobber's comment about ASH above that social marketers are very much on the business community's radar. And just as the tobacco industry will attempt to tackle ASH, so the sugar industry has tried to undermine announcements concerning its products by the World Health Organization (WHO; Boseley, 2003; BBC, 2004) and the advertising industry has tried to avert regulation of food advertising (see Case Study 1).

However, these competitive forces do not need to end in confrontation. The UK food industry, e.g. has cooperated in attempts to reduce salt levels in its products (Food Standards Agency, 2006) and to market healthy foods to low-income groups (National Prevention Research Initiative, 2008). Also in the UK, the alcohol industry has contributed to social marketing efforts by helping establish the Drinkaware Trust (see Case Study 3).

Thus competitive analysis of social marketing and related forces is a reality and has resulted in some useful innovations.

In the face of this attention, it would seem churlish for social marketing not to reciprocate and analyse what our commercial alter egos are doing. The result, as we will discuss in the case studies, is both sensible, well-informed cooperation and, when necessary, tighter regulation. This leads to better social marketing.

It helps us learn from the competition

Critical analysis takes us seamlessly into another extremely useful area of marketing practice: competitive analysis. Competition is a fact of commercial life:

> like the natural world, business is also driven by the law governing the survival of the fittest. However, in this case the forces are not hidden Darwinian genes, but an overt managerial process guided by deliberate planning.
>
> (Hastings, 2007, p. 154)

Crucially, this potential threat is turned into an opportunity by studying the activities of competitors. This enables marketers not only to 'control, influence or at least adapt to the resulting forces' (*ibid*) but, perhaps more importantly, gain greater insights about their customers and, therefore, service them better. Thus McDonald's will carefully analyse Burger King's offerings to help hone their own efforts. They will also maintain a flexible view of exactly who the competition is by asking their customers. It may be that their real rivals are not other burger-sellers, or even fast-food outlets, but recreational venues such as cinemas or play parks. This tells McDonald's that the customer need they are satisfying goes way beyond food and takes in entertainment or childminding.

In this way the analysis of their rivals helps craft their competitive strategy – whether this be combative (perhaps undercutting Burger King's prices) or collaborative (opening an outlet at a cinema complex). This then becomes part of their basic marketing strategy.

Social marketers can gain the same insights about their customers by studying their rivals' successes and failures. For example, Philip Morris's expert stewardship of the Marlboro brand over the last 50 years tells us a great deal about the emotional drivers of teen smoking (see Case Study 2). Similarly their disastrous price-cutting strategy of the early 1990s reminds us that successful brands need sustained and coherent marketing support (see Box 17.2).

It is part of 'moving upstream'

Social marketers have to think beyond the individual. The reasons for doing so take in the theoretical, practical, and ethical (Hastings, 2007).

Box 17.2 The need for sustained and coherent marketing support

Example: The cowboy stumbles

Marlboro is one of the most valuable brands on the Earth. It has enjoyed a premium position in the global tobacco market for over 50 years. This success is driven by excellent all-round marketing: evocative mass media and other commercial communications, a high-quality product that benefited greatly from the early adoption of ammonia technology (to help release the nicotine and give smokers a better 'hit'), wide distribution, a stylish and easily recognized pack and a price that reflects its select market positioning.

The importance of having a coherent strategy was demonstrated in the early 1990s when Philip Morris made a rare marketing mistake by dramatically cutting the price of Marlboro (Klein, 2000). It was seen as undermining not just its brand but the very idea of branding. For a short while the argument gained currency that marketing was finished and business in future would be simply about price. But Philip Morris reversed the decision, Marlboro regained its ascendancy and the uncharacteristic aberration has become a classic business school case study illustrating how important it is to have a consistent and coherent marketing strategy.

Theoretical

Theories of behavioural change (e.g. social cognitive theory, social learning theory, social norms, and social ecology) all emphasize the importance of social context as an influence on individual behaviour.

Practical

On a practical level, marketing planning starts with an environmental scan and goes on to encourage the adoption of the most efficient and effective methods for meeting agreed objectives. Time and again this will include intervening 'upstream' – water fluoridation, flour fortification, and the reduction of salt in processed foods provide obvious examples.

Ethical

Having accepted that individuals are susceptible to their environment, it would be unethical to ignore this when it comes to behavioural change.

This can be illustrated with the story of the baby camel (see Box 17.3)

We are all like the baby camel. We have lots of potential, but as long as we are encaged and restricted by our environment our hopes of fulfilling this are greatly reduced. It is immoral as well as ineffective for social marketers ignore this reality. And the dramatic impact of inequalities on health outcomes, (even in a developed country like the UK, life expectancy in our poorest communities drops 22 years below the average (WHO, 2008)) reminds us that the camel's cage is all too real for many people. If we social marketers keep focussed on the individual – ignoring the environmental determinants of their behaviour – we are effectively making them culpable for their predicament, when in reality it is typically way beyond their control. As social marketers we have to avoid this tendency towards victim blaming.

The key point from a critical marketing perspective is that the commercial sector is an important part of the social context, especially when we come to consider behaviours such as diet, alcohol

Box 17.3 The importance of social context

A baby camel approached his mother one day and asked 'Mummy, why do we have such hard bony tails?' His mother replied 'So that, when we move through the desert, we can protect ourselves from the biting and poisonous insects'. 'Mummy', came a second question, 'Why do we have such big, flat feet?' The mother replied 'So that we can move with ease over the treacherous shifting sands of the desert'. And again the little camel asked 'Why do we have a hump?' The reply? 'So we can travel even into the empty quarter, where no other animal can pass, because we have with us all the food and water we need'.

Finally, the small voice asked: 'Mummy, why are we in the zoo?'

(*Source*: Hastings, 2007, p. 113)

consumption, smoking, and driving. Each of these activities has a raft of commercial actors who are seeking to influence what they characterize as consumer behaviour. However they are also, of course, important health and social behaviours. Overlooking the role Diageo and Land Rover has on them would be as unprofessional and immoral as ignoring the impact of inequalities.

Furthermore, there is a clear overlap between marketing and inequalities. The relationship between disadvantage and smoking has long been noted, and this is matched by an (inevitable) tendency for the tobacco industry to target the less well-off (Devlin et al., 2004). Similar trends are perceptible in fast-food consumption: a study funded by the Medical Research Council showed that the UK distribution of McDonald's outlets correlates precisely with disadvantage (Macdonald et al., 2007).

Proving the power of marketing

Critical analysis of commercial marketing has resulted in the development of an extensive and convincing evidence base showing that marketing can influence behaviour. Rigorous studies and systematic reviews have shown that:

- ***tobacco promotion influences young people to smoke;***

> Longitudinal studies suggest that exposure to tobacco advertising and promotion is associated with the likelihood that adolescents will start to smoke. Based on the strength of this association, the consistency of findings across numerous observational studies, temporality of exposure and smoking behaviours observed, as well as the theoretical plausibility regarding the impact of advertising, we conclude that tobacco advertising and promotion increases the likelihood that adolescents will start to smoke.
>
> (Lovato et al., 2003, p. 10)

Studies also show that other elements of the marketing mix influence young people's smoking (National Cancer Institute, 2008).

- ***advertising for food high in fat, sugar, and salt is implicated in childhood obesity;***

> Beyond knowledge, food promotion influences children's food preferences, and encourages them to ask their parents to purchase foods they have seen advertised. Food promotion has also been shown to influence children's consumption and other diet-related behaviours and outcomes. These effects are significant, independent of other influences and operate at both brand and category level.
>
> (Hastings et al., 2006, p. 2)

- ***alcohol marketing encourages youth drinking.***

> Longitudinal studies consistently suggest that exposure to media and commercial communications on alcohol is associated with the likelihood that adolescents will start to drink alcohol, and with increased drinking amongst baseline drinkers. Based on the strength of this association, the consistency of findings across numerous observational studies, temporality of exposure and drinking behaviours observed, dose-response relationships, as well as the theoretical plausibility regarding the impact of media exposure and commercial communications, we conclude that alcohol advertising and promotion increases the likelihood that adolescents will start to use alcohol, and to drink more if they are already using alcohol.
>
> (Anderson et al., 2009, p. 1)

One result of this impressive evidence base has been the increasing regulation of commercial marketing. In the case of tobacco, which has been most carefully researched, it has resulted in widespread prohibitions on advertising and many other forms of marketing. This has culminated in the Framework Convention on Tobacco Control (FCTC) – the first international treaty designed to protect public health. It adopts an extremely broad perspective on tobacco advertising and promotion, defining it as:

> any form of commercial communication, recommendation or action with the aim, effect or likely effect of promoting a tobacco product or tobacco use either directly or indirectly
>
> (WHO, 2003, p. 4)

In particular, the word 'action' takes the focus way beyond advertising and overt communication efforts and into marketing more generally. This provides social marketers with a much clearer field: it is easier to 'steal' customers if your competitors have got their hands tied behind their backs.

More importantly, this evidence base – and wide-ranging reaction to it – serve to underline the potential power of well-executed marketing campaigns. If marketing by big tobacco companies is so effective and needs such comprehensive controls put upon it, there is all the more reason for public health to start using the same ideas and techniques to combat teen smoking. Like the hefty tether on a prize bull, the very need for a powerful mechanism like the FCTC underscores the effectiveness of marketing – both commercial and social.

Critical marketing in practice

Case Study 1: Food advertising and healthier public policy

The evidence linking the promotion of foods high in fat, salt, and sugar and childhood obesity emerged from a very extended process, comprising several decades of primary research followed by a specially commissioned literature review.

The primary research was conducted by academics throughout the world, but principally in North America. Marketers were at the forefront of research: Marvin Goldberg, a leading social marketer, did some of the most elegant studies; and Ruth Bolton, who went on to edit the prestigious *Journal of Marketing*, did the study that made the crucial link between food advertising and health outcomes. This critical marketing research must have seemed something of a futile exercise at the time because, with one or two exceptions, policy-makers tended to ignore the issue.

Then the obesity epidemic hit. This caused the UK Food Standards Agency (FSA) to commission a review of the evidence (Hastings et al., 2003) that was no ordinary review – it had to be 'systematic', which meant a very complex and rigorous methodology (see Box 17.4).

The Institute for Social Marketing (ISM) review also went through no fewer than seven stages of peer review from the time of the initial protocol to publication of the final report. But from a policy perspective the real work began after the report (which concluded that food advertising

Box 17.4 Systematic methods for reviewing research on the effects of food promotion on children

Three main methods were used to identify potentially relevant research:

- an extensive search of electronic databases;
- searches of the 'grey' literature; and
- personal contact with key people in the field.

The reference list of the original Ministry of Agriculture, Fisheries and Food (MAFF) review (Young et al., 1996) was also examined and an in-house search for relevant literature undertaken at the Institute for Social Marketing (ISM). These search methods yielded 29 946 potentially relevant titles and abstracts that underwent an initial stage of relevance assessment. From this, a total of 201 articles were considered relevant: 79 met the initial criteria for the systematic review of the extent and nature of food promotion to children; 109 met the initial criteria for the systematic review of the effects of food promotion on children's food knowledge, attitudes, and behaviour; and a further 13 articles met the initial criteria for both systematic reviews.

Each of these 201 articles was then assessed against more stringent relevance and quality criteria. In total, 65 articles describing 50 studies passed these criteria for the systematic review of the extent and nature of food promotion to children and 55 articles describing 51 studies passed these criteria for the systematic review of the effects of food promotion on children's knowledge, attitudes, and behaviour. Finally, the included studies were subject to a final quality rating to gauge their relative quality; this was used to help assess which studies' findings should be given more weight in drawing conclusions from the evidence. Studies were categorized, on the basis of their rating scores, as higher, medium, or lower scoring.

was influencing children in an unhealthy way) appeared. This was also when the critical marketing gloves came off.

Publication was greeted with a massive amount of media interest. This was consistently positive and accepting of the findings. The only negative comments were a few mumblings about the conclusion being obvious. Most, however, accepted the need now for solid evidence and for policy-makes to do something about the problem. *The Daily Telegraph* (Uhlig, 2003), for instance, which is a very conservative and staid paper, led with a call for government action (see Fig. 17.1).

The report was also greeted with a rival review, commissioned by the advertising industry, which concluded that:

> [f]ood advertising does not dictate children's dietary patterns but it does have a role to play in food choice at the level of the brand. In addition, television programming offers a generous range of images about food and can shape food choices. Healthy and unhealthy eating with different kinds of foods are represented in all media in a host of different ways
>
> (Young, 2003, p. 2)

In short, it concluded that policy-makers had nothing to worry about.

This put the FSA in a dilemma, which it resolved by convening an academic seminar of leaders in the field to examine both reviews and determine which best reflected reality. and the seminar concluded that the review commissioned by the advertising industry suffered from limited coverage, contradicted a review conducted by the same author in 1996, and seemed to be rejecting virtually all social science research as either too artificial (experimental studies) or having too

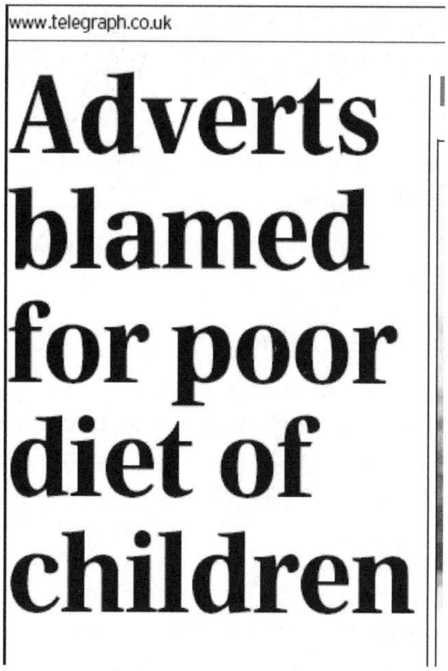

www.telegraph.co.uk

Adverts blamed for poor diet of children

Fig. 17.1 Press coverage of the systematic review of food promotion and childhood obesity

little control (observational studies) (FSA, 2003a). The seminar went on to say that the ISM review: *had provided sufficient evidence to indicate a causal link between promotional activity and children's food knowledge, preferences and behaviours* (*ibid*).

The advertising industry also adopted another approach, commissioning two academics (Paliwoda and Crawford, 2003) to critique the ISM review. The academic seminar was again called in, and Paliwoda and Crawford's commentary was rejected (FSA, 2003b). This time it concluded that the ISM review was *honest to the reality of the research landscape* (*ibid*, p. 3) and that the critique *did not make a sufficiently strong case to warrant re-examination of the conclusions* (*ibid*, p. 8).

A further review of all this reviewing was then commissioned by Ofcom – the UK organization in charge of telecommunications and the regulation of advertising (Livingstone, 2005). This time there was little dispute with the findings of the ISM review, and the way was finally opened for policy options to be considered. Ofcom has now imposed a ban on the advertising of energy-dense foods such as burgers and fried chicken.

> in and around all children's programming and on dedicated children's channels as well as in youth-oriented and adult programmes which attract a significantly higher than average proportion of viewers under the age of 16
>
> (Ofcom, 2006)

Interestingly, the rather defensive reaction of the advertising industry can be contrasted with that of some sections of the food industry, which have seen the controversy about food marketing as an opportunity rather than a threat. The Co-operative, e.g. has become involved in a research project to assess the potential of store-based promotions of healthy eating among low-income groups.

The case illustrates four benefits of critical marketing.

- Critical marketing research is valuable even when there is no obvious social or health problem to address. Research done in the 1970s and 1980s was invaluable in addressing obesity – an issue that did not emerge until this century.

- Whether or not we, as social marketers, get involved in critical marketing, it will impinge itself on us. If commercial marketers think our activities will damage their prospects they will certainly take steps to critique and try and delimit it.
- Critical marketing works. As a result of our review the advertising of food high in fat, sugar, and salt has been restricted, and the social environment of British youngsters is less likely to encourage behaviour that leads to obesity.
- Critical marketing does not have to be negative: the Co-operative has – as marketers so often do – turned it into an opportunity.

Case Study 2: Tobacco marketing

Critical marketing research has also driven the restrictions on tobacco marketing and the FCTC, as discussed above. However, it has another important benefit: it can give us insights into how marketing is used by the tobacco industry to encourage the onset and continuance of smoking, and hence how we can use it to do the opposite. It can inform our direct behavioural change efforts.

The sort of quantitative research summarized by Lovato et al. (*op cit*) which attempts to unpick the causative relationship between tobacco marketing and smoking is important here. It reminds that marketing works. More qualitative and ethnographic studies are also invaluable. They can dig a bit deeper and begin to unpick complex emotional phenomena, like brands.

Perhaps most useful of all in recent years have been analyses of internal tobacco-industry documents. These provide a very clear sense of how customers and marketing managers are thinking. Many of these documents have emerged as a result of legal action in North America, but more recently the UK Health Select Committee conducted an enquiry into the industry's activities and required the industry's leading advertising agencies to provide a selection of their internal marketing documents; from creative briefs to market research. The resulting disclosed documents are available online (www.tobaccopapers.com) and provide fascinating insights into:

- the tobacco companies' use of discount brands to target to disadvantaged groups;
- use of sponsorship;
- the positioning of low-tar brands;
- the promotion of rolling tobacco; and
- marketing to young people.

You will find case studies on each of these at www.tobaccopapers.com/casestudies.

The industry's efforts to market products to young people, e.g. are instructive. First the industry takes great care to get to know its customers using a combination of ethnographic research and detailed segmentation studies.

The ethnographic research reveals that smoking amongst the young is as much about image as it is product attributes. Smoking provides a 'rite of passage', with youngsters 'looking for reassurance' and 'searching for an identity' (see Box 17.5).

The industry caters for these 'needs' with a range of marketing techniques including advertising, which has now been banned, and many others, which have not, such as:

> quality and stylish packaging; peer group endorsement, controlled at first (hopefully spontaneous in time); investment in distribution (the right outlet as a marketing exercise) and "premium pricing"
>
> (Collett Dickenson Pearce and Partners (CDP), 1998, p. 14).

Box 17.5 The emotional drivers of youth smoking

'To smoke Marlboro Lights represents having passed a rite of passage, i.e. it is not something done by immature smokers. Neither is it smoked by older people, unlike Silk Cut which is seen as being fit for all. Silk Cut's universality of appeal is a problem for younger smokers for it means the brand lacks sufficient 'street cred'' (Gallaher Group Plc, 1996, p. 2).

'Young adult smokers are looking for reassurance that they are doing the right thing, and cigarettes is no exception. Any break with a brand's heritage must be carefully considered in order not to throw doubt into the minds of young adult smokers' (Rothmans Inc, 1998, p. 21).

'Young adult smokers are also searching for an identity. Cigarettes have a key role to play as they are an ever-present statement of identity. By inference, if a brand of cigarettes does not convey much in the way of image values, there may well be little reason for a young adult smoker to persist with or adopt the brand. Strong image values can help establish an identity, weak image values are of no use' (*op cit*).

These are built into evocative brands *to engage their aspirations and fantasies - 'I'd like to be there, do that, own that* (TBWA Simons Palmer Ltd, 1997, p. 1). The ideal for an *aspirational lifestyle brand* is to become *[t]he Diet Coke of cigarettes* (Leading Edge Consultancy, 1997, p. 5).

Interestingly, the research to guide and monitor the development of these icons includes competitive analysis:

iii) To track the image of Marlboro and key competitors and develop a measure of brand involvement.
iv) To evaluate smokers' relationships with brands.
v) To separately identify the effect of Marlboro's sponsorship of the Ferrari Formula 1 team on the overall effectiveness of Marlboro advertising

(Taylor Nelson Sofres, 1997, p. 4)

To track the image of Marlboro against a set of key competitor brands using a number of image statements and a measure of brand involvement.

(Hall and Partners, 1997, p. 3)

The industry uses segmentation to focus its efforts on the groups it wants to target or which are most likely to respond to is efforts. Motivations for smoking are mapped against age (see Box 17.6).

These insights are combined with the ethnographic research to create a sophisticated model of youth smoking (see Box 17.7).

The case illustrates how critical marketing research can help social marketers conduct their core business of provoking behavioural change. As well as helping us understand why young people are drawn to smoking (insights that are as useful to the social marketer as the tobacco executive) it reinforces some key marketing lessons.

For example, it reminds us that we need to think about emotional as well as rational drivers of human behaviour. Understanding these will require careful ethnographic research and, because drivers vary between subgroups, segmentation, and targeting. Branding can help meet these emotional needs, and brands are built and maintained not just with communications but the whole marketing effort.

Box 17.6 Mapping motivation for smoking against age

Rejecting	Accepting	Alienated
◆ enjoy disapproval	◆ accommodating perceptions	◆ resent change
◆ sets apart from 'adults'	◆ considerate to others views	◆ feel disapproved of
◆ rebellion/assertive	◆ liberal outlook	◆ need to justify actions
◆ too young to worry	◆ deserve it	
◆ do what I want		
		Age →

Source: Interbrand (UK) Ltd, 1997, p. 13

Finally, all this takes time; Marlboro, Diet Coke, and Lambert & Butler have been around for decades. Good marketing needs sustained effort, reliable funding, and patience.

Case Study 3: The Drinkaware Trust

The UK is a nation of drinkers: per capita alcohol consumption is higher than any other country in Europe. This has resulted in a raft of social and health problems such as:

- children are drinking alcohol in increasing numbers (Fuller, 2007);
- binge drinking and public disorder among young people are rife (Alcohol Concern, 2007; Travis, 2008); and
- chronic conditions such as liver disease are increasing across the population.

The negative effects of alcohol affect not just a minority of problem drinkers, as is sometimes assumed, but the whole population. And the solution needs to be equally wide ranging. Services for problem drinkers need to be combined with reductions in overall consumption levels (Edwards et al., 2004 and 2005).

The Drinkaware Trust has been established as part of the UK's response. It is a charity funded by the alcohol industry to the tune of £12 million for its first 3 years, and its purpose is *to positively change public behaviour and the national drinking culture in the UK in order to reduce alcohol misuse and minimise alcohol related harm* (Drinkaware Trust, 2006). Trustees are drawn from the industry, but the majority come from non-governmental organizations (NGOs) or the academic community.

There are clear concerns that this may just be a convenient corporate social responsibility (CSR) tactic on the alcohol industry's part. Not that CSR is necessarily a bad thing; its just that we have to keep in mind that the watchword in the phrase is 'corporate' – corporations are required by law to put their shareholders first, and this imperative kicks in even when it comes to doing good. Dan Hind (2008, p. 47) writing in the *New Scientist* recently described CSR as a *gold plated contradiction* and given that the UK alcohol industry spends £110 million every year promoting alcohol, the gold plating might seem pretty thin. So maybe participation in the Drinkaware Trust is just a way of currying ministerial favour and staving off harsher legislative measures.

The contrast with tobacco policy has also been highlighted:

> More evidence that health information regarding the dangers of alcohol are being firmly controlled by the alcoholic beverage industry, a rather strange policy for health issues, the phrase chickens and foxes

Box 17.7 Tobacco industry insights into youth smoking

When started

- Starting ages vary

Early (8–9)	With older siblings/friends, lighting parents' cigarettes
In school (11–16)	With friends
In college/uni (16+)	Pub/legal drinking related
	Peer group
Later (20s)	Adult choice

- Little difference between younger and older or social types
- Related to rites of passage

Why started

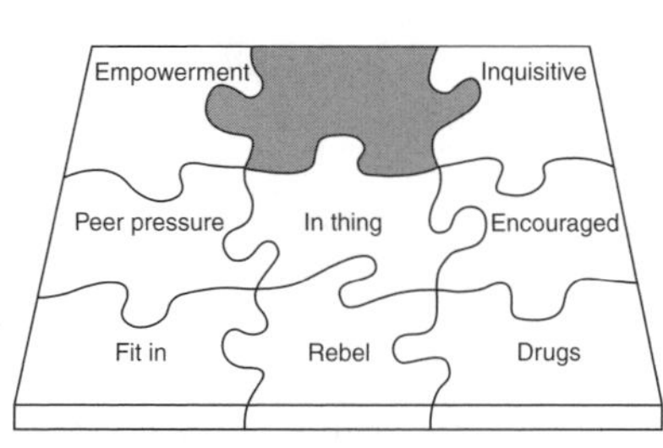

What smoked first

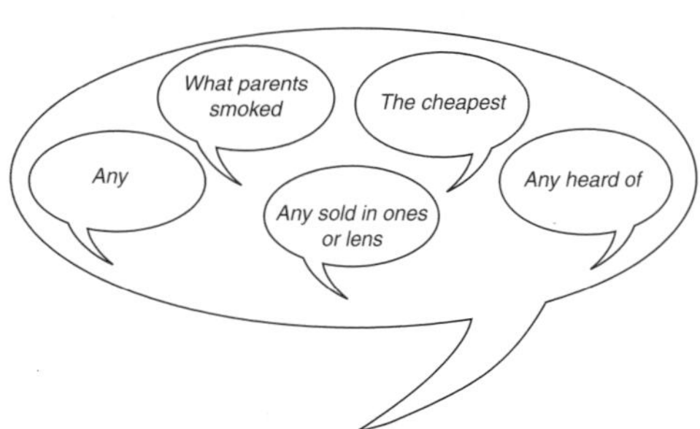

Smoking now

Early adult	Marlboro Lights (Marlboro), Embassy Red, Silk Cut,
Trendies	(B&H)
Early adult	Silk Cut (more females), B&H (more males)
Mid-adult	B&H (strong taste), Silk Cut (lower tar), Marlboro
Older adult	B&H (strong taste), Silk Cut (lower tar), cheapies (L&B)
Mr & Mrs Average	
Older adult	Sovereigns, B&H, SuperKings, L&B (female), Berkeley,
Price	Cheapies

Source: Interbrand (UK) Ltd, 1997, pp. 9–10

> come to mind. Given that health information regarding smoking is controlled by the DH [Department of Health] and not the tobacco industry, is this not a case of double standards?
>
> (O'Loughlin, 2006)

On the other hand, tobacco is not the same as alcohol, the former we simply want to be rid of; the latter we want to learn to use more healthily. A more measured response therefore makes some sense. Also, an additional £12 million for social marketing is surely to be welcomed, and the Drinkaware Trust is, at least on paper, independent. Finally, the pressure is on: the problems presented by alcohol in the UK are prodigious and need tackling, the Drinkaware Trust has to deliver.

The question 'Is the Drinkaware Trust an opportunity or threat?' echoes one of social marketing's classic dilemmas. In these circumstances research is, more than ever, the social marketer's friend. We should welcome and engage with the Drinkaware Trust but insist that it sets clear objects and puts appropriate independent evaluations in place to check on progress. Cooperation, or coopetition, with erstwhile competitors can be a sensible option, but it needs to be handled with care.

Conclusion

Critical marketing is a vital part of social marketing.

Commercial marketers have enormous resources which they invest continuously in attempts to influence our behaviour. We would be foolish if we did not grab the opportunity to analyse, critique, and learn from what they do.

Indeed, social marketing might not exist at all if, 20 years before Kotler stepped up to the plate, another American called Wiebe had not done precisely this. He decided to examine a number of contemporary social change campaigns to see how they measured up to their commercial counterparts. Crucially for us, he concluded that the best campaigns were those which most closely resembled commercial campaigns – or as he pithily expressed it: *Why can't we sell brotherhood like soap* (Wiebe, 1951–1952).

This chapter has simply argued that we should continue to follow in his footsteps.

Review exercise

Case study 2 illustrates some of the benefits of competitive analysis. Think through how you would use these insights to inform a tobacco youth prevention programme. In doing so you might want to consider three questions:

1. What does it tell us about the needs of young smokers?
2. How do tobacco companies cater for these needs?
3. What use do tobacco companies make of competitive analysis?

List the six key characteristics of your programme.

References

Anderson, P. et al. (2009). Impact of alcohol advertising and media exposure on adolescent alcohol use: a systematic review of longitudinal studies. *Alcohol and Alcoholism*, doi: 10.1093/alcalc/agn115. [Advance Access published online on January 14, http://alcalc.oxfordjournals.org/cgi/content/full/agn115?ijkey=1XksNzL37KJyIyJ&keytype=ref]

Alcohol Concern (2007). *Binge Drinking Factsheet Summary*. London: Alcohol Concern, online: http://www.alcoholconcern.org.uk/files/20071029_114336_binge%20drinking%20summary%20July%202007.pdf (Accessed 11 February 2008).

Arnold, M. and Fisher, J. (1996). Counterculture, criticisms and crisis: assessing the effect of the sixties on marketing thought. *Journal of Macromarketing*, 16(Spring): 118–33.

Bartels, R. (1976). The identity crisis in marketing. *Journal of Marketing*, 38: 76.

BBC Online (2004). UN probes sugar industry claims, October 8 2004, online: http://news.bbc.co.uk/1/hi/health/3726510.stm (Accessed 11 February 2008).

Boseley, S. (2003). Sugar industry threatens to scupper WHO, *The Guardian*, April 21 2003, online: http://www.guardian.co.uk/food/Story/0,940574,00.html (Accessed 11 February 2008).

Brownlie, D. and Saren, M. (1997). Beyond the one-dimensional marketing manager: the discourse of theory, practice and relevance. *International Journal of Research in Marketing* 14: 147–61.

Carman, J. (1973). On the universality of marketing. *Journal of Contemporary Business*, 2(Autumn): 1–16.

Catterall, M. et al. (1999). *Marketing and feminism: past, present and future*, online: http://www.mngt.waikato.ac.nz/ejrot/cmsconference/proceedings.htm (Accessed 11 February 2008).

Collett Dickenson Pearce and Partners (CDP) (1998). *Sobranie – examining the opportunities and requirements for a new approach to the UK cigar market*, online: http://www.tobaccopapers.com/PDFs/0200-0299/0288.pdf (Accessed 11 February 2008).

Crane, A. (1997). The dynamics of marketing ethical products. *Journal of Marketing Management*, 13: 6.

Dawson, L.M. (1972). The human concept: a new philosophy for business. In D.G. Kurtz (ed.) *Marketing Concepts, Issues and Viewpoints*. Michigan: DH Mark Publication.

Devlin, E. et al. (2004) *Discount Brands Case Study Prepared for NHS Health Scotland*, Glasgow: University of Strathclyde, Centre for Social Marketing: November.

The Drinkaware Trust (2006) *Board of Trustees*, online: http://www.drinkawaretrust.org.uk/board-of-trustees.html (Accessed 11 February 2008).

Edwards, G. et al. (2004). An invitation to an alcohol industry lobby to help decide public funding of alcohol research and professional training: a decision that should be reversed, *Addiction*, 99(10): 1235–1236.

Edwards, G. et al. (2005). The integrity of the science base: a test case, *Addiction*, 100(5): 581–584.

Firat, A.F. and Venkatesh, A. (1993). Postmodernity: the age of marketing. *International Journal of Research in Marketing*, 10(3): 227–49.

Food Standards Agency (2003a). Outcome of academic seminar to review recent research on food promotion and children (held on 31st October 2003), press release, November 26, online: http://www.foodstandards.gov.uk/multimedia/webpage/academicreview#top (Accessed 11 February 2008).

Food Standards Agency (2003b). *Outcome of the review exercise on the Paliwoda and Crawford paper: an analysis of the Hastings Review 'The effects of food promotion on children'*. London: Food Standards Agency, online: http://www.food.gov.uk/multimedia/pdfs/paliwodacritique.pdf (Accessed 11 February 2008).

Food Standards Agency (2006). New salt reduction targets published, press release, March 21 2006, online: http://www.food.gov.uk/news/newsarchive/2006/mar/salttargets (Accessed 11 February 2008).

Fuller, E. (ed.) (2007). *Smoking, Drinking and Drug Use among Young People in England in 2006*. London: National Centre for Social Research.

Fuller, D.A. (1999). *Sustainable Marketing: Managerial-Ecological Issues*. London: Sage.

Gallaher Group Plc (1996) *Memoranda (1996)*, online: http://www.tobaccopapers.com/PDFs/0400-0499/0438.pdf (Accessed 11 February 2008).

Hall & Partners (1997). *Marlboro: Proposal for Ad and Brand Tracking (1997–06)*, online: http://www.tobaccopapers.com/PDFs/0400-0499/0461.pdf (Accessed 11 February 2008).

Hastings, G. et al. (2006). *The extent, nature and effects of food promotion to children: a review of the evidence*, technical paper prepared for the WHO July 2006. Geneva: World Health Organization, online: http://www.who.int/dietphysicalactivity/publications/Hastings_paper_marketing.pdf (Accessed 11 February 2008).

Hastings, G. and Angus, K. (2004). The influence of the tobacco industry on European tobacco-control policy, in *Tobacco or health in the European Union past, present and future*, The ASPECT Consortium, Luxembourg: Office for Official Publications of the European Communities, pp. 195–225.

Hastings, G.B. (2007). *Social Marketing: Why Should the Devil have all the Best Tunes?* Oxford: Butterworth-Heinemann.

Hastings, G.B. and Saren, M. (2003). The critical contribution of social marketing: theory and application, *Marketing Theory*, 3(3): 305–322.

Hastings, G. et al. (2003). *Review of research on the effects of food promotion to children – final report and appendices*, prepared for the Food Standards Agency, UK, online: website: http://www.food.gov.uk/healthiereating/advertisingtochildren/promotion/readreview (Accessed 11 February 2008).

Hind, D. (2008). What are the true threats to reason? *New Scientist*, 19 January (2639): 46–47.

Interbrand (UK) Ltd. (1997). *Gallaher New Product Development Project Stage 1 and 2 Presentation*, 14 October, online: http://www.tobaccopapers.com/PDFs/0400-0499/0473.pdf (Accessed 11 February 2008).

Jobber, D. (2004). *Principles and Practice of Marketing*. Maidenhead: McGraw-Hill International.

Klein, N. (2001). *No Logo*. London: Flamingo.

Kotler, P. and Lee, N.R. (2008). *Social Marketing: Influencing Behaviors for Good*. Thousand Oaks, California: Sage Publications.

Kotler, P. and Zaltman, G. (1971). Social marketing: an approach to planned social change'. *Journal of Marketing*, 35(3): 3–12.

Lazer, W. and Kelley, E. (1973). *Social Marketing: Perspectives and Viewpoints*. Homewood, IL: Richard D. Irwin.

The Leading Edge Consultancy (1997). *American blends NPD: qualitative debrief Presentation*, May, online: http://www.tobaccopapers.com/PDFs/0400-0499/0479.pdf (Accessed 11 February 2008).

Livingstone, S. (2005). Assessing the research base for the policy debate over the effects of food advertising to children. *The International Journal of Advertising*, 24(3): 273–96.

Lovato, C. et al. (2003). Impact of tobacco advertising and promotion on increasing adolescent smoking behaviours. *Cochrane Database of Systematic Reviews*, (4): CD003439.

Luck, D. (1969). Broadening the concept of marketing – too far'. *Journal of Marketing*, 33: 53–63.

Macdonald, L. et al. (2007). Neighbourhood fast food environment and area deprivation – substitution or concentration? *Appetite*, 49(1): 251–254.

National Cancer Institute (2008). *The Role of the Media in Promoting and Reducing Tobacco Use*. Tobacco Control Monograph No. 19. Bethesda, MD: U.S. Department of Health and Human Services, National Institutes of Health, National Cancer Institute.

National Prevention Research Initiative (2008). *Our research*, online: http://www.mrc.ac.uk/Fundingopportunities/Calls/NPRI3/index.htm (Accessed 28 January 2008).

O'Loughlin, P. (2006). Comment at blog Alcohol Policy UK www.alcoholpolicy.net. December 1, online: http://www.alcoholpolicy.net/2006/11/drinkaware_trus.html (Accessed 11 February 2008).

Ofcom (2006). New restrictions on the television advertising of food and drink products to children, press release, 17 November, online: http://www.ofcom.org.uk/media/news/2006/11/nr_20061117 (Accessed 11 February 2008).

Paliwoda, S. and Crawford, I. (2003). *An analysis of the Hastings Review: reviews of the effects of food promotion on children*. London: The Advertising Association, online: http://www.adassoc.org.uk/fau/hastings_review_analysis_dec03.pdf (Accessed 11 February 2008).

Rothmans Inc. (1998). *Young adult smokers: smoking behaviour and lifestyles 1994–1997*, online: http://www.tobaccopapers.com/PDFs/0600-0657/0626.pdf (Accessed 11 February 2008).

Stead, M. et al. (2007). *Research to inform the development of a social marketing strategy for health improvement in Scotland*, online: http://www.healthscotland.com/documents/1752.aspx (Accessed 11 February 2008).

Taylor Nelson Sofres Plc (RSGB) (1997). *Proposal for Marlboro advertising and brand tracking research: research proposal (1997–06)*, online: http://www.tobaccopapers.com/PDFs/0600-0657/0634.pdf (Accessed 11 February 2008).

TBWA (TBWA Simons Palmer Ltd./TBWA GGT Simons Palmer/BST-BDDP) (1997). *Creative briefs (1997)*, online: http://www.tobaccopapers.com/PDFs/0600-0657/0649.pdf (Accessed 11 February 2008).

Travis, A. (2008). More than half of 13-year-olds have drunk alcohol, says home secretary. *The Guardian*, February 7, online: http://www.guardian.co.uk/uk/2008/feb/07/politics.drugsandalcohol (Accessed 11 February 2008).

Uhlig, R. (2003). Adverts blamed for poor diet of children. *The Daily Telegraph*, September 26.

Wiebe, G.D. (1951–52). Merchandising commodities and citizenship in television. *Public Opinion Quarterly*, 15(Winter): 679–691.

Wilkie, W.L. and Moore, E.S. (2003). Scholarly research in marketing: exploring the 'four eras' of thought development. *Journal of Public Policy and Marketing*, 22(2): 116–146.

World Health Organization (2003). *WHO Framework Convention on Tobacco Control*. Geneva: World Health Organization.

WHO CSDH (2008). *Closing the gap in a generation: health equity through action on the social determinants of health. Final Report of the Commission on Social Determinants of Health*. Geneva: World Health Organization. Online: http://www.who.int/social_determinants/final_report/en/index.html (Accessed 28 January 2009).

Young, B. (2003). *Advertising and food choice in children: a review of the literature*, London: Food Advertising Unit, The Advertising Association, online: http://www.adassoc.org.uk/fau/summary_ofliteraturereview_2003.pdf (Accessed 11 February 2008).

Young, B. et al. (1996). *The Role of Advertising in Children's Food Choice*. London: Ministry of Agriculture, Foods and Fisheries (MAFF).

Chapter 18

Value for money in social marketing

Graham Lister

We can tell our values by looking at our cheque book stubs.
Gloria Steinem

Learning points

This chapter

- Discusses why value for money is an important issue in social marketing;
- Advises on how to prove that your social marketing initiative is a good investment; and
- Sets out practical ways to help show value for money.

Chapter overview

Prevention may be better than cure, but how do we prove that spending money on social marketing to support health and well-being is good value for money? This is the challenge that social marketing must address during every stage of programmes aimed at helping people to change their behaviour and supporting the redesign of services around customers. In this chapter, we examine why this is an important issue not just for social marketing programmes but for the health economy as a whole. We explore the complexities that make it difficult to demonstrate value for money in social marketing and suggest a number of approaches, tools, and resources to address these problems. We also discuss how to apply value for money techniques to local social marketing investment within a national programme.

Introduction

It is generally assumed that the aim of health systems is to improve health, but on closer examination it is not clear that increasing health system expenditure achieves this. While comparisons across the whole range of health system (WHO, 2000) show that countries able to spend more on their health systems achieve better health outcomes than most poor countries, this relationship breaks down when health outcomes and health expenditure are examined in the rich countries with membership of the Organization for Economic Co-operation and Development (OECD), where there is no clear association between health outcomes and expenditure (Nolte and McKee, 2003). In England, a 33% increase in spending on health care from 2002 to 2007 has had only a marginal impact on life expectancy while years lived in poor health continue to rise (National Statistics, 2006).

It could be argued that health-care systems should at least achieve improved customer satisfaction and greater equity in health. At the international level, there is little evidence of this. In England, increased expenditure on health-care services has resulted in higher levels of satisfaction for patients (Healthcare Commission, 2007), but this is not reflected in wider public attitudes. The impact of higher expenditure on health equity in England is not clear, but it appears that health-care improvements tend to be adopted first by higher socioeconomic groups, despite health-equity policies.

Broad scenario planning, as in the Wanless Report of 2002, suggests that spending more on prevention measures could dramatically improve health and reduce long-term health costs. Other reviews such as 'Engaging with Care' (Dawson et al., 2007) suggest that the key to health and care-value for money is public engagement in health and care as customers, co-providers, and as communities, while targetting disadvantaged groups can address equity.

Now that the UK health expenditure is levelling off, after a period of rapid growth, there is even greater focus on value for money. While the general economy achieves an improvement in efficiency of about 2% per year, the health economy has not matched this, indeed it has reduced the level of activity it performs for each pound spent. For some people the idea of efficiency-improvement conjures up images of Charlie Chaplin in 'Modern Times' frantically working faster as the machines speed up. But in fact most economic efficiency improvement comes about as investment moves to products and services that create greater value, improving allocative efficiency. Technical efficiency, i.e. doing the same thing at a lower cost per unit, is a relatively minor contributor to economic performance.

In the health economy, allocative efficiency can be improved by shifting expenditure to activities that produce higher value outcomes at lower cost. Social marketing can achieve higher value for money in health-outcome terms through behavioural change to help customers improve their health and well-being. It is also a lead element in engaging people in the design of health and other services to meet their expectations. It, therefore, holds an important key to improving value for money whether value is defined in terms of health, equity, or customer satisfaction.

The problems of demonstrating value for money

At the national level, successive policy initiatives following 'Our Health, Our Care, Our Say' (Department of Health, 2006) have supported health promotion and measures to promote public and patient engagement. The Health England Committee was asked to produce a 10-year plan for investment in measures to improve health and well-being and to clarify the currently chaotic evidence and evaluation base for health-improvement measures.

But at the local level, commissioners of health and care services face decisions to invest in local services – for which there is often vocal demand from patients and professionals and an immediately visible impact – or to invest in social marketing programmes – for which there may be limited support and an uncertain promise of long-term impact. It is little wonder that these budgets, even when support by national policy, are amongst the first to be raided in difficult times.

The impact of social marketing is difficult to predict or evaluate because it is usually one element of a complex mix of responses to health and behavioural issues, which may have many different causes and consequences. The process of behavioural change is itself uncertain: it depends upon uncontrollable factors, including economic and social conditions, customers' willingness to change, and the competing impacts of commercial marketing and peer pressure. In many cases, people can only be helped to change when they have formed a strong personal motivation to alter their behaviour.

The outcome of behavioural change may only be apparent in the long term, it may have specific consequences for particular health issues, but may also affect peoples lives in many other ways – empowering them to take control of their lifestyle. The benefits of social marketing are therefore likely to accrue to individuals, families, employers, and public services, though in some cases it may increase National Health Services (NHS) costs by recognizing unmet needs and reducing premature mortality, thus increasing the demand for long-term-care.

It is important to focus social marketing interventions on specific segments of the public so that dialogue can be tailored to the specific needs and language of the target groups. This can improve value for money by ensuring that inequality in health is addressed, through a focus on those with greatest needs and least choice. However, social marketing can also have a wider impact on communities and the whole population by raising expectations and norms concerning health and well-being. It may even have an impact on the health of future generations, e.g. parents who smoke have children who are not only passive smokers but tend to become smokers.

The overall impact of social marketing can therefore build expectations and personal responsibility. It must also change the culture of the NHS, developing an understanding of the importance of co-creating health with customers. This demands that social marketing should be a central responsibility of health and care organizations and that a professional approach is taken to delivering social marketing as a high-value element of all health and care services.

Value for money at every stage

To achieve this it is essential to incorporate value for money thinking at every stage in the scoping, development, implementation, and follow-up of social marketing programmes. This does not mean making unrealistic claims about the impact that can be achieved, rather the reverse; it is important to recognize the complexity and uncertainty of the situation and to be clear about the assumptions that are made when assessing investments in and the outcomes of social marketing. The advice on value for money here should be considered alongside the more generic advice on developing and delivering a social marketing initiative contained in Chapters 10–15.

Value for money in scoping social marketing

The scoping of a project involving social marketing must define the target customer-group and establish clear objectives for their behavioural change. It is important to establish how the expected behavioural change will be perceived and valued by the targeted customer-group and what the impact of such changes might be for society.

At the scoping stage a preliminary business case based on outline costing, reasoned assumptions about what might be achieved, and outline values of potential outcomes can guide the design of the project and the mix of interventional methods to be deployed. It is, however, important to be clear that at this stage such estimates will be very uncertain and should not be presented as evidence-based evaluations – they are simply planning assumptions. To paraphrase Donald Rumsfeld, it is important to sort the known knowns (the evidence base) from the known unknowns (including the responses of customers) and to allow for unknown unknowns (including risks of negative consequences, e.g. could increasing alcohol prices lead to increased illicit drug taking). One of the most important factors, that is often unknown, is what would happen without a specific social marketing intervention. This is the 'null hypothesis' against which the impact of any programme should be compared. It requires a baseline study to reflect current trends in behaviour and health and the main factors thought to influence behavioural and health outcomes, including other aspects of social and commercial marketing. The baseline should evaluate the impact of these factors and explain the observed trends in behaviours and outcomes.

Final health outcomes and settled behavioural change may only be apparent in the long term. Thus, in many cases, it is necessary to rely on intermediate measures of behaviour and attitudes as indicators of long-term change. In such cases, allowance should be made for some reversion and the inherent uncertainty of outcomes.

Value for money in development and business planning

The developmental stage should establish a clear project plan, with early feedback from customers aimed at reducing the uncertainty of further phases of the programme and milestones at which decisions can be taken on future steps, including possibly stopping or radically redesigning the project. The plan should recognize that social marketing is a learning process drawing on the insights of the customers targeted by the intervention.

Development planning involves costing the interventional programme and valuing its outcomes to establish an initial business plan or case for the intervention. This is sometimes seen as a chore best left to 'unimaginative accountants', but this is entirely mistaken view, for the essence of costing is the imagination to think through all the actions and resources required by the programme. Business planning always requires careful discussion with all those involved to ensure that all relevant costs and outcomes are captured and that options for saving time and costs are explored (Drummon et al., 2005). It is important to consider the costs and benefits to all stakeholders, including the customers themselves and to respect their view of the exchange involved; what changing the behaviour costs them and how they value the proposed intervention and outcomes. Note that a business plan may change as findings emerge and should be updated throughout the project.

Value for money in implementation

One of the problems of the current evidence-base for social marketing in academic journals is that it tends to focus on the theory and outcome of interventions, without providing sufficient insight into the implementation-management process. It is apparent that even the best designed and potentially most cost-effective interventions can be fouled up by poor implementation.

While the need to monitor findings at project milestone points and to take tough decisions on this basis is clear, in practice it is difficult to change tack in the middle of a programme without this being seen as a sign of failure. It is therefore important to stress that implementation of a cost-effective social marketing programme must allow flexibility to respond to discovery, feedback, and insight gained from customers during the programme, even (or most particularly) where this indicates the need for radical change. This requires a project board able to provide an objective overview of both the emerging findings and management of the project.

One persistent problem in cross-sector public projects is that cost-estimates become entrenched within departmental budgets. Not only is it difficult to monitor expenditure across different organizations, but there is also resistance to the flexible control of expenditure. This requires an integrated progress- and cost-reporting system. It is also essential to plan a contingency reserve for any such project. Again this goes against the grain of public sector practice, but it is easier to control a planned contingency reserve than to try to reassign the padding that creeps into every element of costing without it.

Value-for-money evaluation

Formal evaluation is usually defined as a task undertaken at the completion of a programme, in retrospect. National Institute for Health and Clinical Excellence (NICE) suggests that evaluation should cover: how effective the project was in meeting its objectives, how acceptable the intervention was for the targeted customers, how feasible it would be to replicate the project, the impact on equity, and any possible safety issues as well as value for money (NICE, 2007). Experience suggests that it is also useful to examine how the project was prepared and managed.

The evaluation of social marketing programmes should reflect the values and objectives of the programme. As we have noted, these invoke societal goals of improving well-being and empowering people to take decisions about their lifestyle. For this reason we suggest that social marketing should be evaluated in terms of the full costs and benefits to society and in particular to the customers on whom interventions are focussed.

Just as social marketing initiatives need to take a segmented view of the market, so also evaluation studies must consider their audience. Thus while an overall perspective on societal costs may be taken, it is useful to pick out the specific impacts and costs relevant to different groups to whom the study may be addressed, e.g. to show the costs incurred by employers as a result of avoidable behaviours at work.

It is also important that the evaluation itself should represent value for money. This requires that the scale of investment in evaluation should reflect the value of the project. When small-scale projects are being evaluated it will often be cost effective to support local evaluations with larger scale regional or national reviews that can inform local projects by providing models, outcome targets and measures, and shared lessons. It is particularly important that such evaluations provide practical guidelines for the management and implementation of projects and the basis for evaluating their likely value for money in a way that can be updated and applied to new projects and project follow-up.

As we note, value-for-money evaluation should also be integral to every stage of a social marketing project. The process of and criteria for evaluation need to be thought through at the design stage, planned as part of the programme, and applied to emerging findings as well as at a further stage of formal evaluation.

Value for money in follow-up and dissemination

Often, the most valuable stage of social marketing is the follow-through, which occurs when the values supported by social marketing are picked up and gain momentum and a 'life of their own' in the hands of customers. At this stage, messages become the currency of over-the-fence conversation, or its modern equivalent – the Internet. Frequently, events in the public eye provide the opportunity to reinforce health messages. This may seem like simple opportunism but in fact requires preparation and briefing of media. Action to reinforce such messages and provide resources to opinion leaders can be very cost effective. It is unfortunate if such high-value-for-money opportunities are lost due to a refunding gap between the original project and follow-up. To avoid this it is important to plan for such opportunities for follow-up during the project-development stage.

Approaches to value-for-money analysis

The approach used to evaluate a social marketing intervention should reflect the complexity of the project goals supported by social marketing.

Cost-offset analysis

Project goals may be very simple – e.g. an intervention to remind patients to attend their outpatient appointment may be aimed at saving time and money for the NHS. In this case a simple cost-offset approach would compare the cost of asking patients how they wish to be contacted (phone, text, email, or letter) and using these means to send reminders, against savings to the NHS (reduced postage, missed appointments, etc.). Cost-offset or cost-minimization approaches are appropriate where the goals of the project can be expressed purely in terms of the cost to one stakeholder.

Cost-effectiveness analysis

A social marketing programme with a slightly broader objective might focus on specific disease outcomes. For example, social marketing might be aimed at encouraging the uptake of cervical smear testing by sex workers, applying social marketing and the redesign of services to improve early detection of cancer of the cervix. Such a programme might be evaluated using a cost-effectiveness approach, comparing the cost of the intervention (including social marketing and the capital and revenue cost of redesigned testing and treatment services) with improvement in health outcomes. Cost-effectiveness analysis is appropriate where the objective can be expressed in terms of a single measureable outcome; it is particularly valuable where different methods of achieving the same outcome can be compared in terms of cost per outcome for the target group.

Cost–consequence analysis

Most social marketing programmes have more complex goals. In the case described above it is difficult not to see that empowering sex workers to deal with this health issue would need to address many difficult barriers for them and would have many other outcomes for their health and well-being. A broad range of health issues might be addressed in addition to support for coping with drug addiction, abuse, and other issues. Many different agencies would need to be involved as well as the health workers themselves. Complex multiple goals and cross-sector interventions such as this can be captured by a cost–consequence analysis. This approach sets out the different costs and benefits to each of the stakeholder groups in a pragmatic, layered framework defining costs and benefits for each stakeholder group. Cost–utility analysis is very similar but requires stakeholders to give explicit weightings to the different outcomes to represent their value or utility in non-monetary units. These types of analysis can be evaluated by a panel of stakeholders applying their judgement to evaluate the overall value of the programme.

Cost–benefit analysis

At the societal level, the ideal method for the evaluation of cross-sector social marketing programmes with complex outcomes is cost–benefit analysis (Kelly et al., 2003). This may take the same form as a cost–consequence analysis but applies monetary values to the benefits to produce an overall measure of benefit and value for money. Thus costs and benefits can be expressed in the same way as an investment proposition, that expenditure of £*x* will produce benefits valued at £*y* with a return on investment of *y/x* per cent.

The disadvantage of cost–benefit analysis is that it may go too far in simplifying and hence obscuring a complex programme involving many different agencies and outcomes. For this reason it is important to present a layered framework setting out the costs and benefits to each stakeholder group and to provide a detailed justification of the method used to value the outcomes. We suggest that a layered framework should consider the costs and benefits to: individuals and their families, the NHS, other public and voluntary sector services, employers (where health or other factors impact on productivity), and wider society. Cost–benefit analysis is most helpful when there is consensus on how such outcomes are valued.

Tools for value for money analysis

Assessing health and well-being outcomes

Kurt Lewin, who may be seen as the father of behavioural change theory, noted, *there is really nothing so practical as a good theory*, and there are many to choose from including: the Health Belief Model, the Theory of Reasoned Action, Social Cognitive Theory, the Stages of Change Model, and the Trans-Theoretical Model (May et al., 2005; McQueen et al., 2007). These general theories map out the path from attitudes and knowledge to the ability to change and maintain behaviour. While these can be helpful starting points, it is important to set out a model for each project to explain how the intervention is intended to support behavioural change and to note points at which progress in raising awareness, addressing barriers to change, and intermediate or final behavioural outcomes can be assessed.

The point of this exercise is not to derive some grand model to explain all behaviour, but to develop specific testable propositions for each project. This can be most helpful when assumptions based on initial theory prove wrong, so that it is necessary to re-examine the model and adapt strategies to reflect customer behaviour as it is found in practice.

It is important to be able to relate specific behavioural changes to avoidable health outcomes. Again this will vary for each project; however, a helpful baseline for many behavioural risk factors is provided by the World Bank work on health attribution fractions (Lopez et al., 2006). This provides an estimate of how common risk factors relate to health outcomes. The estimates for high-income European countries can be applied to UK data to derive an estimate of the incidence of disease attributable to risk-behaviours.

Where different types of health outcome are expected, it may be helpful to apply a consistent measure of their impact. The most commonly used measures of health outcomes are quality-adjusted life years (QALYs). Essentially QALYs apply a weight to years of life lived between 1 for full health and 0 for death. Weights for different conditions are determined from public surveys. Thus, e.g. a certain behaviour may, on average, reduce the quality of life by 50% over 10 years and reduce life expectancy by 10 years. Behavioural change in such a case could therefore produce a benefit of 15 QALYs.

This relatively simple concept is more complicated in practice because the weights people ascribe to conditions depends upon which groups of respondents are surveyed, when and how they are asked, the age of those with the condition, and the 'dread' factor associated with the disease and, in particular, risk of death. The most common QALYs used in the UK are EuroQols which are based on an assessment of the quality of life using five dimensions – mobility, self-care, ability to perform usual tasks, pain/discomfort, and anxiety/depression (Euroqol website: http://www.euroqol.org). Disability-adjusted life years (DALYs) are a similar measure of burden of disease, and thus equivalent to QALYs lost. In this case, disability weights are created based on judgements made by a panel acting as health commissioners (Arnesen and Nord, 1999).

While there are complex questions as to where the economic and social impacts of ill health fall and how they are measured, current research (Lister et al., 2008) indicate that the value of a QALY to society may be assessed at between £20 000 and £70 000 in 2005 values. This, fortuitously, is the range of values suggested by the NICE as the cut-off point for the economic assessment of new interventions with a norm of £30 000 in 2005 values.

Assessing costs and benefits

As previously noted, costing plays an important and creative part in social marketing projects. It is generally found that it is only at the point at which detailed cost-estimates and budgets are prepared that the full processes and resources required to manage, deliver, and evaluate the project are clarified. This can be assisted by setting out process-charts describing each task to be undertaken and the relationship with every other task. The direct costs of each task and any applicable support or time costs can then be estimated. Using the same charts the value added by each task can be assessed and options for improving value by combining or cutting out tasks and or reassigning how they are done and by whom. This approach can greatly improve value for money, particularly when customers are involved in the project-design process.

The costs included in an economic appraisal may be different to the budgeted costs as, for economic evaluation, resources should be evaluated at their marginal or alternative use value. In general, staff costs should be allocated on a time basis. They will usually include an allocation of overheads, though it could be argued that central support costs are not likely to change as a result of a small redeployment of staff time. Capital costs for equipment are included in economic evaluation when they are incurred (rather than as an equipment depreciation charge as in accounts), a residual value may apply at the end of the project. Costs of premises may not be applicable if an underused space in existing premises is allocated (because there is no alternative use value) but if additional premises are used they should be included as a capital cost (with a residual value). Running costs should be included as they are incurred.

Project costs and income should be discounted to net present values using the discount rate applicable to the funding organization – for the NHS this is currently 3.5% in real terms, before adding inflation, though before 2003 it was set at 6%.

Benefits and disbenefits should be discounted at the social time preference rate and should be netted off if they are expressed in common value terms. The social time preference rate reflects the extent to which social goods are preferred now rather than at a later date. Currently the social time preference rate is estimated by the Treasury at 3.5%.

Uncertainty

It is unrealistic to ignore the uncertainty inherent in a social marketing, after all we will probably never fully understand what motivates human behaviour. It is therefore important to attempt to show how the outcome of the intervention might be changed by a range of factors including how the intervention was delivered, the customers targeted, and their predisposing factors. In order to do this it is necessary to revisit the model of behavioural change developed for the study and examine what would happen if the assumptions about the cause and effect of these factors were varied. This so-called 'sensitivity analysis' can be helpful to other practitioners trying to replicate the intervention. There are also many cases in which the long-term outcome will be uncertain. In these cases it is important to evaluate a range of possible outcomes covering realistic optimistic and pessimistic assumptions about the final outcomes. It may be useful to show the minimum outcomes required to justify an intervention, for example to show that an intervention would be justified even if only *x* per cent of customers succeeded in changing their behaviour in the long term.

Scaling up and scaling down

It is sometimes assumed that the approaches suggested in this chapter apply mainly (or only) to large-scale national programmes, whereas many social marketing programmes may be small scale and local in character. We would argue that the concepts and tools suggested here are equally applicable to all social marketing projects, though clearly the scale of investigation needs to be matched to the level of investment proposed. If you are working on a small-scale intervention, as well as adhering to the advice in this section, you will need to also follow guidance in Chapter 16.

At the local level it is important to identify and evaluate a social marketing programme involving local health, local authority, and voluntary and private sector organizations. Such a programme can make best use of regional and national as well as local resources and is a vital link between social marketing programmes and local delivery of services. Local programmes should include appropriate monitoring, value-for-money evaluation, and feedback to regional and national networks.

Regional-level social marketing networks can provide mutual support, shared learning, and resources. At this level it is helpful to share best practice and develop targets and coordinate cross-sector action. A national social marketing network can provide a link to policy and establish agreed guidelines and targets, drawing on these regional networks to identify the best ways of achieving value for money. Evaluation can be supported for both large-scale programmes and social marketing initiatives which, though widespread, are too small in scale to carry the cost of detailed evaluation. This should establish a detailed guidelines and justification for investment based on the impact on societal costs. These in turn should provide the basis for simple measures and targets such as the 'cost per quitter' for smoking to be applied in local evaluations.

Professional management of social marketing for health does not mean central control but it does place a responsibility on those working in this field to work together to apply approaches to achieving value for money from social marketing for health.

Conclusion

In this chapter we have argued that while there are many factors that may make it difficult to measure the cost effectiveness of social marketing, it is nevertheless an essential discipline. Practitioners need to consider value for money at every stage in a social marketing programme in order to apply the lessons learnt to improve outcomes and reduce costs. Moreover it is important to be able to demonstrate value for money to encourage and guide further investment in the field. Approaches to value for money measurement and tools such as sensitivity analysis need to be used selectively depending upon the nature of the project. But even when projects are relatively small in scale and local in application, thinking through costs and outcomes and measures of cost effectiveness will help. Larger scale regional or national projects should establish guidelines for local investment in social marketing along the lines of 'cost per quitter'.

Review exercise

Consider a practical example of a social marketing intervention,

- Describe how value for money was ensured during the:
  - scoping,
  - development,
  - implementation,
  - evaluation, and
  - follow-up stages.
- What form of economic evaluation was applied?
- What costs and health outcomes were measured? and
- How was uncertainty recognized?
- How did the project share lessons with other regional or national projects?
- What would you do differently in future projects?

Limit yourself to no more than five bullet points for each response.

References

Arnesen, T. and Nord, E. (1999). The value of DALY life: problems with ethics and validity of disability adjusted life years. *British Medical Journal*, November, 319:1423–1425.

Dawson, S. et al. (2007). *Engaging With Care: a Vision for the Health and Care Workforce of England.* London: The Nuffield Trust.

Department of Health (2006). *Our Health, Our Care, Our Say.* London: Department of Health.

Drummon, F. et al. (2005). *Methods for Economic Evaluation of Health Care Programmes.* Oxford: Oxford University Press.

EuroQol web site at http://www.euroqol.org/ (Accessed 15 January 2009).

Healthcare Commission (2007). Patients give vote of confidence in overall care provided by NHS in largest national survey, press release, May 16.

Lopez, A.D. et al. (2006). *Global Burden of Disease and Risk Factors.* New York: The World Bank and Oxford University Press.

Lister, G. et al. (2008). Measuring the societal impact of behaviour choices, *Social Marketing Quarterly*, 285060, XIV(1).

National Statistics (2006). *Health Expectancy: Living Longer: More Years in Poor Health*, archived National Statistics see http://www.statistics.gov.uk/CCI/nugget.asp?ID=934&Pos=1&ColRank=2&Rank=1000 (Accessed 15 January 2009).

May, G. et al. (2005). *Guidance for Evaluating Mass Communication Initiatives: Summary of an Expert Panel Discussion*, sponsored by CDC, online: http://www.healthcommunication.net/Evaluating_Mass_Comm.pdf (Accessed 15 January 2009).

McQueen, D. et al. (2007). *Health and Modernity: the Role of Theory in Health Promotion.* New York, NY: Springer.

Kelly, M.P. et al. (2003). *Economic Appraisal of Public Health Interventions*, Health Development Agency briefing paper, online at: http://www.chsrf.ca/kte_docs/Economic_appraisal_of_public_health_interventions%5B2%5D.pdf (Accessed 15 January 2009).

National Institute for Health and Clinical Excellence, Behaviour Change Programme Development Group (2007). *Behaviour Change at Population, Community and Individual Level: Public Health Guidance 6.* Available at: http://www.sussedprofessionals.net/files/PH006quickrefguide.pdf (Accessed 15 January 2009).

Nolte, E. and McKee, M. (2003). Measuring the health of nations: an analysis of mortality amenable to healthcare, *British Medical Journal*, November, 327:1129.

Wanless, D. (2002). *Securing Our Future Health: Taking a Long Term View.* London: HM Treasury.

World Health Organization (2000). *Health Systems: Improving Performance*, The World Health report 2000. Geneva: World Health Organization.

Chapter 19

Capacity building, competencies, and standards

Paul White and Jeff French

When planning for a year, plant corn.
When planning for a decade, plant trees.
When planning for life, train and educate people.
Chinese proverb

Learning points

This chapter

- Highlights the issues contributing to the development of standards for social marketing;
- Provides an insight into the challenges of developing skills in social marketing, both as an integrated skill-set within other disciplines and as a dedicated capacity;
- Sets out core competencies for social marketing;
- Highlights the principles of 'team competencies' versus 'individual competencies'; and
- Examines the opportunities to integrate social marketing practice and principles into existing professional frameworks.

Chapter overview

As discussed in Chapters 1 and 5, the Unite Kingdom (UK) has been witnessing a growing trend towards more citizen-centric social policy in recent years. There is increasing interest from policy-makers in the potential of social marketing to positively influence public behaviour and improve people's lives – most notably in the areas of health, environment, and physical activity. However, such sustained cross-governmental support comes with an increased expectation of delivery against a very challenging agenda, and at a time when, arguably, specialist skills and training capacity in social marketing are in short supply. A great deal of work is in progress to address this shortfall, as this chapter will demonstrate. Maintaining momentum and progress will be crucial if the current level of political support is to be maintained.

Building a sustainable infrastructure is the key factor. We need to be able to help both those coming into the field and those already in the field to achieve the skills, competence, and confidence in their ability to elicit positive behaviour through interventions and research (Thorpe et al., 2008). This means taking a holistic approach to capacity development; recognizing skill-sets which are fundamental to delivery and which should be common to the whole workforce, in addition to skills more specialist in nature and scope. This chapter reflects on the work that is in progress in the UK to advance this agenda. It highlights in particular the diversity of issues that are being considered as part of this process.

Introduction

Mapping the current provision

Social marketing is not a new concept in the UK: high-quality work has been in progress in discrete pockets of the country for many years. However, 2005 research by the National Social Marketing (NSM) Centre revealed that within the marketing industry 'only a relatively small number of organizations profess to be social marketing specialists' (NSM Centre, 2006a).

A brief trawl of the Internet suggests the number of social marketing initiatives is growing, with a proliferation of new organizations offering social marketing services to the unsuspecting, and increasingly demanding, public sector. However, the evidence suggests that there is significant variation in the skill-sets and understanding of these organizations. Much of the work undertaken to date has not adhered to social marketing best practices. Examples have emerged of organizations planning and delivering so-called social marketing services that do not meet the discipline's expectations or produce behavioural outcomes. Social advertising or purely communications-focussed solutions – which only seek to raise awareness – fail to achieve the behavioural impact sought by clients. In an increasingly busy marketplace, it is crucial to ensure consistency and high standards in the use of social marketing and to share widely the results of interventions so that other social marketers can use them in their work.

The NSM Centre found that the situation was much the same in the academic sector:

> Social marketing in the academic sector in this country can be described as still in a nascent period, and scope for real social marketing learning and implementation is still currently limited.
>
> NSM Centre, 2006b

With some studies and interventions, the label 'social marketing' is a misnomer, as their activities bear more resemblance to social advertising than social marketing (Health Challenge England, 2006). But there are social marketing initiatives that exhibit the benchmark criteria (see Chapter 3) and which do not use the social marketing label at all. As NSM Centre (2007a) noted, 'the resulting evidence base, if it relies entirely on intervention approaches which are labelled "Social Marketing", is likely to be limited and flawed'.

Such findings are a cause for concern. With a potential market demand for over 10 000 social marketing practitioners in the UK alone over the next 5 years (Hastings, 2007, p. 164), there is an urgent need for a consistent framework in social marketing to support the development of social marketing skills and understanding at all levels. For example:

- policy strategists and public service managers need to understand the benefits and core principles;
- programme, campaign, and intervention designers need a deeper range of skills and understanding to research, scope, and plan;
- delivery practitioners need skills in the use of research techniques, tactical tools, and methods and evaluation techniques;
- procurers need to ensure that they are commissioning accredited social marketing skills; and
- training developers need a consistent framework within which to operate.

If social marketing is to progress as a field of applied study, there is a need for a set of occupational standards and a common understanding of what social marketing is and can deliver. This will also help avoid misrepresentation of social marketing and social marketing professionals, which could undermine attempts to engage people with the discipline and communicate what it can genuinely achieve.

However, the basic infrastructure to support this skills development may be lacking at present in the UK. An initial mapping exercise carried out in 2006 found that only 15 of the UK's universities were teaching social marketing (NSM Centre, 2006a). In universities teaching social marketing, the subject was an optional module on courses such as undergraduate and postgraduate qualifications in marketing, communications and public health. That number is rising rapidly, and there is growing interest in social marketing as a discrete field of practice within continuing professional development (CPD) courses, and undergraduate and masters study.

Skills for effective social marketing

Individual and team skills

A broad range of understanding and skills is needed to ensure successful behavioural outcomes through scoping, planning, and delivering a social marketing intervention. These include:

- social research and theory;
- strategic intervention planning;
- piloting techniques;
- partnership development;
- segmentation and targeting;
- the social marketing mix (top-down and community-based approaches); and
- measurement techniques.

It is unlikely that a single individual will possess this broad spectrum of skills. Any social marketing initiative will need a team of generalists and specialists working with a common purpose. It is important that each member of the team understands the role and relationship of their particular skills within the social marketing process. They (in particular, the team leader) will need to have a fundamental understanding of the core principles and planning process to secure successful outcomes.

An organizational issue

At a higher level, an organizational appreciation of the benefits and core principles of social marketing makes for much more effective delivery. This is as true for the health services facing the challenge of local health improvement as it is for businesses facing the challenge of delivering sustainable products to customers. To effectively deliver behavioural outcomes through social marketing, campaigns will need to draw on a wide range of public health, management, research, and communication skills locally or regionally. All parts of your organization, particularly the executive, must understand:

- the people-centred approach;
- how they can contribute to your social marketing programme; and
- how to overcome the organizational barriers that stand in the way of effective delivery.

For example, in the health sector the application of social marketing skills is highly relevant to:

- community and social care practitioners;

- communications and health promoters;
- procurers of clinical and community services; and
- service strategists and managers.

The key fundamental concepts of social marketing (customer insight, setting behaviour goals, designing an approach, and segmenting your audience; see Chapter 7) can help all these workers. A customer-centric focus is key, as it benefits all members of staff in their interaction with patients and members of the community. The level of content can be set appropriately to types of staff. For example, for general staff, this could be a conceptual understanding of what social marketing is and the benefits of a customer-focussed approach. For more involved staff, such as those above, as a minimum this could comprise of:

- how to apply customer insight to their work;
- how to set behaviour goals; and
- how to design a segmented approach to the target group.

At the executive level, the chief executive or board needs to develop a supportive culture. Social marketing will flourish in organizations that have a long-term and sustained approach to mobilizing resources and assets, creating a learning and reflective culture. Therefore, understanding at this level is of vital importance.

Understanding the sector context

It is important that social marketers have a deep understanding of the sector context in which we are influencing behaviours, be it in health and well-being in the community or in the workplace, environmental lifestyles, crime-reduction, or sporting activity, for example. All these require an understanding of the policies, social theories, stakeholders, and factors which influence existing behaviours. Much of this will be assimilated during your initiative's scoping stage (see Chapter 11), but if your team has sectoral experience, it can provide greater insight into the challenges you face and help inform the design of your intervention.

Managing the diversity

Implicit in a team approach is the bringing together, blending, and managing of diverse people, skills, and values. Managing this effectively requires particular personal qualities and a recognition that this may lead to differences in perspectives, values, and approaches. For example, differences over the ethics of partnership with businesses often leads to tensions and debate within a team.

A good starting point

Recognizing the need for consistency in social marketing, the NSM Centre developed National Benchmark Criteria (see Chapter 3) as the foundation for best practice. Whilst not undermining flexibility, the benchmarks provide a:

> simple and easy way to check whether what is being described as social marketing, really is consistent with social marketing: the bottom line being that if there is not a strong customer and behavioural focus, then it is not social marketing.
>
> (NSM Centre, 2007b, p. 38)

At the same time, recognizing the need for a systematic approach in social marketing, the Centre developed its Total Process Planning (TPP) framework (see Chapter 10) to describe best practice in the execution of programmes and campaigns. In particular, the independent review,

It's Our Health! (NSM Centre 2006c) had identified the limited evidence of a scoping stage, which is so crucial to effective outcomes. The TPP framework considers the important management processes such as team development, stakeholder and partner engagement, behavioural analysis, and evaluation metrics.

The combined benchmark criteria and TPP framework provide invaluable guidance for practitioners and have helped to lay a firm foundation for developing standards and competencies in social marketing.

Standards and competencies in social marketing

In the UK, there has been increasing interest over recent years in the development of common standards of practice, which will:

- provide employers with a substantive description of the required functions of social marketing; and
- enable the identification of the skill-sets and competencies required of prospective employees to enable the team to deliver on every aspect of this map (see Box 19.1).

The standards do not just work to support the employer. They also support the employee by identifying learning and development needs to perform their function within the overall framework.

For social marketing, common and consistent occupational standards have an additional advantage which relates to the sustainability of the profession into the future. There is a potential lack of understanding about the scope and focus of social marketing amongst many people. Misrepresentation of social marketing, or poorly articulated or incomplete codification, has the potential to undermine the growing consensus about what social marketing is. Following the publication *It's Our Health!* (NSM Centre, 2006c), setting out a set of occupational standards enables the development of a functional map for social marketing and a way to define a set of measures of quality and competencies for those delivering social marketing. There is also the potential to use national standards to inform curriculum development, although, as previously mentioned, it is unlikely that a single person would possess all the skills necessary for an end-to-end social marketing programme.

Box 19.1 Working definitions of standards, competency, and competence

- **Standards** provide the means to express scope and best practice within a profession.
- They are defined through core **competencies** which describe the outcomes, behaviours and knowledge required in functions which are required to achieve the key purpose of the profession (the functional map).
- **Competence** is the ability to perform consistently in line with the standards relevant to the job.
- A person is considered **competent** if they can demonstrate they consistently perform in line with the standards relevant to their job.
- To be competent a person needs to:
  - know the **standards** relevant to the job;
  - possess the **knowledge**, **skills**, and **personal qualities** required; and
  - be **motivated** to perform to the required standards.

For social marketing, with its broad base of practitioners in the UK, there are a broad range of pre-existing national occupational standards which have relevance to both practice and professional outcomes. During 2008, the Marketing and Sales Standard Setting Body (MSSSB) undertook a project to develop a distinctive set of specialist standards that reflect the key purpose, areas, and core competencies of social marketing, yet continue to iterate with the broader, generalist competencies reflected within these frameworks. These standards were formally approved by the UK Commission for Employment and Skills in March 2009. They form a fundamental building block for the development of a sustainable infrastructure for social marketing, and will support the development of career pathways for the practitioners. Before we examine these standards, it is worth taking a brief look at the pre-existing marketing occupational standard framework.

The marketing national occupational standards

In 2006 the MSSSB published a new set of world-class, national standards for marketing and marketing communications.

A functional map of these standards is shown in Box 19.2, which describes the key functions of the profession. A cursory examination of these functional areas indicated a strong resonance with best practice functions of social marketing, but questions remained. Were they, e.g. sufficiently representative to capture the full dimensions of social marketing? Should the application of social behavioural theory be represented? Should due diligence in ethical considerations be more prominently represented? These pre-existing standards were referred to in significant depth during the development of the social marketing standards, and many of the marketing competencies have been retained in the final version.

The social marketing national occupational standards

The fundamental concepts of social marketing are valuable across the public and private sectors and to all social policy, not just health. We have shown that although there are areas in which

Box 19.2 The MSSSB functional map of marketing

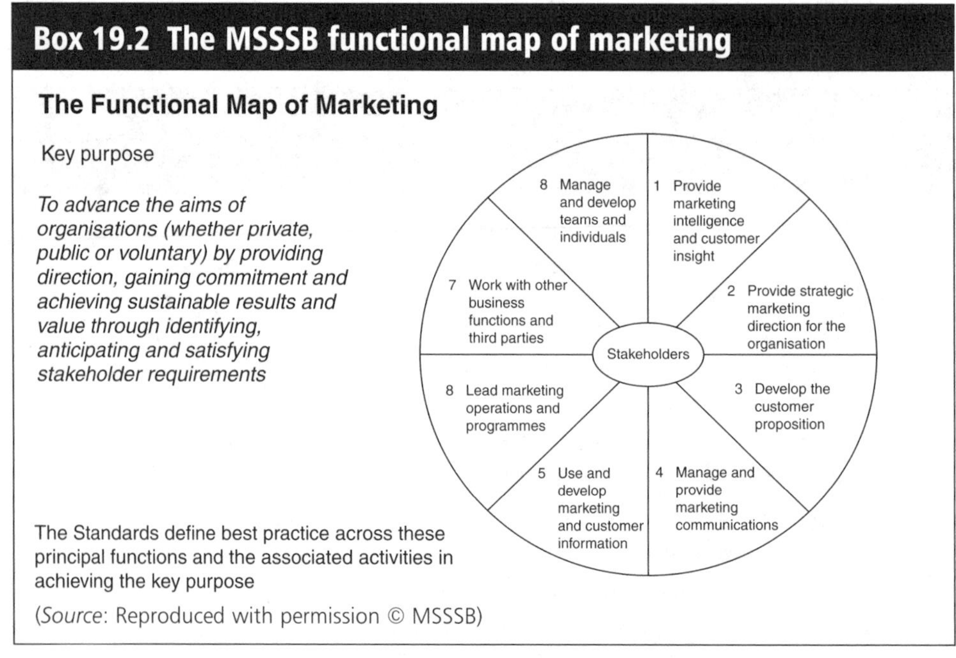

The Functional Map of Marketing
Key purpose
To advance the aims of organisations (whether private, public or voluntary) by providing direction, gaining commitment and achieving sustainable results and value through identifying, anticipating and satisfying stakeholder requirements
8 Manage and develop teams and individuals
1 Provide marketing intelligence and customer insight
7 Work with other business functions and third parties
2 Provide strategic marketing direction for the organisation
Stakeholders
8 Lead marketing operations and programmes
3 Develop the customer proposition
5 Use and develop marketing and customer information
4 Manage and provide marketing communications
The Standards define best practice across these principal functions and the associated activities in achieving the key purpose

(*Source*: Reproduced with permission © MSSSB)

national frameworks link to social marketing best practices, there are also important omissions. For social marketing to achieve its potential, frameworks must acknowledge and respond to its customer focus, which would benefit all members of staff in their interaction with the public, patients, and wider engagement with the business and private sectors. However, the extent to which people must be familiar with social marketing principles will depend on their role. Some will require specialist knowledge, whereas others will be able to fulfil their duties with a broader knowledge. For example, people operating at an organizational level with a broader knowledge of social marketing will still contribute to more effective delivery, but they will not need the specialist knowledge required of somebody who is heading a social marketing initiative.

These organizational issues and others referred to earlier have been considered fully in the development of the social marketing standards. The UK is leading the field internationally in this area. There are currently no formal standards anywhere else in the world, even though social marketing has been practised for many years in other countries. For further information on the social marketing standards visit the MSSSB website (www.msssb.org/SocialMarketing.htm).

Dr Chahid Fourali, head of MSSSB, explains why the UK has taken this course of action and the benefits the project is likely to bring.

Box 19.3 National occupational standards

National occupational standards are the currency that enables professionals to communicate and understand the vocational relevance of their profession. For too long, debates about best practice were monopolized by academic/theoretical conceptualizations rather than addressing the practical issues that marketers face on the job on a daily basis. Practitioners ask questions such as 'Is what I am doing right?' 'If not how can I improve my skills in order to achieve the outcomes that I want?' Such perspectives also reflect the voice of businesses and industries that are limited by time and resources and want to maximize the effectiveness of their work.

Social marketers are no different. They have limited budgets and want to maximize the effect of their work by adopting best practice. National occupational standards aim to offer just that. They distil the expertise of many established professionals/organizations and make it available to the future social marketing stakeholders in a simple but comprehensive language covering the key facets of competence: outcomes, behaviours, and underpinning knowledge.

Successful national occupational standards not only benefit practitioners but also the educational industry and beyond. The standards will benefit candidates, teachers, qualification designers, and policy-makers as they will have an impact on all their work. As a minimum here are four key useful benefits of the standards.

- They describe good practice in particular areas of work.
- They provide managers with a tool for a wide variety of workforce management and quality control.
- They offer a framework for training and development.
- They form the basis of National Vocational Qualifications (NVQs), Scottish Vocational Qualifications (SVQs), and an increasing number of Vocationally Related Qualifications (VRQs) recognized nationally by UK regulatory bodies.

The concept of vocational competence is very old and can be related to best practice in established sectors such as dentistry and medicine. The challenge is to extend this concept to all sectors including and especially to such important fields as social marketing.

The 12-month long consultation process with numerous groups of social marketing experts and practitioners, conducted by MSSSB, has led to the formulation of a specific set of standards for social marketing. The functional map is illustrated in Box 19.4.

The functional map shows the 'Key Areas' of social marketing, and at a more detailed level, the 'Areas of Competence'. Taking Key Area A (*Carry out social marketing research)* by way of example, the Key Areas of Competence and the Units of Performance are shown in Box 19.5 to provide a more detailed picture of the functions identified in the framework.

Each of the Units are then further defined in greater detail in terms of 'Outcomes of Effective Performance', 'Behaviours', and 'Knowledge and Understanding'. The 'Outcomes' describe what a social marketer needs do to be considered competent. For example, SMA1.5 *Develop and define segments within target groups* has nine outcomes of effective performance, two of which are provided here for illustration;

1. Use valid analysis and interpretations of data and research findings to identify the characteristics which are common to, or distinguish between, members of the target groups.
2. Identify segments within the target groups with characteristics which are sufficiently similar to allow them to be accessed by, and potentially responsive to, targeted social marketing activities.

In this way, a social marketing research-team can be described as competent, if between the individuals in the team, they can demonstrate all of the outcomes of effective performance, along with the appropriate behaviours, knowledge, and understanding, for all Key Area A Units.

Box 19.4 The MSSSB's functional map of social marketing

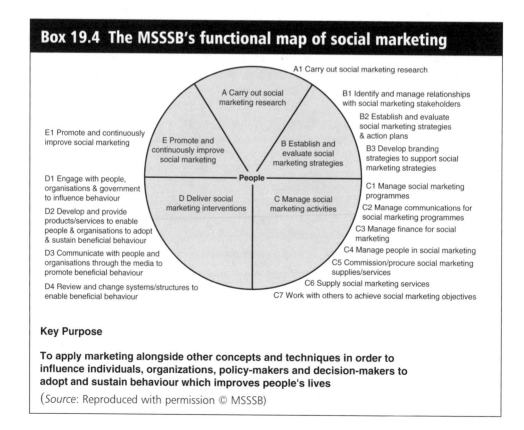

D3 Communicate with people and organisations through the media to promote beneficial behaviour

D4 Review and change systems/structures to enable beneficial behaviour

Key Purpose

To apply marketing alongside other concepts and techniques in order to influence individuals, organizations, policy-makers and decision-makers to adopt and sustain behaviour which improves people's lives

(*Source*: Reproduced with permission © MSSSB)

Box 19.5 Key Area A – areas of competence and units of performance

Key Area A: Carry out social marketing research

Areas of competence	Units
A1 Carry out social marketing research	SMA1.1 **Plan, manage, and evaluate social marketing research programmes**
	SMA1.2 **Collect data** on the knowledge, attitudes, and behaviours of target groups
	SMA1.3 **Develop understanding of theories and evidence** about what might influence the behaviour of target groups
	SMA1.4 **Analyse, interpret, and synthesize** data and research findings to inform social marketing strategy
	SMA1.5 **Develop and define segments** within target groups to inform social marketing strategies
	SMA1.6 **Develop social marketing propositions and test their potential to influence the behaviour** of target groups

(*Source*: Reproduced with permission © MSSSB)

This emphasizes an important point. The functional map describes the full range of functions necessary to achieve the 'key purpose'. No single organization, and particularly no individual worker, will possess all of these skills. Rather, to achieve effective social marketing outcomes, organizations and workers with complementary skill-sets must work together to achieve the Key Purpose.

Applying the standards

The national occupational standards for social marketing will be able to be applied in a number of ways. They will be:

- a framework for developing training and qualifications;
- a means for accreditation of individuals and training courses;
- a template for commissioning social marketing services;
- a tool for developing job descriptions; and
- a device for integrating social marketing into other professional standards, career, and skill-set frameworks.

They will also provide a means of reviewing and redefining best practices over time, capturing innovation as new concepts and techniques (e.g. social networking media) emerge. Box 5.2 in Chapter 5 illustrates the areas where national social marketing standards can be applied.

Conclusion

The demand for social marketing skills is high and will grow in coming years, but so too is the expectation of delivery. One of the aims of this book is to set out explicitly what social marketing is and how it can be put into practice. There is confusion amongst some people in the public sector about what is meant by social marketing and how it fits within the social policy arenas and other forms of social policy intervention such as public health and health promotion. Against such a backdrop, the codification of social marketing is key to its being used effectively. Codification is also essential to achieve a sustainable system for developing capacity and capability within the field. The setting out of clear occupational standards will help the development of recognized skill-sets and competencies for those working in the field.

The situation is eloquently summarized in the words of Dr Chahid Fourali, Head of MSSSB:

> No professional area can become established unless its practitioners have developed what constitutes best practice. The national occupational standards for social marketing represent the first international point of rally for all social marketing practitioners to develop professional practice and gain the status they deserve.
>
> (Dr Chahid Fourali)

The standards will also help shape the development and delivery of educational and training programmes for those people who wish to practice social marketing. This does not mean that a set of occupational standards is fixed and immutable. Like all vibrant areas of study and application social marketing is a developing field and, therefore, it will be necessary to periodically review and adjust the codification of social marketing based on emergent theory and evidence.

References

Hastings, G. (2007). *The Potential of Social Marketing: Why Should the Devil Have All the Best Tunes.* Oxford: Butterman-Heineman.

Department of Health (2006). *Health Challenge England.* London: Department of Health.

National Social Marketing Centre (2006a). *Social Marketing Capacity in the UK: Commercial Sector and Social Marketing Related Work*, Report 5. London: National Social Marketing Centre.

National Social Marketing Centre (2006b). *Social Marketing Capacity in the UK: Academic Sector and Social Marketing Related Work*, Report 4. London: National Social Marketing Centre.

National Social Marketing Centre (2006c). *Its Our Health*! London: National Social Marketing Centre.

National Social Marketing Centre (2007a). *Business Success and Employee Wellbeing. The Case for a New Cross-Government Approach.* London: National Social Marketing Centre.

National Social Marketing Centre (2007b). *Big Pocket Guide: Social Marketing*, Second Edition. London: National Social Marketing Centre.

Thorpe, A. et al. (2008). Social marketing superman, or a sustainable system, *Social Marketing Quarterly*, special edition, publication pending

Chapter 20

Partnerships in social marketing

Jeff French

Coming together is a beginning, staying together is progress, and working together is success.
Henry Ford

Learning points

This chapter

- Discusses the importance of establishing and managing partnerships as part of social marketing interventions;
- Sets out some of the differences between partnerships with the not-for-profit sector, communities, and non-governmental organizations;
- Defines the differences between partnership development and stakeholder management and explains how to manage both within social marketing initiatives; and
- Advises on how to select appropriate partners and develop an appropriate partnership management system.

Chapter overview

This chapter sets out the rationale and processes for developing effective partnerships, an important component of many social marketing initiatives but one with which care needs to be taken. It sets out a number of common principles for establishing and maintaining partnerships across different sectors. The chapter also reviews the differences between stakeholders and partners and the gives advice on how best to manage partnerships.

Introduction

Building and sustaining a dynamic, productive, and a culturally rich and healthy society presents real challenges that no single sector or organization alone can tackle. This is true even for the government. Indeed, we know that in many circumstances interventions that are perceived to be led by the government or governmental agencies are seen as intrusive or a turn-off to some potential target audiences. The task, therefore, requires the release and coordination of all relevant resources held by communities and organizations across all sectors, and so many social marketing programmes start by building delivery coalitions amongst all those who can help.

If social marketing is to successfully tackle issues such as health inequality, one of the most important types of partnership it needs to develop is between the private and public sectors. Although there are many examples of social marketing initiatives that have relied on partnership between these sectors, many public sector staff are still reluctant to work with the private sector due to ethical considerations or fears that the private sector will take advantage of public sector endorsement. In extreme cases, public sector workers believe that the private sector is the 'enemy' and that capitalism and consumerism sit at the root of many of society's problems. There are also real challenges in developing partnerships with non-governmental organizations (NGOs) and local communities and between developed and developing countries (Crisp, 2007).

The basic actions that need to be taken to empower people to choose positive behaviours include:

- building a supportive social network and strong communities;
- ensuring people are protected by laws that reflect fundamental human rights and responsibilities;
- providing appropriate information at the right time and place;
- ensuring that people have access to the resources they need;
- providing goods and services that meet people's needs;
- markets that work for the benefit of both people and those who profit from them; and
- ensuring that the environment people live in is safe, healthy, and inspiring.

Clearly the public, voluntary, and private sectors all have key roles to play in these activities. Nationally and locally, cross-sector partnership can increase the impact of social marketing initiatives and deliver support for behavioural change in areas and in ways that the public sector alone cannot.

There have always been partnerships for social good. The public sector relies on businesses to supply it with goods and services and is itself an important customer for the private sector, enabling it to create wealth and employment opportunities, which in turn contributes to well-being and social development. The public sector also relies on the voluntary sector and the communities it serves to supply volunteers and programmes that complement public sector initiatives. NGOs and foundations supply funding for research and support thousands of local community interventions. Communities themselves supply cultural, spiritual, educational, and support services, as well as economic goods and services that make for vibrant social environments that are the very stuff of social capital (Putman, 2000).

The 2004 Global Corporate Citizenship Initiative survey showed that over 90% of the chief executives surveyed believed that the world's development challenges cannot be met without partnership (World Economic Forum, 2005). The respondents felt that partnerships between business, government, and civil society would play a major role in addressing key developmental challenges.

However, official government or public sector agency guidance about working with the private sector, and sometimes the voluntary sector, is often framed defensively and seeks to minimize risk (World Health Organization (WHO), 2000; DH, 2000; NHS Scotland, 2003; NHS Management Executive, 1993; and The Audit Commission, 2005). Whilst it is appropriate to minimize risks, there is also a need to harness the power, influence, and know-how of all potential partners if we are to make progress in tackling the huge social challenges that we face.

There is a need to move away from passive forms of partnership that merely seek funding for government-shaped initiatives towards more active and jointly developed initiatives. Sustained, active partnerships need to be developed that encourage sharing of expertise and resources and that build trust.

One of the first challenges is to begin to build a dialogue between potential partners around areas of mutual concern. A second challenge is to agree how we can work together.

Partnerships with the private sector

An important opportunity for those leading social marketing interventions is the increasing enthusiasm of many sections of the private sector for supporting social marketing initiatives. Companies are increasingly interested in corporate social responsibility (CSR), which can be defined as:

> business taking account of their economic, social and environmental impacts, and acting to address the key sustainable development challenges based on their core competences wherever they operate.
>
> (Department for Trade and Industry (DTI), 2004)

Whilst there have always been commercial drivers for effective partnerships, there are now additional compelling social drivers concerned with tackling some of the key challenges facing the world today (as discussed in Chapter 1). Developing a sustainable economy, a pleasant and productive environment, and a healthy population are all key goals of the public sector, but they also represent the best long-term strategy for the private sector in its mission to benefit shareholders in a social responsible way. In short, the key challenges facing society today (including poverty, poor health, sustainable consumption, inequality, and climate change) require coordinated effort between the state and the private sector. A full discussion and guidance about how social marketing can be enhanced by working with companies as part of the CSR agenda can be found in *Corporate Social Responsibility: Doing the Most Good for your Company and your Cause* (Kotler and Lee, 2006).

The Ministry of Foreign Affairs of Denmark has instigated a public–private partnership (PPP) programme to promote sustainable PPPs. It recognizes that private sector involvement is crucial to achieve the development goals of the international community (Ministry of Foreign Affairs of Denmark, 2006, visit www.pppprogramme.com). PPPs are also currently being promoted as an innovative policy by institutions such as the UN (2003) and UNAIDS (2007).The private sector is increasingly being seen as a route to reach and connect with different societies or specific communities, as stated by Ban Ki-Moon, Secretary-General of the UN: *We need business to give practical meaning and reach to the values and principles that connect cultures and people everywhere* (online at http://globalcompact.org.ua/en).

There are many examples of successful PPPs, such as in the Netherlands, where the public sector partnered supermarkets to run a 'Fat Watch' campaign. This campaign reduced consumption of saturated fats from 16.4–14.1% of energy intake over a 5-year period (Edition, 2000). Another good example is the Big Noise Snack Right campaign, which aims to improve the healthy snacking behaviours of children under the age of 4 in deprived areas of North West England (visit http://www.nsms.org.uk/public/CSView.aspx?casestudy=37).

The increasing importance of PPPs can partly be partly attributed to the growing emphasis that governments are placing on CSR, as demonstrated by the following quote from Gordon Brown during his time as Chancellor of the Exchequer:

> Today, corporate social responsibility goes far beyond the old philanthropy of the past – donating money to good causes at the end of the financial year – and is instead an all year round responsibility that companies accept for the environment around them, for the best working practices, for their engagement in their local communities and for their recognition that brand names depend not only on quality, price and uniqueness but on how, cumulatively, they interact with companies' workforce, community and environment.
>
> (DTI, 2004)

However, as previously stated, the private sector is also increasingly keen to get involved in achieving public sector objectives. Reasons why companies might want to partner the public sector include a desire to:

- strengthen brand position, company reputation, and corporate image;
- increase customer loyalty;
- attract and motivate high-quality employees;
- differentiate themselves form competitors;
- meet corporate social responsibility targets;
- increase their appeal to investors;
- be altruistic; and
- increase the size of their target market if public sector objectives are met.

Other reasons that are more sensitive from a public sector perspective include opportunities to:

- enter a specific market;
- increase sales;
- influence public sector policy; and
- promote products or services.

Ethical considerations

There are obviously many benefits to using PPPs in social marketing initiatives. However, they should not just be the default intervention when seeking to influence behaviour for social good.

The European Commission's guidelines (2003) set out a range of recommendations to be considered before creating a PPP:

- There should be detailed analysis of the costs and benefits of private sector involvement versus public alternatives.
- Both parties should appreciate the appropriateness of working together in a partnership – this could be through their organization type or the subject matter.
- Detailed analysis of the full costs should be calculated before the partnership starts.
- There needs to be a sufficient structure and ability to effectively implement an intervention.
- The relationship should achieve the objectives of both parties.
- Finally, a PPP should only be used if it can be clearly demonstrated that it will add additional value to other approaches.

Another consideration before embarking on PPPs is to ensure that the process is open to scrutiny by public agencies and is independent of commercial interest (National Institute for Public Health and the Environment, 2006). This will help to enable transparency in the process and can help prevent future issues arising.

Partnerships with communities

The World Bank defines empowerment as: 'The expansion of assets and capabilities of poor people to participate in, negotiate with, influence, control, and hold accountable institutions that affect their lives'.

In their report on the social determinants of health (2004) Wilkinson and Marmot state that societies where people play an active role in the social, economic, and cultural life of society will

Box 20.1 Working with the private sector to improve health opportunities

Example 1: Clubs that count

In 2004's *Choosing Health* White Paper, the UK Government acknowledged the importance of sport in improving the nation's health. Research showed that sports clubs are good mechanisms for engaging some groups of young people in disadvantaged areas: 64% of professional football and rugby league clubs in England are located in deprived neighbourhoods and 61% of football league clubs are in areas with significant or high minority ethnic populations. Business in the Community (BITC) is a government-funded organization that works to create partnerships between business and communities. BITC has over 20 years' experience of helping companies improve their positive impact on society and meet their goals for corporate social responsibility. BITC used DH funding to create 'Clubs that Count'. Clubs that Count measures how well sports clubs are implementing their corporate social responsibility strategy, identifies gaps in delivery, and gives advice on how the club can improve – with a focus on getting tangible results in the poor areas.

In its first year the initiative exceeded its target of working with 20 clubs, bringing on board nine premier rugby union clubs, eight premier league football clubs, seven football league clubs, one rugby league club, and one Welsh football club – a total of 26 clubs.

One example member is Saracens national league rugby club. It provides schools with a range of activities such as tag rugby, teacher training, and cross-curriculum themed lessons. Professional players visit schools to deliver key messages on health, diet, and exercise. These visits prove to be the highlight of the programme for nearly all children, and help to give them positive role models. During 2005–06, the programme worked with over 25 000 children and young people, trained 400 teachers, and donated 600 h of first-team player time. Evaluation demonstrated that 99% of teachers said they felt that the quality of their teaching had improved, while 85% witnessed an increase in children's activity levels. In addition, there has been a 10% increase in the number of children who participated in the scheme bringing fruit or vegetables to school. (DH, 2007)

Example 2: School Food Trust Partnership with Walt Disney Motion Pictures International

In 2008 the School Food Trust – the organization charged with transforming school food – partnered with Walt Disney Motion Pictures International on High School Musical 3 to encourage more children to eat healthy school food.

By working with a brand phenomenon the Trust was able to engage with children at Primary and Secondary school using a variety of communications channels. Through interactive competitions and carefully targeted public relations (PR), the campaign activated children by offering them a chance to win a ticket to the premier of the film if they ate a school meal. Over 70 000 children entered the 'Magic Meal ticket' competition.

Working with an international, long established film company brought with it superb benefits of strong brand allegiance and media engagement however the multi-layered sign-off processes and contractual arrangements of the film's stars resulted in regular delays and changes to the overall project brief. Taken as a whole the campaign was a significant success and the benefits far outweighed the difficulties encountered.

be healthier than those where people face insecurity, exclusion, and deprivation. Wallerstein (2006) furthers understanding of the nature of empowerment by describing how it is both an outcome of and an intermediate step towards a healthier life status. As such, it can be seen as a goal to achieve and also as a mechanism for achieving healthier life goals and impacting in areas such as disparities in health outcomes. Wallerstein's report recommended that effective empowerment strategies that health promotion could use are:

- Increasing citizens' skills, control over resources and access to information relevant to public health development;
- Using small group efforts, which enhance critical consciousness on public health issues, to build supportive environments and a deeper sense of community;
- Promoting community action through collective involvement in decision-making and participation in all phases of public health planning, implementation and evaluation, use of lay helpers and leaders, advocacy and leadership training and organizational capacity development;
- Strengthening healthy public policy by organizational and inter-organizational actions, transfer of power and decision-making authority to participants of interventions, and promotion of governmental and institutional accountability and transparency;
- Being sensitive to the health care needs defined by community members themselves

(*ibid*)

Other reviews have reported that health-development initiatives based on participatory approaches are more likely to be successfully implemented (Bonnefoy et al., 2007). Some have also shown that community-based approaches which combine many different risk factors into one 'package' tend to be more effective (Ministry of Health Planning, 2003).

Community-based approaches can follow a similar path to empowerment. For example, an intervention may seek to empower a community. A review of randomized control trials (Giles, 1998) found that the greater the representation of the local community in health promotion programme design and delivery, the greater the impact and the more sustainable it is. Activities that help to increase community engagement include:

- volunteer activities;
- peer programmes; and
- durable structures to facilitate planning and decision making, such as the use of local committees and councils.

In February 2008, the National Institute for Health and Clinical Excellence (NICE) released guidance on community engagement. It argues that approaches which allow communities to work as equal partners, delegate some power to them, or give them total control may lead to more positive health outcomes. Box 20.2 sets out the guidance's four recommendations.

Setting out degrees of participation

Whether you are applying a community development or social marketing approach, you need to set out explicitly the degree to which you will allow your target audience to participate and the degree to which you will give them access to power. Arnstein's ladder of citizen engagement (1969) is a useful tool for doing so. As Fig. 20.1 shows, it sets out a graded movement upwards through eight 'rungs' – from manipulation of citizens to citizen control.

The ladder depicts participation as essentially a power struggle between citizens trying to move up the ladder and controlling organizations and institutions, intentionally or otherwise, attempting to limit their movement up the ladder. The metaphor of the ladder has become an enduring part of policy, academic enquiry, and practice. However, Mayo (2005) has put forward an

Box 20.2 NICE recommendations for community engagement

1. Prerequisites for success

There is a need for:

- coordinated implementation of the relevant policy initiatives;
- a commitment to long-term investment;
- openness to organizational and cultural change;
- a willingness to share power; and
- the development of trust and respect among all those involved.

2. Infrastructure

Once the prerequisites have been met, it is easier to set up the infrastructure required to implement effective practice. There is also a need:

- to provide support for appropriate training and development of those working with the community – including members of that community; and
- for formal mechanisms which endorse partnership working and support for effective implementation of area-based initiatives.

3. Approaches

To support and increase levels of community engagement, 'agents of change' and a range of other approaches such as community workshops and resident consultancy can be used to encourage local communities to become involved in activities and area-based initiatives.

4. Evaluation

Finally there is a need to invest in evaluation of community-engagement programmes and processes in order to increase understanding of how community engagement and the different approaches used impact on health and other social outcomes.

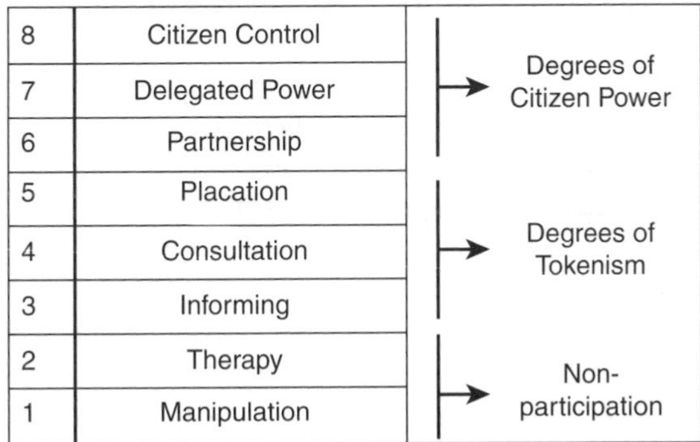

Fig. 20.1 Arnstein's ladder of citizen engagement.

Source: Reproduced from A Ladder Of Citizen Participation, Arnstein S., *Journal of the American Planning Association*, 1969, 35: 216–224, reprinted with permission of Taylor & Francis group.

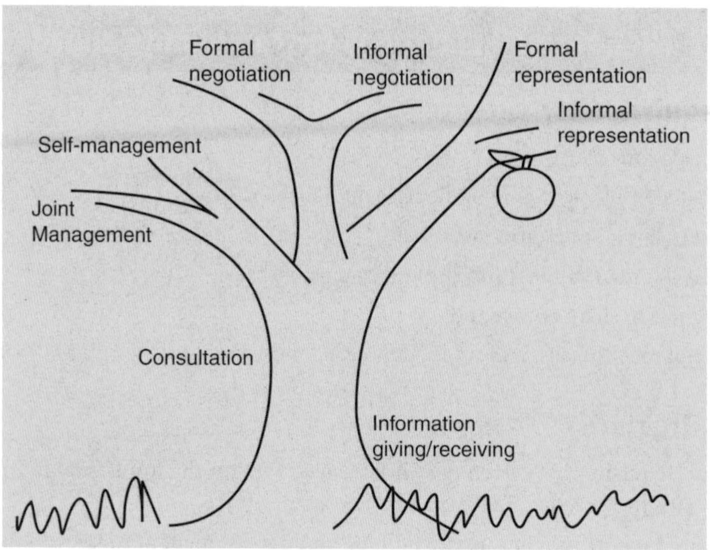

Fig. 20.2 Mayo's fruit tree of participation.
Source: With permission from Mayo E (2005) A playlist for public services. London: National Consumer Council.

alternative metaphor: that of a fruit tree (see Box 21.4). Mayo asserts that whilst most engagement strategy might be based on a core trunk of information provision and consultation, there are in fact many legitimate reasons for engagement. These can be conceived as separate branches that bear different fruits or desired outcomes that have explicit levels of power transfer that have been set out at the beginning of the process. The point is that it is important to be clear about why organizations are seeking to engage or partner with citizens and how much power is being transferred prior to embarking on the engagement process.

Comparing social marketing, community empowerment, and community development

The links between community empowerment, community development, and social marketing are often not clearly articulated. There is some degree of overlap in terms of the principles of practice between these approaches. Social marketing shares with empowerment and community development a focus on developing a deep understanding of individual and community beliefs, values, environmental, and social factors. It also shares the basic democratic principles of community development and empowerment approaches: goals need to be supported by the majority of the general population and the target audience. However, social marketing differs form these approaches in that it moves earlier to define specific behavioural goals and it applies a more consistent approach to initiative development, implementation and evaluation. Community development and empowerment approaches, in contrast, adopt a more reflexive approach to their implementation, one characterized by a willingness to shift the goals and objectives of the initiative in response to community needs and wants. Social marketing, as outlined in Chapters 1 and 3, is ultimately concerned with achieving measurable behavioural goals. Community development and empowerment programmes may have this as a focus, but they may also be concerned with informing, educating, and creating attitudinal and belief change as end-points in themselves. Social marketing programmes often involve information and attitudinal change, but these are steps towards the ultimate goal of measurable behavioural change, and are not ends in themselves. So although it is desirable that social marketing programmes be informed by what is known about successful empowerment and community engagement programmes, and community engagement programmes and empowerment programmes can gain much form an understanding of social marketing principles, the key imperative is to understand what the end-point of the intervention is and what approaches are best deployed to achieve those end-points.

Partnerships with NGOs

Voluntary organizations, foundations and charities all provide a huge amount of local national and international social programmes. Many such organizations also sponsor and deliver a wide range of social marketing interventions. NGOs are increasingly well-managed and highly efficient organizations that can be effective partners in many social marketing programmes. As partners, therefore, they offer a range of advantages.

- They are usually driven by strong ethical and humanitarian motives that are similar to those of social marketing.
- They are fast on their feet and can often make decisions and take action more rapidly than some public sector or private sector organizations.
- They often have a very well developed structure and delivery chain that can enable local initiatives to be developed quickly.
- They usually have good relationships and ready access to groups of the population that some businesses and public sector organizations might view as being 'hard to reach'.
- NGOs often have strong brands and good reputations, so they can be very useful as the face of social marketing initiatives rather than a government or government agency, whose branding or endorsement can sometimes limit the extent or success of an intervention.
- NGOs that are foundations or research institutes often offer grants and funds to support social marketing initiatives and they are a source of knowledge about what works and what does not.

For these reasons, when you are developing your social marketing partnership or coalition strategy you should consider which NGOs should be approached.

How partners differ from stakeholders

In this chapter the term 'partners' and 'partnerships' is used in a positive sense to reflect the way different organizations can agree to come together around a shared commitment to a particular endeavour or cause. Partners bring different resources, skills, and expertise to a partnership to achieve things that they could not achieve alone.

Although there tends to be a great deal of rhetoric about creating conditions where partners can come together 'as equals', the reality is rarely this straightforward, and acknowledging this from the start is an important factor if a partnership is going to work.

Stakeholders are typically people or organizations who have an interest in the issue that the social marketing programme is seeking to influence but who are not formally engaged in developing or delivering the programme. For example, this interest may be because they are in a group affected by the issue, or because they are currently trying to do something about the issue or serve a community affected by the issue. Stakeholders are typically identified and classified using a matrix with two parameters: their power and influence; and their level of support for the social marketing initiative. This is illustrated in Box 11.9: The Stakeholder Matrix, in Chapter 11: their power and influence; and their level of support for the social marketing initiative.

Box 20.3 How do partners differ from stakeholders?

Partners:

- are actively involved in the scoping, development, delivery, and evaluation of social marketing interventions;
- contribute resources, such as know-how, information, facilities, or finance; and
- make a commitment, usually in the form of a written agreement, to actively contribute.

Stakeholders:

- can be involved in a range of ways, from wishing to be informed through to some level of support;
- may not have an active interest in an initiative but would be offended if they were not informed or consulted; and
- are not subject to any form of written commitment to participate or deliver.

Stakeholders in each quadrant of this matrix require different management strategies. Most stakeholder management strategies involve stetting out clear aims and objectives for each quadrant and sometimes for specific named stakeholders. These objectives depend on the characteristic of each stakeholder and can range from keeping stakeholders informed through to attempts to get them to become partners. Action at the opposite extreme can include focussing on managing stakeholders who oppose the social marketing initiative to either reduce their impact or to encourage them to be positive in their attitude. Typically, stakeholder management is evaluated by assessing how much progress has been made against each of the agreed objectives on a regular basis.

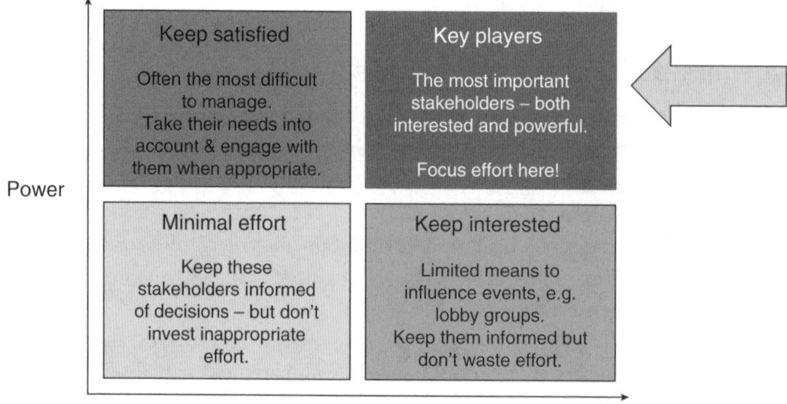

Fig. 20.3 The Power and Matrix tool.

Source: Reproduced from Gardner, J.R., Rachlin, R., and Sweeny, H.W.A. (1986). *Handbook of Strategic Planning*. New York: John Wiley & Sons Inc, with permission.

Although stakeholder management is a vital component of all social marketing initiatives, it will not deliver the impact that a fully engaged and well managed partnership coalition can. Successful joint working with partners means moving away from a situation where a stakeholder may have a passive or reactive relationship with the social marketing programme to one that is active, evolving and long term.

A true partnership approach:

- enables partners to work together to set objectives that are owned by all partners;
- recognizes that no one organization has all the answers;
- mobilizes partners to deliver appropriate, sustainable solutions for citizens;
- acknowledges that complex, sensitive issues require a long-term approach that works through cultural, rational, and emotional influences;
- provides appropriate support to facilitate, maintain, and evaluate the partnership;
- provides feedback and evaluation about the work of the partnership to all who are involved; and
- listens, respects, and forgives minor mistakes.

Finding the right partners

Finding the right partner or partners is critical to developing and delivering effective sustainable partnerships. When seeking partners, you will need to ask a series of questions.

- What are we trying to achieve?
- What is in it for the partner?
- What do we hope they can bring or help us with?
- What do we not need from them?
- What can we give them?
- What can we not give them?

By answering these questions, you will ensure that the needs of partners are considered and contributions fully integrated from the planning stage. Investing the time and effort at the outset to bring the right organizations on board, and to create win–win outcomes for all partners, will help lay the foundations for a strong, mutually beneficial partnership.

Where to start

Building a successful partnership takes time and effort. Be clear about the goals of your initiative and target group, as this will help you shortlist potential partner organizations. As discussed in Chapter 11, it is preferable to map out potential stakeholders during your initiative's scoping stage and to determine those who will become actual partners and what role they will play.

Define the desired outcomes

A clear statement of the desired outcomes from a partnership initiative lays the foundation for developing an effective partnership. A clear statement of purpose should:

- include clear aims and objectives that put the citizen at the centre of the initiative;
- include key performance indicators, deliverables, and milestones from the citizen's perspective;
- outline the scope for partners to help deliver the outcomes as a starting point for a conversation with potential partners.

In assessing the role of an organization that you may want to partner, it is essential to keep in mind:

- the desired outcomes;
- the way the target audience responds to different influences; and
- the comprehensiveness of the support the partners provide to the target audience.

Ultimately, your choice of partners will be influenced by many factors. Table 20.1 shows some considerations that may help your prioritization.

The process of assessing the strengths and weaknesses of organizations as partners should help formulate a delivery matrix that maps out the roles of preferred partners. Such a matrix can be market-tested with the target audience to validate the choices from their perspective.

An active partnership should evolve and develop organically in response to the changing needs of the target audience. Different partners may have important roles at different times. It is essential that before a partnership begins everyone is clear about what is being offered, what is not or cannot be delivered and how any conflicts that might arise will be settled.

Table 20.1 Assessing potential partners

Shortlisting criteria	Acceptance criteria
A good track record and sound management and stable financial position.	◆ Evidence from annual reports and accounts of organizational health and past good work in the area you are interested in.
Good standing with their own sector.	◆ A strong reputation as a for profit or not-for-profit organization. ◆ Recognized as a market leader. ◆ Recipient of sector awards and other forms of recognition.
Access to the people you are seeking to help or could they develop it.	◆ User or customer profile indicates that they are serving or seeking to serve the intended target audience. ◆ Evidence from the target audience indicates that the organization already influences and supports their lifestyle choices. ◆ The organization has established links to key social networks within the target audience or specific segments.
Access to relevant technical, research, or other facilities that will help with the social marketing programme.	◆ Existence of the forms of technical skills and insights and or facilities sought. ◆ Willingness to make these available.
Are they attractive partners? Are they like minded? Are they reputable?	◆ The organization have a good reputation within the target audience. ◆ More widely it seen as reputable and will withstand scrutiny for conflicts of interest.
Credibility: does the organization's brand, services, or products complement your brief?	◆ The organization is known as an advocate and supporter of the issue.
There is an obvious role for the organization.	◆ There is a clear, well-defined opportunity and the partner has the necessary resources.
Capacity for partnering	◆ Support from senior managers and leaders. ◆ Staff with good interpersonal skills and wiliness to partner. ◆ Time will be allocated to engage in active partnering.

Managing partnerships

The mechanisms for joint working with partners outlined in Box 21.8 are tried and tested, but they should not be taken as the only acceptable solutions and should not limit your imagination. In developing a partnership with any organization a focus, on win–win outcomes are more important than precedent.

Developing a mutually beneficial and active partnership takes time, understanding, and respect for all parties' positions. The path to an agreement may be smoothed by introducing a participative approach from the outset. Engaging partners early, ideally at the scoping stage, ensures there is time for:

- constructive discussion and negotiation with regards to the desired outcomes of the partnership, how they might best be achieved, and the contributions of the partners;
- thorough consideration of the implications of the partnership, the risks involved and the attendant benefits;
- development of a shared, realistic vision based on common goals; and
- involvement in the planning and risk-management processes.

Participation encourages an open, honest approach that builds goodwill and confidence between potential partners, so that there is natural progression towards an agreement. A for-profit organization will almost certainly require a senior management or board-level decision in order to commit significant resources to a partnership.

Early engagement means that decision-makers can be fully briefed on the partnership and can include the resources required in the business planning process. Moving from the scoping phase to implementation means building the right active partnerships to deliver the desired outcomes. It is important to try and keep as many options for joint working open as possible at this stage.

In many circumstances, information, know-how, networks, branding, or facilities can be more important than money in achieving the partnership's objectives. There are many ways of matching these opportunities to preferred partners, or, where market research has revealed gaps, to finding new partners.

The core principles for partnerships are:

- be legal and above suspicion, e.g. by being non-exclusive and based on a formal contract;
- be fair and equitable;
- benefit society, be cost effective, and in accord with the available evidence;
- do not jeopardize the integrity and reputation of members of the partnership; and
- do not compromise the independence and impartiality of the partnership, e.g. through a real or perceived conflict of interest or the endorsement (actual or implicit) of an organization or its products and services.

Establishing a management framework

Successful partnerships are those with effective management frameworks. An effective management framework is one that:

- is proportionate to the scale of the partnership;
- ensures all partners have a voice while providing overall leadership and accountability; and
- is efficient and non-bureaucratic.

Table 20.2 Proven mechanisms for joint working

Joint promotions	For-profit organization will invest its resources in joint working with partners to raise awareness of the need for change (e.g. in promoting sensible drinking).
Joint marketing	The partner will invest its resources and lend its brand to raising cash to support actions to bring about changes. The partner's understanding of the target audience demographics, their influence, and their reach can be of immense value here, ensuring that key messages are presented in ways that strike home.
Provision of financial incentives	Partners may offer financial or other forms of incentives to encourage the desired behaviour being promoted by the coalition (e.g. free exchanges of energy efficient light bulbs for older less efficient ones in the cause of reducing energy use).
Provision of non-financial incentives	Partners may offer non financial incentives such as a healthy menu choice in support of a healthy-eating programme
Sponsorship in kind-coalition programmes	Rather than straight financial contributions a partner will provide endorsements via the use of its logo, its outlets it staff time and effort, etc., to promote the programme's aims. For example, use of locations to act as collection points for good to be recycled or to dump unused and unwanted out of date medicines.
Financial sponsorship	A partner will donate cash to the partnership. This is the most traditional approach. The sponsor may reasonably expect co-operation, loyalty, and active PR from the partnership. The cash may or may not be tied to a particular activity. Again, it is essential any finance is clearly separated from the public coffers and care must be taken to ensure the sponsor has integrity.
Corporate volunteering and use of staff time.	Many businesses now encourage skilled staff to help by the voluntary public sector. Partners can also offer to train their staff to assist with interventions by providing information or signposting.
Socially responsible business practices	The corporation conducts its discretionary business practices and investments in ways that support the partnership or the underlying cause.
Acting as examples of good practice	Employers can have considerable influence with a target audience and can play an important role within a partnership. Employer participation ensures that the work culture emphasizes the desired goals of the partnership. By throwing their weight behind the message and being seen to 'walk the talk' employers ensure that the target audience receives consistent signals about making healthy choices and active support. In addition, the workplace may be one of the few routes to reaching some members of the target audience. Employers can give support in a variety of ways ranging from providing information to supporting activities.
Advocacy	A partner will act as an advocate for the desired issue and may include references to the programme issue in its own marketing or service delivery. It may run informational campaigns to raise awareness about the issue as part of its contribution
Access to partner's promotions	Partner offers the use of existing promotions and channels to the partnership to support the programme. For example, allowing informational materials to be inserted into direct mail shots.
Funding research	The for-profit organization may sponsor research activity. It is important that any such research activity is independently monitored and evaluated and is subject to strict governance.

Creating a partnership agreement

Every partnership should be founded on a written agreement that sets out the terms and conditions of the partnership and its objectives. You should set out clearly the expected duration of the partnership, the contribution of each partner, and any timescales for delivery. Agreements should ensure that there is a leadership and management structure for the partnership and that there are clear lines of accountability. Performance-management mechanisms – including key success factors, performance indicators, monitoring arrangements, and evaluation criteria – all need to be set out. The partnership's first year business plan should also ideally be included, setting out the source and application of resources, key milestones, and objectives to be delivered.

At the very least, agreements should contain:

- details of the partners and responsible officers;
- a statement of intent: what is to be achieved, what each partner will do, and what partners will not be required to do;
- structures and procedures for managing the partnership including roles and responsibilities, administrative arrangements, decision-making processes, and accountabilities;
- details of what resources are being committed by partners and what influence they and all partners have over these;
- a review and audit of the processes that will be put in place to monitor progress, the functioning of the partnership and how adjustment will be made if necessary.
- caveats: these may include the use of intellectual property, use of copyright materials, including logos, use of confidential information, and permissions that may be needed for the use of information or resources;
- legal status of the agreement and its implication; and
- the timeframe for the partnership and the delivery of any specific areas of work or commitment.

The agreement should also be signed by an officer with the authority to represent the partner organization. It is a good idea to get the most senior person possible to sign the partnership agreement, as it is a public declaration of commitment that staff within the organization can refer to as the programme develops.

The importance of flexibility

Partnerships that seek to sustain and support change are usually long-term commitments. Over the duration of the partnership, the target audience will be continually exposed to new stimuli and influences. Effective monitoring procedures help:

- demonstrate the partnership is fulfilling its purpose;
- ensure the partnership remains responsive to change, so that it continues to be effective and influential; and
- develop an evidence base for continuous improvement.

References

Andreasen, A.R. and Drumwright, M.E. (2000). *Alliances and Ethics in Social Marketing*. Washington DC: Marketing Institute.

Arnstein, S. (1969). A ladder of citizen participation. *Journal of the American Institute of Planners*. 35: 216–24.

Audit Commission (2005). *Governing Partnerships: Bridging the Accountability Gap*. London: Audit Commission.

Ban Ki-Moon, speech by Secretary-General of the United Nations, available at: http://globalcompact.org.ua/en (Accessed 13 March 2008).

Barket, L. (2001). *Customer-Focused Government: from Policy to Delivery*. London: Public Services Productivity Panel.

Bonnefov, J. et al. (2007). *Constructing the evidence base on the social determinants of health*. The Measurement and Evidence Knowledge Network of the World Health Organization. Commission on Social Determinants of Health. Geneva: World Health Organization.

Business in the Community (2006). *The Market Place: Responsibilities, Principles*. December. London: Business In the Community.

Cogman, D. and Oppenheim, J.M. (2002). Controversy incorporated. *McKinsey Quarterly*, 4: 57–65.

Davis, I. (2005). What is the business of business? *MckKinsey Quarterly*, 3: 105–13.

Department of Health (2000). *Commercial Sponsorship: Ethical Standards for the NHS*. London.

Department of Health (2004). *Guide to Non-Commercial Contracting for Primary Care Trusts*. London: NHSFT Implementation Branch. Contracting and Partnerships.

Department of Health (2004). *Choosing Health: Making Healthier Choices Easier*. London.

Department of Health (2005). *Delivering Choosing Health: Making Healthier Choices Easier*. London: Department of Health.

Department of Health (2007). *Partnerships for Better Health*. London: Department of Health.

Crisp, N. (2007). *Global Health Partnerships: the UK Contribution to Health in Developing Countries*. London: COI available at: http://www.dh.gov.uk/en/Publicationsandstatistics/Publications/PublicationsPolicyAndGuidance/dh_065374 (Accessed 23 February 2009).

Department for Trade and Industry (2004). *Corporate Social Responsibility: a Government Update*. London.

MacDonald, G. (1999). *The evidence of health promotion effectiveness: shaping public health In a new Europe*. Paris: International Union for Health Promotion and Education/Commission of the European Union.

European Commission (2003). *Guidelines for Successful Public-Private Partnerships*. Brussels: Directorate-General Regional Policy. European Commission.

Gillies, P. (1998). Effectiveness of alliances and partnerships for health promotion. *Health Promotion International*,13: 2.

Hunter Centre for Entrepreneurship (1980). *Building a sustainable and ethical business in the 21st century: people, planet and profit*, Golden Jubilee Queen's Awards for Enterprise Research Initiative, University of Strathclyde.

Hutton, J. (2005). Making public services serve the public, speech to the Social Market Foundation, August. London: Cabinet Office.

Innovation and Development Agency (2005). *Communicating Sustainable Development: 10 Ways to Make a Difference*. London: I&DeA.

International Business Leaders Forum (2006). *Facing the Facts: Realities of Partnering in Practice*. London.

Kotler, P. and Lee, N. (2006). *Corporate Social Responsibility: Doing the Most Good for your Company and your Cause*. New York: John Wiley and Sons.

LaVake, S. and Rosen, J. (2003). *A Handbook for Assessing the Potential for Youth Reproductive Health and HIV/AIDS Program Interventions in the Private Sector*. Arlington, VA: YouthNet.

Markwell, S. et al. (2003). *The Working Partnership*. London: Health Development Agency.

Mayo, E. (2005). *A Playlist for Public Services*. London: National Consumer Council.

Ministry of Foreign Affairs of Denmark (2006). *Corporate Social Responsibility: Support Facilities in the Public Private Partnership Programme*. Denmark.

Ministry of Health Planning (2003). *Prevention that Works: a Review of the Evidence Regarding the Causation and Prevention of Chronic Disease*. Consultation draft, November. Victoria.

National Cancer Institute (2004). *Making Health Communication Programmes Work*. London: National Cancer Institute.

National Consumer Council (2005). *Better Business Practice: How to Make Self-Regulation Work for Consumers and Business.* London: National Consumer Council.

NHS Management Executive (1993). Standards of business conduct for NHS staff. HSG(93)5. London: Department of Health.

NHS Scotland (2003). A common understanding: guidance on joint working between NHS Scotland and the pharmaceutical industry. Edinburgh: NHS Scotland.

National Institute for Public Health and the Environment (2006). *Report on the contributions to the Green Paper "Promoting healthy diets and physical activity: a European dimension for the prevention of overweight, obesity and chronic diseases"*. The Netherlands.

National Institute for Clinical Excellence (2008). *Community Engagement to Improve Health.* Available at: www.nice.org.uk/PH009 (Accessed 5 January 2009).

Putnam, R.D. (2000). *Bowling Alone: the Collapse and Revival of American Community.* New York: Simon and Schuster.

Reed, M.H. (2001). *IEG Legal Guide to Cause Marketing.* Chicago: Intl Events Group.

Tennyson, R. (2003). *The Partnering Tool Box.* London: International Business Leaders Forum.

Tennyson, R. (2003). *The Brokering Guidebook: Navigating Sustainable Development Partnerships.* London: International Business Leaders Forum.

The World Economic Forum report (2005). *Partnering For Success: Business Perspectives on Multi Stakeholder Partnerships.* Geneva: World Economic Forum.

United Nations (2003). *Enhanced Cooperation between the United Nations and all Relevant Partners, in Particular the Private Sector.* Report of the Secretary-General.

UNAIDS (2007). *AIDS is Everybody's Business, Partnerships with the Private Sector: a Collection of Case Studies from UNAIDS.* Geneva: UNAIDS.

Wallerstein, N. (2006). *What is the Evidence on Effectiveness of Empowerment to Improve Health?.* Copenhagen: World Health Organization Regional Office for Europe. Available at: http://www.euro.who.int/Document/E88086.pdf (Accessed 21 February 2008).

Walt, G. (2001). *Using Private Money for Public Health: the Growing Trend Towards Partnership.* Seminar Report, Health Action International Europe.

Wilkinson, R. and Marmot, M. (2004). *Social Determinants of Health: the Solid Facts.* Second Edition, Geneva: World Health Organization.

The World Bank. *What is Empowerment?* Available at: http://siteresources.worldbank.org/INTEMPOWERMENT/Resources/486312-1095094954594/draft2.pdf (accessed 21 February 2008).

World Business Council for Sustainable Development (2004). *The Business of Health, the Health of Business.* London: International Business Leader's Forum.

World Economic Forum (2005). *Partnering for Success: Business Perspectives on Multi-Stakeholder Partnerships.*

World Health Organization (2000). Executive Board EB107/20 107th Session. Provisional agenda item 8.3, Guidelines on working with the private sector to achieve health outcomes, Report by the Secretariat, Geneva: World Health Organization.

Chapter 21

Social marketing in developing countries

William A Smith

If you talk to a man in a language he understands, that goes to his head.
If you talk to him in his language, that goes to his heart.
Nelson Mandela

Learning points

This chapter

- Provides lessons about social marketing to low-income rural populations;
- Uses examples from developing countries to show that social marketing can work when targeting poorer communities;
- Provides valuable lessons that social marketers can learn and apply in their own local interventions.

Chapter overview

Social marketing in much of the West, Britain, America, Canada, and Australia, has focussed on creating campaigns to reduce smoking, increase seat-belt use, and prevent obesity. The hallmark of these programmes has been their messages: carefully developed with segmented audiences, positioned to break through the clutter of advertising-saturated markets and resulting in compelling television, radio, and print executions which garner their creators fame, if not fortune.

The use of messages as surrogates of social marketing in the West is well documented. Despite all the theory and academic guidance by specialists such as Kotler, Andreasen, and Roberto, the promotion P rules. Forty years after Kotler's (1971) first article, a participant on the US Social Marketing Listserv (http://www.social-marketing.org/aboutus.html) asked incredulously 'does social marketing sell things?'

Well, the truth is social marketing does sell things. It also designs products or services to meet the special needs of poor people.

- It packages them so poor people can use them.
- It distributes them in places poor people can get them.
- It prices them so that poor people value them.
- And, yes, it advertises and educates poor people about why and how to use them.

This chapter focusses on this unique contribution of social marketing, developed out of the necessity to compensate for dysfunctional public systems. Social marketing in the poor countries of the world faces three challenges rarely met by programmes in the developed West. First, there is no reliable health system to deliver anything. Second, funding of most health programmes are highly dependent upon the unreliable largesse and political priorities of international donors. Third, there is a desperate need for jobs coupled with the same enormous creativity that exists in the West.

It might be argued that social marketing in the West has served the middle class better than it has served the poor. Health disparities in America, Britain, Canada, and Australia continue to be a national embarrassment, even where socialized medicine is the standard. It may be that we all have a lot to learn from the experience of developing countries about the power of social marketing, not just to motivate and educate, but to create social systems that serve their peculiar needs. That, at least, is the intention of this chapter.

Introduction

The special conditions of developing countries

Developing countries represent a unique context for social marketing. Governmental health services are inadequate to meet the health needs of many developing countries. Private sector health systems (with the exception of some faith-based health centres) service a small minority of the population. The major health problems (reproductive health, infant mortality, HIV/AIDS, and malaria) are infectious rather than chronic diseases and are caused by the lack of basic infrastructure (e.g. clean water, adequate sanitation, a reliable food supply, refrigeration, and the delivery of basic health services such as immunizations, epidemiology surveillance, and effective treatment). The lack of basic education, the exclusion of women, a brain-drain of trained professionals, rapid population growth, and political instability compound these problems. Despite these formidable barriers, considerable progress has been made in the developing world, although the progress varies widely from one country and one health problem to another.

For the exclusive purposes of this chapter, we will define social marketing as:

> Any deliberate programme of large-scale behavioural change which creates and markets new products and services designed to improve the quality of society, with a specific focus on public health.

Our purpose in using this narrow definition is not to redefine the field, but simply to place emphasis on the one unique contribution of social marketing to social change – that is the creation and marketing of physical products and social services for the purpose of societal benefit. We recognize and accept that many social marketing programmes in the literature do not create new products or services, but rather use strategies to realign attitudes towards benefits and barriers based upon a people-centred planning model.

This definition makes the importance of product, place, and price in the selection of examples and case studies for this chapter more specific. There are hundreds, perhaps thousands, of examples of health communication programmes which we will not review in this chapter, focussing instead on this narrower and more marketing-centred definition.

We recognize that there is a debate among leading academics as to whether 'communication' includes social marketing, or 'social marketing' includes communication. Rice and Paisley in their book *Public Communication Campaigns* (1981), e.g. include social marketing as a practice of communication. Marketing textbooks, however, consistently view communication as either an integrated function across product, place, price, and promotion, or as a function primarily managed by promotion. This debate is critical to understanding the contributions of social marketing to international development. In the West, this debate remains masked by the prevalent practice of describing almost all modern mass communication campaigns as social marketing, so that 'campaign' and 'social marketing' are synonymous in many practitioners' minds.

Both communication and social marketing share important tactical approaches. For example, both:

- emphasize the importance of consumer research in programme development;
- segment audiences;
- promote benefits; and
- integrate various media in strategic ways to reach and influence audience segments.

The fundamental differences we focus on in this chapter rests in two areas. First, social marketing creates environmental changes by creating new products and/or services that make access easier, increase benefits desired by audiences, and reduce barriers audiences consider important. Second, it uses persuasive communication to promote those changes. Communication programmes focus principally on the role of messages in promoting benefits, reducing audience concern over barriers, and creating a widespread sense that social norms are changing in the direction of the desired behavioural change.

Advocacy approaches to large-scale behavioural change, like social marketing, also focus on creating new benefits and reducing barriers, but their focus is largely through legislation, rather than designing and marketing new products and services. These three approaches (social marketing, communication, and advocacy) share many tactics and are often confused for each other, leading to pointless debates about which is better. What we hope to do here is avoid that debate and simply focus on the unique strength of social marketing in a developing country to create and market new products and services.

This narrow definition also allows us to include public/private partnership as a social marketing model. Here, commercial companies cooperate with public agencies and non-profit organizations to deliver subsidized products to low-income markets. Pricing these subsidized products to promote both sustainability and access by the poor is a critical social marketing challenge. Indeed, the sales of subsidized products to the poor has recently attracted criticism from some Western economists, who consider the sale to the poor of vital social products such as malaria bed-nets to be both immoral and ineffective. Advocates of social marketing argue, however, that stimulating private sector participation in delivering social services to the poor:

- helps relieve the burden to serve everyone on embattled public sector institutions;
- increases the likelihood of long-term sustainability in resource-scarce environments; and
- stimulates the creation of businesses and well-paying jobs locally.

In the West, the integration of the private sector in social marketing programmes is much less common. Indeed, certain private sector industries, notably the tobacco industry, have been identified as the leading focus of social marketing attacks. Industry generally has been considered an unnecessary and somewhat suspect partner in the promotion of social good. Internationally, corporations often suffer from the same suspicion, but the practical needs to deliver services in countries where the public sector is weak has helped overcome and innovate in the creation of effective public private partnerships.

Examples from developing countries

Social marketing emerged in developing countries as one away to address the complex barriers to achieving adequate public health. It was designed to complement and support a public sector that was unable to meet the demands made of it. Social marketing programmes in countries like India, Bangladesh, Thailand, Brazil, the Philippines, Ghana, and others were created by local talent with little control or aid from Western experts. But there has been a small cadre of Western organizations which have been active in international social marketing. These including the Academy for Educational Development (AED), The Futures Group, DKT International, and Population Services International (PSI). The largest single funder of social marketing in developing countries has been the United States Agency for International Development (USAID). Beginning with family-planning programmes in the 1970s, USAID has provided the funds to expand and sustain the application of social marketing to other social problems around the world. Its commitment to measurement has provided our field with some of the most convincing data that social marketing works. The range of products and services successfully promoted in dozens of cultures, under conditions we cannot even imagine here in the West, is the best evidence we have to show the robust and sustainable impact of social marketing on human health and development.

Social marketing in developing countries has focussed on the creation of new products, the creative use of unexpected distribution channels, clever pricing of subsidized products, and some compelling and exciting promotional communication. From elephants in Thailand, to Carnival floats in Rio de Janeiro, social marketing has been serious business with a funny face. Although social marketing has been used for a wide variety of health problems, four health sectors (reproductive health, infant mortality, HIV/AIDS, and malaria) have received major attention and will form the organizational structure of this chapter. Rather than providing a comprehensive review of each health sector, we will discuss the sectoral issues broadly and provide one or two of the most important and evaluated examples of social marketing in each sector.

Sexual health in India

India has the largest social marketing capacity in the world. It was one of the first countries to introduce social marketing for family planning, with sales of condoms today reaching over 1 billion condoms a year. The sophistication and creativity of India's programme represents something of the enormous challenge the country faces in providing voluntary alternatives to female sterilization.

India's population growth rate is 1.74%. It accounts for about 20% of all new births worldwide. One-third of India's population is under 15 years of age and 50% are of reproductive age. The norm of a smaller family has been adopted in India with family size down from six children in the 1960s to just under 2.85 today. Condom use accounts for 3.1% of the contraceptive market, female sterilization for 34.5%, and traditional and natural methods 5.4%. India's large rural population (70%), the large number of languages and religions, and the traditional beliefs about women's role in society make the distribution, sale, and use of condoms an enormous challenge.

Nirodh, India's most widely known condom, was introduced in 1968 by the Department of Family Welfare. It is a high-quality condom that is manufactured in India and the price subsidized by the government. Social marketing is used to develop innovative distribution channels, organize community action and advertising, and promote the brand.

DKT India is one of the Indian government's social marketing partners in promoting the use of condoms for both contraception and HIV/AIDS prevention. It works in 18 of India's 29 provinces and reaches some 599 million people. About 30% of condom sales take place in rural areas of the country. A variety of condom products are offered to meet various segments of the marketing. Packaging emphasizes the sensual qualities of the product and makes the product more desirable. Prices remain stable at less than $0.01 per condom.

Emphasis has been given to developing a local distribution network to meet the special challenges of a country of India's size and complexity. A system of one hub, six agents, 500 stockists, and 80 000 retailers provides reliable channels through which to deliver a variety of contraceptive products. Sales representatives not only provide face-to-face promotion to retailers but monitor stocks of contraceptives to ensure consumers have reliable access.

Creative point-of-purchase materials stimulate retailer and consumer interest. Discounts and contests for customers provide a promotional push for selected products. Communications to doctors and private family-planning clinics include meetings, leaflets, and newsletters. Mass media campaigns also play a major role in promoting the brand. And mass media is complemented with community education programmes that are coordinated by government and other players.

Educational activities are conducted in villages at the *Mandi* (weekly market) and include interactive sessions with married men and women to demonstrate condom use. Barbers and adolescents are also educated on HIV/AIDS awareness as part of the programme. Young women serving and dancing in local bars are at particular risk of contracting HIV. Training sessions for small groups of these women provide them with information but also sensitizes local bar-owners to the need for protection.

The DKT programme is one of many which complement the government's massive family-planning effort. Branding, consumer choice, multiple distribution points and systems, and promotion of condoms from multiple sources have been key factors in meeting India's enormous reproductive health challenges. Further information with regards to the programmes can be found on the DKT International website (http://www.dktinternational.org).

Infant mortality in Honduras

In 1978, the WHO, United Nations International Children's Fund (UNICEF), and USAID embarked on a crusade to combat infant mortality in the developing world, which at this time averaged more than 200 per 1000 live births. Children in developing countries were dying in large numbers from such preventable diseases and illnesses as diarrhoeal dehydration, measles, and respiratory infections, all of which had long been under control in the rest of the industrialized world. Inadequate medical resources and facilities and the lack of effective immunization programmes in developing countries allowed diseases such as these to persist, and kept infant mortality inordinately high.

The Mass Media and Health Practices project was the first major test of social marketing applied to infant mortality in developing countries (AED 1982). The project soon outgrew its name and became a full-fledged social marketing programme as data poured in from grassroots consumer research to reveal the need for new products, lower complexity and costs, and massive teaching of new skills. Mothers were being asked to adopt a new product – an oral rehydration solution – that required them to learn when it was needed, how to find and prepare it, and how to administer it safely to their child. The product was differentiated in the two test-sites: home-mix sugar, salt, and water in Africa and pre-packaged salts in Latin America. In Africa a mass mobilization strategy was driven by the use of a radio course that involved thousands of women learning and then practising to mix the home-mix safely. In Latin America the programme evolved from package salts to a broader childcare diarrhoea product. In Latin America, infant mortality due to diarrhoeal dehydration dropped from 47.5% to 25% in the first year. Both programmes became models for a decade of child-survival initiatives that successfully attacked infant mortality in a dozen countries around the world.

As part of this movement to significantly reduce infant mortality in developing countries, USAID contracted a number of non-profit development organizations to take the lead in developing and implementing customer-oriented social marketing programmes. One such programme was the Mass Media and Health Practices Program, initiated by the AED to address the growing epidemic of acute diarrhoeal dehydration in infants in Honduras.

Before the start of the USAID-funded programme, diarrhoeal dehydration accounted for 24% of all infant deaths in Honduras and represented the single leading cause of infant mortality. In 1977, the year before the programme began, diarrhoeal dehydration caused the deaths of 1030 infants. Treatment at this time was expensive and limited, both in scope and availability. The only treatment available to Hondurans was intravenous therapy – which required trained medical personnel and a sterile environment – and was offered exclusively in fixed health facilities serving only a small percentage of the country's rural population.

The existing product of oral rehydration therapy had been developed by UNICEF as a packet of salts, wrapped in a high-quality aluminum foil envelope with instructions for use printed in various languages. Field testing of this product in rural areas of Honduras demonstrated that not only were the instructions unintelligible, but that illiterate women did not even recognize them as instructions. Tests also showed that women mixed the treatment as they would a headache medicine. They used an eight-ounce glass of water rather than the required litre. Administration of this dense concentration of salts would lead to severe shock and death.

It was clear another packet design was necessary if oral rehydration therapy was to become recognized as the primary treatment for early-onset diarrhoea. Extensive field tests were developed using a prototype methodology rather than focus groups or survey research. Here, various formats were shown to women and they were asked to use the new packet to mix the salts. Verbal instructions were kept to a minimum in order to simulate the conditions under which women would use the packets – often alone in their home with a sick child and no coach. Again, testing showed that even carefully designed visual instruction went unrecognized as instructions. The culture of illiteracy had accustomed women not to look for instructions on medicines, but rather to mix them intuitively.

This insight led to an approach that was much more marketing based than originally anticipated. A series of radio programmes were designed to 'teach' the mother to look for the instructions by looking at the pictures on the packet. Radio messages constantly repeated the mixing volumes, saturating the country with the 1 litre message.

A second problem was encountered when women said they understood the litre message but did not believe that a medicine could be given to a small child in a litre volume. It just seemed too much liquid to give. The solution was to market the product as a tonic rather than a medicine, which fitted comfortably into mothers' mental model of health products. The packet was also designed to be colourful and fun – contrasting greatly with the UNICEF look of a serious complex medicine.

The programme operated in a carefully chosen site that included a representative population of 400 000 individuals. The campaign began by providing 900 health-care workers with 4–8 h of training in oral reyhydration therapy. The training programme concentrated on teaching the proper mixing and administration of salts and instructing other village assistants, who would ultimately have to conduct the same exercises directly with rural families. Using props and training dummies, the trainees repeatedly practised each step of the mixing and administration processes. The health workers and village trainees then began instructing mothers and grandmothers in oral rehydration therapy and other health behaviours, such as breastfeeding, food preparation, and personal hygiene. When rural families completed their oral rehydration therapy training, a flag was posted at their house to let other mothers in the area know where they could obtain health advice and instruction.

As the training programme was being carried out, a media campaign was implemented to reinforce the health-care instructive effort. The campaign developed print materials and radio advertisements to issue basic messages related to the diarrhoea rehydration therapy and the AED training programme. The messages emphasized the correct administration of oral rehydration salts and the importance of continuing breastfeeding during infantile diarrhoea periods, and it encouraged mothers to seek medical assistance if a child's condition deteriorated. Posters and flipcharts were also created to demonstrate oral rehydration therapy and communicate supportive messages. The radio advertisements were placed in announcements of 30–60 s and often included some form of jingle, slogan, or song. Many of the advertisements included a familiar announcer, Dr. Salustiano – the programme's spokesman for technical information – who subsequently became a nationally known figure.

The tone of the campaign was serious, straightforward, and caring. It successfully promoted a mother-craft concept, where a mother's current actions and beliefs are supported and the programme's health techniques become an added complement to her care-giving regimen. Oral rehydration therapy training was presented as a new development in modern medicine: the latest remedy for lost appetite and a recovery aid. With a high rate of literacy (87% of each household with at least one literate member) and 71% of all households owning a functional radio, the media campaign became an effective communication and educational tool.

A year after the programme's implementation, Stanford University carried out an evaluation to chart the project's impact (Rice and Paisley, 1981). Consisting of a data sample collected from 750 randomly selected families from more than 20 communities, the study showed that the diarrhoeal dehydration project in Honduras had achieved significant results in both disseminating important health information and in fostering specific changes in behaviour related to treating infantile diarrhoea.

Decreased mortality

Between 1981 and 1982, mortality rates for children under 5 years of age had decreased from 47.5–25%.

Significant campaign awareness

After little more than a year, 93% of mothers sampled from rural Honduras knew that the programme's radio campaign was promoting Litrosol, the brand name of the locally packaged oral rehydration salts; and 71% could recite the radio jingle used to promote the administration of liquids during diarrhoeal affliction.

Increased health knowledge and changed behaviour

Of the mothers sampled in the study, 42% had knowledge that the use of Litrosol prevented dehydration; and 49% had actually used the product. Of those that had used Litrosol, 94% were accurate in describing the correct mixing volume, and 96% knew that the entire package of salts was to be used in treatment. Sixteen months after the programme started, 39% of all of the cases of diarrhoea within the previous 2 weeks among the sampled families had been treated using Litrosol.

HIV/AIDS in Brazil

Brazil shocked the world when it broke the patent on anti-retroviral drugs (ARVs) and began to provide anti-retroviral therapy (ART) universally and for free. The average cost of ART per patient in 1998 was around $4459 in Brazil. By 2000, Brazil had reduced treatment costs by 72.5% through local manufacture, while prices of imported drugs dropped only 9.6%. The number of deaths due to AIDS is reported to have dropped by 80%. Some 125 000 people were in treatment, and another 300 000 were having their T-cell count checked constantly.

But behind this highly publicized political manoeuvre, the Brazilian national AIDS programme has been a model of social marketing. Focussing on the two audiences most at risk (men who have sex with men and female sex workers), Brazil rejected international funding that required they condemn prostitution. Recognizing that stigma would drive those most at risk underground, it launched a consumer-centred programme that provided the target groups the support they needed to avoid infection. Brazil has criticized countries that preach celibacy and fidelity as the primary means to fight HIV/AIDS.

The intervention also included a prevention campaign for young people. Street-youth in Brazil fight a daily battle for survival. They live for the day and have no sense of a future, and so do not plan for prevention. They are often rounded up by private police, attacked, and sometimes killed. They trust few people. Sex is one of their few joys and high-risk sex is all that is open to them. A local non-governmental organization (NGO) – working with a team from Porter-Novelli and AED – began to ask what might be done to help these children protect themselves. Street conversations with the kids showed that condoms were too expensive and not a viable solution to gangs of kids on the move. These children were proud of their ability to survive. They called themselves 'streetwise rascals'. Working with this image, the social marketers developed a series of tee-shirts which promoted non-penetrative sex and masturbation as a way to beat AIDS. The message was that the 'rascals' had beat the system, beat the police, beat all the adults that tried to trap them, and now they would beat AIDS by being smart.

This small project is just one example of the enormous creativity of the Brazilian programme. Its ability to understand different audiences, create solutions that work for them, and execute the solutions in creative ways was a key to its overall success. If there is one lesson from the Brazil programme for social marketers, it is that people know what they need. Social marketing is not only a way to listen to the disenfranchised; it is a way to create services and products that help them within the context of their own reality.

HIV prevention in Cameroon

The AIDS Control and Prevention (AIDSCAP) programme in Cameroon (1992–96) was designed to address unmet needs in HIV prevention. Available HIV prevalence information in 1992 indicated that Cameroon still had a relatively low HIV prevalence rate, estimated between 0.5% and 1% of the general population. However, surveillance studies suggested that the epidemic was increasing rapidly among specific populations, specifically, urban youth, commercial sex workers, sexually transmitted infections (STI) patients, and the military.

The programme focussed on improving behavioural change communication for targeted groups, increasing condom availability and affordability through social marketing, and assisting the Ministry of Public Health to establish a national STI control service. It was funded by USAID through a cooperative agreement with Family Health International. The programme's final report be accessed online at http://www.fhi.org/en/HIVAIDS/pub/Archive/aidscapreports/FinalReportAIDSCAPCameroon/ExecutiveSummary.htm.

The programme's strategy included peer health education, community-based outreach programmes, and the development and distribution of educational materials and alternative media such as theatre. The heart of the programme was its pioneering behavioural change interventions that have inspired the peer education models currently used around the world. Interventions with the military, university students, STI patients, and sex workers and their clients were implemented by the National AIDS Control Service (NACS) in collaboration with the ministries of defence, higher education, and health. CARE/Canada and Save the Children, USA – two international NGOs – respectively implemented the in- and out-of-school youth project and a community-based intervention project in the East and Far North Provinces of the country. The interventions focussed on adoption of risk-reduction behaviour, including promotion of abstinence for young adults, fidelity for couples, partner reduction, condom use, and treatment for STIs. They used multiple, reinforcing communication channels and information, education, and communication activities.

Specific approaches included counselling, educational techniques such as formal education sessions, drama and informal chats, and mass and traditional media. The projects also focussed on building capacity for sustainability through training, and the development and production of peer health-educator manuals for sex workers, the armed forces, youth, and university students. Over the course of the programme, more than 2000 peer educators and leaders were trained, and they in turn educated more than 700 000 women, men, and youths about HIV prevention. Over 1.18 million educational materials that reinforced communication activities and behavioural change were produced and distributed, and they were supported by radio and television spots.

The strategy was complemented and reinforced by a specific condom social marketing programme. Condom programming was implemented by AIDSCAP's subcontractor, PSI. Under AIDS Control and Prevention (AIDSCAP), the condom social marketing programme expanded countrywide to reach additional target-group populations. As part of its strategy, PSI established officially recognized and supervised distributors in all major urban centres, using specific marketing techniques and advertising to cover all of Cameroon's 10 provinces. Over 9500 condom sales locations were established for Prudence condoms. The programme also used peer educators, especially sex workers, to serve as condom sales agents in nontraditional venues, while contraceptive social marketing sales staff supplied the more traditional commercial outlets. In Yaoundé alone, sex workers sold over 3 million condoms. A number of sex workers were so successful as condom sales agents that they were able to leave the sex work profession. Over the lifetime of the AIDSCAP project, the social marketing programme sold over 24 million condoms and distributed close to 1 million for free.

At the initiation of the AIDSCAP/Cameroon programme, no national STI control programme existed. AIDSCAP/Cameroon efforts led by an AIDSCAP subcontractor, the Institute of Tropical Medicine, concentrated on supporting the NACS in the development of national STI guidelines. As a result of these efforts, a national STI control plan and standard diagnosis and treatment guidelines were adopted by the Ministry of Health.

Over the lifetime of the programme, there were other significant achievements:

- There was a substantial increase in the capacity of the Ministry of Health to plan, manage, and evaluate comprehensive STI/HIV/AIDS programmes.
- More than 700 000 men, women, and youths were educated about how to protect themselves from HIV and STIs.
- Over 2000 individuals working in professional and/or volunteer capacities were trained in the skills they need to sustain HIV-prevention activities in their communities.
- Over 1 million educational and promotional materials that reinforced behavioural change communication efforts and condom use were distributed.

The final evaluation was completed under a grant with the *Institut de Recherche et des Etudes de Comportement* (IRESCO) – a local research institute. IRESCO conducted the end-of-project knowledge, attitudes, beliefs, and practices surveys among all the target groups.

- **Knowledge of two correct methods of preventing HIV has increased among all the target groups.** One of the most dramatic increases was evidenced among youth in the Eastern Province. In 1993 only 37% were able to cite two correct methods of HIV prevention. By 1996 this had increased to 70%.
- **Reported safer sexual behaviour related to condom use increased among several target groups.** The percentage of commercial sex workers reporting to have used a condom has risen steadily from 28.3% in 1988 to 65% in 1990, to 68% in 1994, and finally to 88% in 1996. The percentage of clients who reported ever having used a condom also rose significantly, from 55.5% in 1990 to 81% in 1996. Consistent condom use by sex workers with non-regular clients increased from 52% in 1994 to 75% in 1996.

Fighting malaria across Africa

NetMark is a unique cross-sector partnership created to fight malaria in sub-Saharan Africa, where the disease kills more than 2 million people each year. NetMark was initiated by USAID and developed under the management of AED, its website is www.netmarkafrica.org.

NetMark's mandate is to increase demand for, and expand the availability of, insecticide-treated nets (ITNs) – a simple but effective way to prevent the mosquito bites that cause malaria. To accomplish this task, AED has developed a market-based approach of shared risk and investment dubbed Full Market Impact™ (FMI™),based on the premise that as demand grows within a competitive market, customers will benefit from improved quality, lower prices, and wider availability. Further information on FMI™ is available online at https://pshi.aed.org/fmi.htm.

FMI™ provides an operational model that creates common ground between the private and public sectors. Partners from both sectors agree on common objectives while observing their respective roles across each of the five factors: supply, distribution, affordability demand/appropriate use, and equity/sustainable markets.

The model was intentionally designed to reflect the way businesses thought about the market, which is why it dovetails with the classic four Ps of marketing: product, place, price, and promotion. In this way, FMI™ demonstrates how meeting the needs of the poor can translate into good business that promotes expansion into new market segments. AED believes that FMI™ challenges the way businesses think about market opportunity, taking a broader view of the role their products play and the consumer behaviours they influence, whilst addressing critical public health issues and serving the needs of the poor.

In the 6 years since its inception, the NetMark programme has shown that international and African companies are willing to invest in producing, marketing, and distributing ITNs when working in partnership with the public sector.

Data from household surveys conducted by NetMark in 2004 show considerable gains since the baseline research in 2000 and the first country launch in late 2001. In all NetMark countries, awareness and use of nets and ITNs increased dramatically, and more nets are being treated or purchased pre-treated. For example, the percentage of households that owned a net or ITN in Nigeria rose from 12% in 2000 to 27% in 2004; in Senegal the figures were 34% and 56%; and in Zambia 27% and 50%. Moreover, NetMark's commercial sector-consumers approach resulted in increased use among all socioeconomic groups. Net coverage rates are increasing equitably, and vulnerable groups are being reached in both urban and rural areas.

By 2004, ITN sales by NetMark's formal partners neared the 2 million mark. While this represented only 62% of the ambitious projection total made by the various commercial partners for 2004, it did represent a 132% increase over 2003 sales. Progress is being made in a sustainable manner, and the market appears to be poised for rapid growth now that supply issues are being addressed. Overall commercial sales in NetMark countries have reached 9 million based on reports from partners and estimates of additional sales made by NetMark based on market research conducted in 2004.

There have been other important achievements.

- More than US $18 million has been invested by private sector partners in developing the commercial ITN market in Africa.
- In total, nearly 15 million more people are protected from malaria by ITNs.
- More than 100 million people have been educated about malaria, the importance of ITNs, and how to use them effectively.
- More than 350 000 pregnant women and children under 5 have received discount vouchers for ITNs, of which 243 000 have been redeemed.
- Treated nets now cost from between 30% to 75% less than untreated nets did in 2000, due to competition fostered by NetMark.
- NetMark has increased the supply of ITNs in eight African countries, with the number of ITN distributors increasing from two in 1999 to 29 in 2005.

There are still challenges ahead. Public policy must continue to support ITNs, and there must continue to be a role for the commercial sector. Free and subsidized ITN programmes must be fully targeted to the poorest and not totally undermine commercial investments. NetMark and partner marketing efforts must continue to build sustainable demand, and NetMark's commercial partners must expand their investment in ITNs to replace the support provided by NetMark. Under these conditions, the ITN market will continue to grow while serving the public health fight against malaria.

Conclusion

What lessons can we learn about social marketing to the poor?

There are perhaps three important lessons that can be gleaned from the experience of social marketing to the poor.

1. The poor need more than messages.

To tell a woman to use a condom when she cannot find one, afford one, or convince her partner to use one is nonsense. Social marketing has proven very efficient at listening to the poor, designing contraceptives that meet their needs, making them widely available, pricing them, and promoting them in ways that are compelling and credible to people who have little trust of authority.

2. The poor are willing to pay for services they value.

The poor are like everyone, except they have less money. Like the rest of us, the poor are not all alike. Some know that you do not get much for nothing. Those who are so poor that they have no choice but to depend on hand-outs often become trapped in a vicious cycle of dependency. For others, paying as much as one-third of their income to a traditional healer is a price they are willing to pay for health services they trust. Others distrust anything free from the government. Social marketing does not meet all the needs of the poor, but the subsidized creation and marketing of useful goods and services to the poor relieves financially stretched governments and provides quality services the poor desperately need.

3. The poor can be just as creative and entrepreneurial as the rich.

Social marketing to the poor is not only about price and subsidized products. It is about understanding who the poor are. It is about understanding that street-kids in Brazil are not going to read a pamphlet, see a television spot, or buy a condom. It understands that many rural women in Africa have come to believe that cleanliness is next to godliness. Therefore, they want to wash the dirt off a malarial bed net that has become infested with dirt and insects. They do not need a lecture on how the insecticide washes off: they need a net that can be washed without ruining it. Social marketing is also about bringing fun into the lives of people with precious little of it. It is about contests instead lectures, parades instead of pamphlets, and participation instead of preaching. Social marketing to the poor has released the inherent creativity of communities across the world and shown that you do not need an MBA to be a business person.

References

Academy for Educational Development (1982). *Mass Media and Health Practices Implementation: Project Description*. Washington, DC: Academy for Education Development Jun. 14, [17] p.

Family Health International *Final Report for the AIDSCAP Program in Cameroon:* Available at: http://www.fhi.org/en/HIVAIDS/pub/Archive/aidscapreports/FinalReportAIDSCAPCameroon/ExecutiveSummary.htm (Accessed 21 January 2009).

Kotler, P. and Zaltman, G. (1971). Social marketing: an approach to planned social change. *Journal of Marketing*, Jul; 35(3):3–12.

Rice, R.E. and Paisley, W.J. (eds.) (1981). *Public Communication Campaigns*. Beverly Hills: Sage Publications.

Chapter 22

Learning from the experts: Interviews with leading social marketers

Dean Hanley and Allison Thorpe

Never doubt that a small group of thoughtful, committed citizens can change the world. Indeed it is the only thing that ever has.
Margaret Mead

Learning points

This chapter

- Gives an insight into the thinking of some of the world's leading social marketers;
- Highlights some of the major challenges and opportunities facing social marketing today; and
- Draws on the experts' advice as to how you can approach these challenges and opportunities in your day-to-day work.

Chapter overview

Although, as we explained in the initial chapters of this book, social marketing began life as the offspring of commercial marketing and social sciences, it has evolved into an independent discipline in its own right, retaining links to the many schools of thought that have influenced its development. But if evidence of these diverse influences can be found in social marketing theory, it can also be found in the professional credentials of those promoting the discipline and those putting theory into practice 'on the ground': from academics to frontline health professionals, from policy-makers to interventional project managers, from commercial marketers to public sector professionals seeking to change behaviour for social good.

This chapter provides an opportunity to learn from these diverse influences, drawing on interviews with expert social marketers from across the globe and from a range of professional backgrounds. As well as painting a picture of where social marketing is at today – and what it is achieving – it sets out what our expert social marketers think will be the major challenges and opportunities in the discipline's future and gives you access to specialist advice on how you can approach these challenges and opportunities in your day-to-day working life. A full list of the experts taking part in interviews for this chapter can be found in Appendix 1, along with a list of the interview questions. Transcripts of face-to-face interviews and complete written responses can be found online at http://www.nsmcentre.org.uk/images/CoreFiles/NSMC_Effectively_engaging_people_conference_version.pdf.

Introduction

No publication aiming to paint a picture of the current state of social marketing would be complete without the voice of those working in the field: it is practitioners and specialists, after all, who can tell us first-hand what social marketing is achieving across the world, what works and what does not and how we can improve things in the future. With this in mind, we conducted interviews with 18 specialists from across the globe who are closely involved with social marketing. Interviewees included representatives from commercial marketing and social science backgrounds. They included academics, social marketing project managers, policy-makers, consultants, and directors of social marketing centres. Where possible, the interviews were conducted face to face. However, some interviewees provided written responses. In addition to obtaining expert advice for readers, we wanted to demonstrate the diverse and sometimes contrasting voices that contribute to the discipline and to show that social marketing is a vibrant school of thought that is very much in touch with, and evolves in response to, broader societal concerns. The views expressed by interviewees by no means provide conclusions to some of social marketing's key debates. On the contrary, they very much keep those debates alive, and you will no doubt add to them in your work and conversations with colleagues and stakeholders. Whatever your opinion on the debates, as this chapter shows, as a social marketer you are participating in an emerging and increasingly important discipline that offers possible solutions to some of society's most important problems – health related and otherwise.

Why did our experts get involved in social marketing?

In spite of their diverse backgrounds, many of our interviewees, when asked why they first got involved in social marketing, answered that it was the discipline's focus on people that first interested them. Some, such as Fiona Adshead (then Deputy Chief Medical Officer at England's Department of Health), were drawn by social marketing's *interest in people and what motivates them and how to inspire them to change.* The opportunity, then, to gain insight into the drivers of human behaviour and to use them to influence lifestyle choices was deemed to be too powerful to miss – particularly for interviewees whose professional background was in public health. For example, one interviewee described how she realized that social marketing would be a practical tool for encouraging her depressed clients to take up and stick to treatment, while another saw opportunities for improving the efficacy of his work when he realized that the health-promotion materials he was creating were just not getting results. But if the desire to help improve people's health and lifestyles was a key driver, so was the desire to apply the principles of commercial marketing for social good. After all, in the words of Michael Rothschild (Emeritus Professor at the University of Wisconsin, USA), *There should be better things to do with marketing than selling shoes or beer.* This desire was not just reflected at an individual level. Often, organizations or governments took the initiative: e.g. Jim Mintz (Director at Centre of Excellence for Public Sector Marketing in Canada) describes how he was hired to bring a marketing approach to Canada's federal health department in the early 1980s. In fact, the joint role of commerce and social sciences in social marketing's development was acknowledged by most of our interviewees, many of whom, when asked to define social marketing (for the National Social Marketing Centre's formal definition, see Chapter 3) replied in the same manner as Professor Susan Dann (Australia's Bond University):

> Social marketing involves the use and adaptation of the same types of marketing techniques that makes companies like McDonalds so successful to 'sell' positive changes in attitudes and behaviours.

In addition, if the applicability of a marketing approach to social problems was increasingly being realized by both the public and private sectors, it was also being acknowledged by academia.

Susan Dann describes how she was *asked to develop a course in social marketing at Griffith University* in 1994. We see, therefore, in the professional provenance of our social marketing experts, evidence of the discipline's multifarious influences and applications (see Chapter 2 for more information about social marketing's origins). But it is important to acknowledge that just as influential as personal and professional interest in social marketing is, so is the impact of attempts to promote the discipline. Several of our interviewees mentioned how conferences, individuals, or social marketing books had played an important part in capturing their attention.

How can we respond to the challenges of integrating marketing and social sciences?

Perhaps inevitably, our interviews touched on one of the major challenges facing social marketing today: the merging of marketing and social sciences may create a new, powerful discipline, but the two schools of thought often make uncomfortable bedfellows, and, as Susan Dann points out, this can lead to a mutual distrust or selective uptake of social marketing principles:

> Both sides of the equation ... have a tendency to cherry pick what they like about each other's areas rather than taking a fully integrated approach ... One of the keys to resolving the conflicts is to acknowledge the difference between 'social' marketing and social 'marketing' so that an integrated body of 'social marketing' can be developed ... Without a clear understanding and recognition of the alternative ideological frameworks underpinning the marketing discipline and the different social sciences an integrated and agreed 'social marketing' framework is difficult to develop.

But what exactly are the problems created by social marketing's hybrid nature? There may be suspicion on the part of those from a social science background, e.g. that marketing's commercial nature renders it unsuitable for use in public health interventions. One interviewee mentioned that those from a marketing background might not understand the work environment of people working in public services, who often have to elicit behavioural change on smaller budgets than those used for commercial campaigns. Iain Potter (Chief Executive at New Zealand's Health Sponsorship Council) also highlighted the perceived risk of *bringing the largely unrestricted practices/opportunities and experiences available in the commercial sector into the far more risk conscious government agency environment.*

But if there is wariness on the part of those from a social science or public health background, there is a similar level of concern amongst marketing professionals, some of whom are concerned, e.g. that non-marketers will pick up on.

> trappings of social marketing (doing research, having a 'marketing mix') without understanding the underlying philosophy of a customer orientation and holistic and systematic nature of the marketing process
>
> (Ken Peattie, Director, BRASS Research Centre, Wales)

There is also the worry that because much of the social marketing activity has been in health, the experience might not translate perfectly into other social marketing issues.

But these concerns need not be divisive – a point made by our consecutive interviewees. As Fiona Adshead advises, one of social marketing's strengths is that it learns from different disciplines:

> A futurologist can have as much to teach us as the core disciplines. The challenge is to co-ordinate the input from across the disciplines and make everyone feel valued without creating a competitive environment. Social marketing strength will come from its intellectual diversity.
>
> Fiona Adshead

"When we work together the results are amazing", says Michael Rothschild. "We all have much to offer to create a synergy that is much greater than the sum of its parts"

It is important, therefore, to see the above concerns as opportunities for growth, rather than threats, and to encourage an understanding of the contribution of different schools of thought to social marketing. For interviewees such as Stephen Dann (Senior Lecturer at the Australian National University), it is imperative that social marketing moves on from discussions about whether to drop *the M word ... If there's no marketing, its not social marketing, and it's not what we do*. Others believe that social marketing has, in its own tools and processes, the solution to its own challenges. Ray Lowry (Senior Lecturer at England's Newcastle University) stresses the importance of conducting market research to gain insight into social marketing's contrasting 'audiences' before using that insight to plan convergence. Of course, overcoming these challenges is vital if social marketing is to promote itself as a cohesive discipline that can influence human behaviour for social good. If we get it wrong, we will find it increasingly difficult to promote the benefits of our work not only to each other but to 'outsiders' who might be cynical as to social marketing's worth.

How can we help high-level decision-makers to understand the benefits of social marketing?

Our interviewees were clear that although overcoming its internal disagreements will help with promoting the discipline's practical benefits, there will still be other obstacles to overcome. Box 22.1 lists 10 ways in which the experts feel we could improve promotion of social marketing to communicate its practical application and ensure that policy-makers and decision-makers include it as an integral part of efforts to elicit behavioural change for social good.

Box 22.1 Ten ways to promote social marketing's benefits

1. Have a clear and consistent definition of social marketing.
2. Be clear about what we do and don't do – stress the differences between social marketing and social advertising.
3. Develop a marketing strategy to market social marketing: apply the discipline's own tools and follow its own processes.
4. Build a robust evidence base of cases in which social marketing has achieved significant successes (see below).
5. Disseminate guidance on best practice.
6. Stress that social marketing helps engage individuals and communities in social change, linking policy to the very people it aims to reach.
7. Improve professional capacity and training opportunities (see below).
8. Never overpromise on what we can deliver.
9. Demonstrate that social marketing has a foundation in strategic planning and contributes to strategy and policy development.
10. Find ways to better calculate and communicate social marketing's economic benefits.

How can we improve capacity and build the social marketing workforce?

If targeting high-level decision-makers and policy-makers is vital to the promotion of social marketing, so too is improving capacity and building a social marketing workforce. But how can we go about achieving this? It is evident that our experts feel that much more could be done in academia, the workplace, and beyond.

> For a long-term sustainable capacity development, I think academia is key. Social marketing should be a key element of the syllabus on a variety of courses: public health masters, undergraduate and postgraduate business and marketing, and medical and nursing [courses] ... we need the top universities ... to start including it on a number of their courses. That way, the top academics will be attracted to the topic area.
>
> Dr Rowena Merritt (National Programme Manager at England's National Social Marketing Centre)

It is a popular opinion. The role of education in expanding the reach of social marketing was a major theme of our interviews. In addition to the subjects listed by Rowena Merrit, one expert felt that social marketing should also be a required course for all degrees in social work, public administration, political science, and environmental studies. Another felt that social marketing experts should be proactive in providing guest lectures, while others drew attention to the importance of work experience in social marketing for students and the quality of educational resources, which must, of course be first rate and reflect the latest developments in social marketing thought.

However, it will not be enough to merely wait for those educated in social marketing to take their newly developed skills into the workplace. We must push for greater professional development and, as Jim Mintz puts it *training, training, training!* A range of training opportunities is needed, from hour-long casual seminars to more formal training courses that equip participants to get the most from social marketing in their day-to-day work. Who should we be targeting? The views of our interviewees included:

- practitioners who are not qualified marketers and who need skilling up in marketing;
- anyone working in the public sector with marketing in their job title;
- public sector workers working on social marketing interventions;
- those who are involved in social advertising but should be applying a social marketing approach;
- communication experts (who play an important part in social marketing interventions) and community development leaders (who have a powerful influence at a local level);
- intervention managers in public health, injury prevention, and environmental protection and stewardship; and
- marketing managers in agencies – who are, it seems, much more difficult to find than creatives, researchers, and account managers.

You will, of course, have your own views on where resources should be focussed, but it would be difficult to argue against the promotion of social marketing training.

In addition to training, our experts argued that salaries must be competitive enough to attract high-quality, skilled workers into social marketing positions and that employers should consider granting sabbaticals to employees interested in studying or getting experience in social marketing. 'Social marketing' should also appear more often in job titles. There should also be increased interaction between commercial and social marketers, and a sharing of experience between potential and experienced social marketers, so that practitioners and specialists stay abreast of marketing theory and best practice. Alan Andreasen (Professor of Marketing at the McDonough School of Business of Georgetown University, Washington DC, USA) stressed the importance of providing methods for practising social marketers to communicate with each other, e.g. through blogs, listservers, and other media.

However, there were words of caution: it was deemed important that in building capacity and promoting social marketing, we should try to prevent conventional consultants and practitioners from 'hijacking' the term 'social marketing' and applying it to their existing agenda. And, as with promoting the discipline to policy-makers and decision-makers, we must have a robust evidence base that we can develop into case studies, checklists, tools, and other important resources for increasing social marketing's impact.

How can we develop a robust shared evidence base?

> We need a comprehensive knowledge exchange mechanism, ensuring that we are capturing learning and continue to evaluate national campaigns and also develop ways to capture the learning and experience in local communities.
>
> (Fiona Adshead)

But what should an evidence base consist of?

> First we need to debate what we mean by evidence. It is unlikely to be as defined as, say, the outcomes of pharmaceutical research, as it is more difficult for us to be as precise in social marketing. We need a more flexible approach that learns from experience and intuition.
>
> Gerard Hastings (Professor of Social Marketing, University of Stirling, UK)

Others are clearer about what they think an evidence base needs to achieve: we must develop metrics to measure behavioural change, and we must also track the societal benefits of our interventions. This re-emphasizes the importance of the evaluation stage of social marketing initiatives (see Chapter 14), during which you will measure how well your intervention has performed: what has worked and what has not?

Just as important as the collation of data to demonstrate the effectiveness of social marketing interventions is the communication and dissemination of findings. François Lagarde (Social Marketing Consultant and Trainer at Canada's University of Montreal) stresses the importance of publishing findings in the most creditable journals, such as *Social Marketing Quarterly*, whereas other experts iterate that negative findings are just as important as positive, and that these should be communicated so that others can learn from your mistakes. Current reports of evaluatory findings often neglect to mention what has not worked, thus holding back vital information.

However, Ken Peattie argues that there already exists a wealth of studies demonstrating the effectiveness (or ineffectiveness) of social marketing interventions. The challenge now, he believes, is to collate and make these studies more accessible and to help practitioners find those that are most relevant to them. We also need to disentangle those cases that are pure examples of social marketing from those that only embody some social marketing principles – should information on both kinds of intervention be included in the evidence base or should we exclude those that do not adhere completely to the social marketing model? One important move towards creating an international, accessible, and easy-to-use evidence base would be the establishing in every country that has social marketing a centre in the same mould and with the same responsibilities as England's National Social Marketing Centre.

What advice can our experts give to newcomers to social marketing?

We asked our social marketing experts for advice to those conducting their first social marketing initiative. Interestingly, much advice concentrated on the importance of investing in research at the start of your initiative to obtain an in-depth understanding of the problem you are addressing, its context and the people whose behaviour you are trying to influence. This forms an important part of what is termed the 'scoping stage', and you will find more detailed guidance about it in Chapter 11. If you fail to conduct sufficient research early on in your initiative, you could be decreasing your chances of success, as any interventions you create may not be based on genuine insight into what you need to achieve.

Box 22.2 sets out examples of our experts' comments.

What is the best way to make a business case for social marketing?

At some point in their career, all social marketers will need to put a business case for a social marketing intervention. But what is the best way to convince stakeholders or funders that your intervention is financially viable and able to get results?

One of the most important messages to get across is that a failure to elicit the targeted behavioural change will have consequences for society. *Ask them what the cost of failed behaviour change is to society*, suggests William A Smith (Executive Vice President at the USA's Academy for Educational Development), *But listen to them, speak their language and target their self-interest.* Robert Marshall (Assistant Director at RI Department of Health, USA) develops the argument:

> I would point out that whatever we are [currently] doing is clearly not working! And if business can successfully use marketing to change the behaviours of target audiences to promote fast-food

Box 22.2 Tips for conducting your first social marketing initiative

- You must invest as heavily as possible in research (primary and secondary) before you do anything.
- Live with your audience for a week and make your intervention fun and easy for them to take part in.
- Get inside your target audience's heads. See the world as they see it before you make any decisions and before you produce any materials.
- Forget communication. Think about barriers to and benefits of behaviour, and address those.
- Make sure that you are trying to influence very precise behaviour or a set of behaviours, because many interventions try to tackle too much or focus on attitude change – they are educational programmes rather than social marketing interventions.
- Do not cheat. If your intervention does not work, find a viable alternative and do not fall back on relying on government policy to enforce change.
- Find someone with practical experience and get them to help you.

> consumption and sedentary lifestyles, then we have to use the same approaches to changing those behaviours. I would also add that social marketing is also a useful approach to policy development – probably the only way we will be ultimately successful in changing these health behaviours.

It is a good idea to set out how your intervention will have a positive impact, as Alan Andreasen sets out:

> Putting the case for the positive aspects of the behaviour outcome. The extent to which the campaign focuses on the behavioural outcomes, the framework and way of thinking, profile targeting of behaviour and targeting context makes it likely that one can measure programme efforts and justify budgets and therefore encourage larger budgets.

Give examples of similar successful campaigns and outcomes – if you do not have an example of an intervention that targeted the same behaviour you are targeting, can you at least provide an example of how an intervention with a similar approach has elicited behavioural change? Or can you provide something to show that funders or stakeholders will have something tangible as proof of success within a given period of time? However, as Iain Potter iterates, *Make sure you stress it's on ongoing process* and that your intervention does not just have a short-term focus. Gerard Hastings, e.g. points out that:

> for obesity you need to think in terms of at least five to ten years. The public sector needs to take its cue from the commercial sector which engages in real long-term strategic thinking.

Of course, at the end of the day it is imperative to demonstrate cost-effectiveness. You may start with the argument that it is generally more cost-effective to prevent a bad outcome than it is to fix a bad outcome, but you will ultimately need to demonstrate a return on investment analysis to show the value to the community. You might work with health economists, e.g. to quantify what it will mean to the community if your intervention does not go ahead.

What are the challenges of conducting social marketing with a limited budget?

When it came to discussing social marketing on a shoestring, our interviewees were unanimous in the view that limited budgets do not stand in the way of social marketing success. *Funds are not the issue*, advises William A Smith, *Expectations are.* It is important, therefore, to be realistic about what you can achieve and to set achievable goals, and you can also make sure you learn as much as possible from other social marketers and about interventions that might have succeeded or failed in the field in the past. Importantly, you should never use a limited budget as an excuse to cut corners – social marketing is a cohesive model, and an initiative that uses only part of that model is not a social marketing initiative. Jim Mintz advises concentrating on working with all of marketing's 4Ps (see Chapter 12) and perhaps, if relevant for your target audience and behaviour, some of the more cost-effective new media techniques. Try not to see social marketing as an isolated budget item but consider your whole budget as the social marketing budget.

However, we must face reality and admit that there are important implications when working with restricted financial resources. Iain Potter points out that it might be difficult to conduct formative research on a shoestring budget so, as discussed, you will need to look for existing information and casual research opportunities. Similarly, you will need to find inexpensive evaluation techniques. Ken Peattie suggests you call on volunteers to help with research so that you get to talk to your target audience for free, or you could always try to obtain sponsorship from a private sector company. In fact, partnership (see below) with the private sector, or indeed with any other organization, will be of utmost importance in initiatives that have smaller budgets, as it is a great way of increasing the impact of your resources. *Find allies to work with you so you can develop some level of scale*, suggests Alan Andreasen. But he goes on to suggest that you be as:

> narrow as possible in your behaviour objectives and target market. The more micro you can be in your objectives and audience the more likely your budget will be well spent.

For more detailed guidance on conducting social marketing initiatives on a limited budget, see Chapter 17.

What are the challenges of conducting social marketing with a significant budget?

You could be forgiven for thinking that working with a larger budget removes a lot of the stresses that working on a shoestring budget brings, and to some extent you would be right. But the truth is that large-budget initiatives introduce a whole new set of challenges that social marketers would be careless to ignore. It would be wrong to think, for example, that a large budget precludes the need to form partnerships and that it means an intervention can achieve change alone. As François Lagarde stipulates, *Reach and sustainable change needs a range of stakeholders, partners and influencers.*

Similarly, large budgets do not equate to immediate results. Money in social marketing does not necessarily mean power, and the multifarious forces that determine the success of low-budget interventions can be just as powerful with larger interventions. It is a mistake to 'throw money' at a target problem, just because money is there – it must still be invested wisely. For example, there may be a temptation to focus on expensive solutions rather than small-scale options: television advertisements rather than research; or activity to please stakeholders rather than evaluation to demonstrate how an intervention has performed. If you are working with a large budget, remember that this does not necessarily mean you have to make more noise: rather than throw your finances straight into an expensive advertising campaign, apply the social marketing model as you would normally, to gain insight into the problem you are tackling and the target audiences and to shape a suitable intervention that is more likely to get results.

Nonetheless, it is important to bear in mind that with larger budgets comes greater public scrutiny of how money is being spent. *The larger the intervention the greater the pressure to prove that it worked*, says Susan Dann. As with any social marketing initiative, it is important to set aside adequate budget for formative research at the 'scoping stage' (see Chapter 11). Gerard Hastings stresses the importance of thinking long term: *The big danger with being given £5m is in blowing it because you have to spend it.* So you should be asking how sustainable the funding is and how long you have to deliver your intervention.

How can we coordinate effective public–private sector partnerships?

As Robert Marshall points out, partnerships between the public and private sectors can be *both extremely rewarding and entirely frustrating. … It takes a lot of partnership management and maintenance to make this work.* And yet partnership is a key tenet of social marketing, extending the reach of an initiative's resources and potentially increasing impact. It is a mistake to think that your intervention will succeed if you rule out the possibility of working without partnership of any kind, and just as much a mistake to think that the private sector will be unable to add anything to your work. Box 22.3 sets out our interviewees' advice for negotiating partnerships and making them work to their full potential.

Box 22.3 Tips for effective public–private sector partnerships

- Define the self-interest of your potential partner before you start negotiations.
- Make sure that all parties get more than they give up in the partnership.
- Have a clear understanding of mutual obligations and responsibilities as well as limits to the partnership.
- Start negotiating partnerships early in the planning process and keep dialogue going – even when it appears there is no progress.
- Identify potential barriers and have a strategy for overcoming them.
- Use a social marketing approach: research your target audience and see negotiations as a marketing activity.
- Do not court partnerships just for the sake of public relations (PR).
- Do not be overly suspicious of commercial companies' motives – many do want to go good, although some do, of course, just want the PR.
- Develop a 'network' of partnerships to increase their power.
- Go beyond short-term sponsorships and engage in dialogue about longer-term strategies.

What are the key ethical issues in trying to influence people's behaviour?

In Chapter 9 of this book, we discussed some of the ethical issues involved in social marketing. In our discussions with our social marketing experts, we experienced first-hand iterations of why these ethical issues are so important in our day-to-day work. Gerard Hastings, e.g. highlighted one of the most important ethical dilemmas a social marketer faces: the choice of target behaviour.

> We have to ask why has this behaviour been chose and why do we want to change it? Does it need changing in this way and in this direction? Are there other issues that are more deserving? Whose behaviour is it and who is deciding that it needs changing? We have to consider these issues, otherwise we are no better than mercenaries. We must remember the old Hippocratic oath of no harm.
>
> (Gerard Hastings)

Stephen Dann argues that social marketers are inherently prone to utilitarian ethics based on the idea of social marketing being about improving the welfare of society and the target individual. *No social marketing campaign sets out to do evil, yet evil can easily be done in the name of improving society.* In your choice of target behaviour, e.g. are you in danger of imposing middle-class values on other section of society, or might you be promoting behaviour that is beneficial to government but not to your target audience? You need to check that you are not pursuing big headline benefits at the expense of less high-profile but just as significant matters. Similar issues arise in our choice of target audience: e.g. what happens to the people we do not focus on?

But if social marketing is beset with so many ethical dilemmas, what can you do to make sure your work is as ethical as possible? It is important to be aware of the validity of the decisions you make and to be aware of their potential consequences. If you are conducting a mass media campaign, consider its effects on people other than your target audience who see it. What can a perpetrator of domestic violence learn from advertisements encouraging his spouse to report abuse, for example? And ask if your intervention could have unpredicted effects on minors who come across it.

Mike Newton-Ward (Social Marketing Consultant at the North Carolina Division of Public Health, USA) argues that ethical decisions are about

> ensuring that one honours the dignity and right to self determination of the individual and balancing the right of people to make 'bad' choices (in our eyes), with the interests of the 'state' to mitigate the impact these choices have on the larger whole

It is, however, ultimately impossible to provide comprehensive ethical guidance for social marketers, as issues will evolve along with the discipline. You and your colleagues will need to allow for discussions about the ethics of your decisions throughout the social marketing process and to bear in mind that there will inevitably be consequences and implications to your decisions that you may not ultimately be able to mitigate.

Conclusion

Although the interviews for this chapter may have been short, they brought to light some of the most important issues facing social marketing today. These are issues that inevitably will affect you in your working life, and they will be issues about which you are likely to have strong views, particularly as social marketing becomes part of your everyday practice. But if social marketing in its current state poses challenges to practitioners, they are not challenges that are insurmountable – as the advice contained in this chapter shows. We need to draw on the experiences and views of those who have pioneered the discipline and to ensure that social marketing is cohesive, relevant and is successful in eliciting behavioural change for social good. Only if we meet these challenges will we be able to promote the discipline successfully, create a resource base of case studies and build capacity so that social marketing achieves its potential at an international level.

Social marketing experts interviewed for Chapter 22

Fiona Adshead, Deputy Chief Medical Officer, Department of Health, London, UK.

Alan Andreasen, Professor of Marketing at the McDonough School of Business of Georgetown University and Executive Director of the Social Marketing Institute, Georgetown, Washington DC, USA

Stephen Dann, Senior Lecturer, Australian National University, Canberra, Australia.

Susan Dann, Professor, Bond University, Brisbane, Australia.

Jeff French, Director, National Social Marketing Centre, London, UK.

Gerard Hastings, Professor of Social Marketing and Director of the Institute for Social Marketing and the Centre for Tobacco Control Research at University of Stirling, UK.

François Lagarde, Social Marketing Consultant and Trainer, University of Montreal, Montreal, Canada.

Nancy Lee, President, Social Marketing Services Inc., Mercer Island, USA.

Ray Lowry, Senior Lecturer, Newcastle University, Newcastle upon Tyne, UK.

Robert Marshall, Assistant Director, Rhode Island Department of Health, Providence, USA.

Rowena Merritt, National Programme Manager, National Social Marketing Centre, London, UK.

Jim Mintz, Director, Centre of Excellence for Public Sector Marketing, Ottawa, Canada.

Mike Newton-Ward, Senior Marketing Consultant, North Carolina Division of Public Health, Raleigh, USA.

Ken Peattie, Director, BRASS Research Centre, Cardiff University, Cardiff, UK.

Sue Peattie, Lecturer in Marketing, Cardiff Business School, Cardiff, UK.

Iain Potter, Chief Executive, Health Sponsorship Council (HSC), Wellington, New Zealand.

Michael Rothschild, Emeritus Professor, University of Wisconsin, Madison, USA.

William A Smith, Executive Vice President, Academy for Educational Development, Washington DC, US.

Appendix
NSMC TEXT BOOK

Resources

Websites and online tools and resources

National Social Marketing Centre
A strategic partnership between the Department of Health and Consumer Focus (formerly the National Consumer Council), founded to build skills and capacity in social marketing in the United Kingdom
http://www.nsmcentre.org.uk

ShowCase
The National Social Marketing Centre's case examples database of social marketing programmes from the United Kingdom and beyond
http://www.nsmcentre.org.uk/public/CSHome.aspx

Institute for Social Marketing
An institute committed to the study and dissemination of social marketing theory and practice, based at the University of Stirling, Scotland
http://www.ism.stir.ac.uk

Social Marketing Institute
A Washington DC-based organization with the aim of advancing the science and practice of social marketing
http://www.social-marketing.org

Centers for Disease Control and Prevention
Health information from the US government
http://www.cdc.gov/

Turning Point
A US public health improvement agency
http://www.turningpointprogram.org

Social Marketing Downunder
Designed by the Health Sponsorship Council for social marketers in New Zealand, Australia, and the South Pacific
http://www.socialmarketing.co.nz

Social Marketing.com
Social marketing online resources from Weinreich Communications, based in Washington DC
http://www.social-marketing.com/SMLinks.html

Cases in Public Health Communication & Marketing
A journal intended to advance practice-oriented learning in the fields of public health communication and social marketing
http://www.casesjournal.org

Social Marketing Quarterly
International journal covering theoretical, research, and practical issues in social marketing
http://www.ingentaconnect.com/content/routledg/gsmq

On Social Marketing and Social Change
A social marketing weblog
http://socialmarketing.blogs.com

CDCynergy
A CD-ROM-based tutorial and planning tool designed to help organizations plan, implement, and evaluate best practice social marketing interventions
http://www.cdc.gov/healthmarketing/cdcynergy/editions.htm

Health Canada E-learning Tool
A tutorial designed to assist the development of a complete social marketing plan
http://www.hc-sc.gc.ca/ahc-asc/activit/marketsoc/tools-outils/index_e.html

Social Marketing Listserv
An email listserv run by Alan Andreasen from Georgetown University, which is a very useful resource for keeping up to date and for sharing information on social marketing
http://www.social-marketing.org/aboutus.html

Tools of Change
Methods for promoting health, safety, and environmental citizenship
http://www.toolsofchange.com

The websites listed here are just a small selection of the social marketing resources available online. For a more complete list of materials, including books and reports, please refer to the resources section of the National Social Marketing Centre's website www.nsmcentre.org.uk

Index

Since "social marketing" is the subject of the entire book, entries under this topic have been kept to a minimum, and readers should look for more specific aspects.